# Encyclopedia of Wellness

# Encyclopedia of Wellness

## From Açaí Berry to Yo-Yo Dieting

### Volume 2: F–O

### Sharon Zoumbaris, Editor

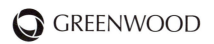 GREENWOOD

AN IMPRINT OF ABC-CLIO, LLC
Santa Barbara, California • Denver, Colorado • Oxford, England

**Library of Congress Cataloging-in-Publication Data**

Encyclopedia of wellness : from açaí berry to yo-yo dieting / Sharon Zoumbaris, editor.
         p. cm.
    Includes index.
    ISBN 978-0-313-39333-4 (hardback) — ISBN 978-0-313-39334-1 (ebook)
1. Health—Encyclopedias.    2. Medicine, Preventive—Encyclopedias.
I. Zoumbaris, Sharon, 1955–
    RA776.E524   2012
    613.03—dc23        2011045406

ISBN: 978-0-313-39333-4
EISBN: 978-0-313-39334-1

16  15  14  13  12    1  2  3  4  5

This book is also available on the World Wide Web as an eBook.
Visit www.abc-clio.com for details.

Greenwood
An Imprint of ABC-CLIO, LLC

ABC-CLIO, LLC
130 Cremona Drive, P.O. Box 1911
Santa Barbara, California 93116-1911

This book is printed on acid-free paper ∞

Manufactured in the United States of America

This book discusses treatments (including types of medication and mental health therapies), diagnostic tests for various symptoms and mental health disorders, and organizations. The authors have made every effort to present accurate and up-to-date information. However, the information in this book is not intended to recommend or endorse particular treatments or organizations, or substitute for the care or medical advice of a qualified health professional, or used to alter any medical therapy without a medical doctor's advice. Specific situations may require specific therapeutic approaches not included in this book. For those reasons, we recommend that readers follow the advice of qualified health care professionals directly involved in their care. Readers who suspect they may have specific medical problems should consult a physician about any suggestions made in this book.

# Contents

# *Alphabetical List of Entries*

# Entries Arranged by Broad Topic

**Alternative Health Care and Complementary Medicine**

Acupuncture
Ayurveda
Biofeedback
Chelation
Dance Therapy
Dietary Supplements
Dream Therapy
Guided Imagery
Homeopathy
Hypnosis
Macrobiotics
Medical Marijuana
Meditation
National Center for Complementary and Alternative Medicine
Naturopathic Medicine
Pauling, Linus
Probiotics
Qigong
Reflexology
Reiki
Rodale, Jerome
Spas, Medical
Tai Chi
Therapeutic Touch
Traditional Chinese Medicine

## Nutritional Health

# F

## FAST FOOD

In a typical year the average American spends $500 dollars on fast food ("Did You Know," 2008). Fast food isn't healthy eating to be sure, but just how bad is it? What is fast food and can healthy choices be made? Most importantly, how can Americans eat healthy and still enjoy such favorite foods as burgers, fries, pizza, and tacos?

Fast food—foods like hamburgers, French fries, shakes, and tacos—are high in saturated fat, calories, salt, and cholesterol. On the plus side, they also contain protein and some other nutrients. While it's not clear whether fast food was ever supposed to replace home-cooked meals, it is certain that today's youth cannot imagine a world without hamburgers and fries served in bright cardboard containers and without drive-through service for quick meals.

White Castle is considered the first U.S. fast-food operation. Its major product was hamburgers, which had been sold as a sandwich by street vendors since the 1890s, but hamburgers were not a particularly popular food when White Castle opened in the 1920s. In fact, many Americans were leery of them. Because hamburgers consisted of ground beef, it was easy to adulterate them, and many Americans were concerned with the sanitary conditions at hamburger stands. White Castle convinced Americans that its products were pure and thus tapped into the American concern with hygiene. White Castle also proved that hamburgers could be inexpensive, good tasting, and quickly prepared. This success plowed the ground for other hamburger chains, such as White Tower, White Huts, Little Kastle, Royal Castle, and many others.

Other chains emerged during the 1920s, such as A&W Root Beer and Nathan's Famous; the latter was launched as a hot dog stand on Coney Island, New York, in 1915. Many small, regional chains developed during the 1920s. When the Depression hit in the 1930s, fast food not only survived but thrived. Thousands of fast-food outlets dotted the urban landscape and the nation's highways, selling hundreds of thousands of low-cost hamburgers annually. Most were based on

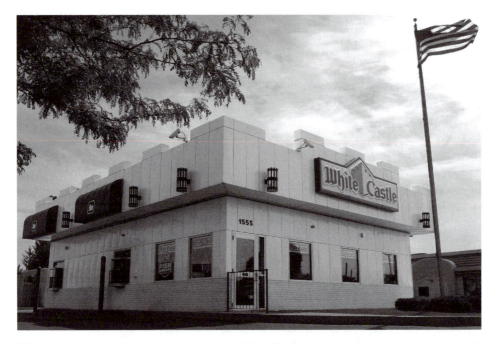

White Castle is considered to be the first U.S. fast-food operation and its food is now available from its food outlets and can also be found in grocery and wholesale stores. (AP/Wide World Photos)

franchising, wherein local entrepreneurs usually paid a fee to and bought goods or equipment from a franchisor. In turn, franchisees gained visibility though the promotional activities carried out by the franchisor, and they benefited from the consistency of the products and the methods of preparing them.

The early success of fast food can be directly linked to automobiles, which became common during the 1920s. Travelers needed places to eat, and fast food was offered through chains. Travelers were familiar with chains: they offered low-cost food, quick service, and chain outlets were easily and conveniently accessible on highways. The years during World War II were difficult for fast-food operators, because meat was rationed and many employees went into the military. Fast food chains barely survived by developing new products, such as French fries and egg sandwiches.

A robust self-confidence emerged in the United States after World War II that encouraged entrepreneurs to try new ideas. The construction of the new interstate highway system created a need to satisfy popular expectations for reliable roadside food. The highway system encouraged the growth of suburban communities, which had no established culinary infrastructure. Fast-food restaurants jumped in to meet this need. Fast-food chains initially catered to automobile owners in suburbia.

The baby boom after World War II encouraged middle-class families to purchase homes, and families meant young children and parents who preferred low-cost food. Also, the notion of fast food reflected U.S. culture in which speed and efficiency were highly prized. As a result, many fast-food operations emerged during the 1940s and 1950s. Ice cream chains were the first to develop. Dairy Queen (1940) and Baskin-Robbins (1948) expanded rapidly during their early years. The nation's first doughnut chains emerged at about the same time. Dunkin' Donuts in Quincy, Massachusetts, and Winchell's Donut House in Los Angeles both started in 1948.

Chicken-based fast-food chains began during the early 1950s. Kentucky Fried Chicken's first franchise was established in Utah in 1952, the same year that Church's Chicken was launched in San Antonio, Texas. But it was the hamburger chains that dominated the fast-food industry in the United States. Jack in the Box (1950) was launched in San Diego, Burger King (1954) was launched in Miami, and Wendy's (1969) started in Columbus, Ohio.

The most important fast-food chain was McDonald's, which was launched in San Bernardino, California, in the 1940s, but it did not take shape until 1954. Founded by Richard and Maurice McDonald, it was greeted with wonder by the public. Its golden arches were modern; its facilities were bright and clean; its service was fast; and its food was inexpensive. Like White Castles, McDonald's were lined with white tiles to emphasize cleanliness and, like other drive-ins, McDonald's architecture featured outlandish (but eye-catching) golden arches. The front of each store was glassed-in, putting food preparation into a fishbowl so the customers could see firsthand the sanitary conditions of food preparation.

Ethnic fast food (specifically pizza) also matured during this time. Shakey's (1954) was started in Sacramento, California; Pizza Hut (1958) was launched in Wichita, Kansas; and three years later, Domino's was created in Ypsilanti, Michigan. Mexican-type fast food emerged later, with Taco Bell (1962).

As competition grew, so did the need for advertising and promotion. Fast food chains spent millions on television advertising, much of it targeted to youth. As competition grew, so did the need for innovation. Fast-food chains adapted to the changing needs of the buying public. While a limited menu, low-cost food, and eating in the car were important components of the early chains, each of these elements changed during this period. The appeal of eating in the car declined, especially in cold winters or hot summers, and fast food operations opened indoor dining facilities.

Menus became more complex as new items were tested and incorporated if successful. Many new items, such as Burger King's Whopper, were more expensive but they attracted a wide following, and other chains began to develop more costly items. McDonald's began serving chicken; Burger King offered croissants; and the pizza chains began serving hot and cold sandwiches and pasta dishes.

**Globalization**   Fast-food establishments in the United States were built on the notion of standardization; every restaurant was the same, as were menus and procedures. Fast-food customers behaved in certain ways: they stood in line, paid in advance, picked up their own utensils and napkins, ate quickly, cleaned up after themselves, and left promptly, thereby making room for others. While these assumptions are understood in the United States, they are not necessarily understood in other countries. Russian and Chinese customers, for example, needed guidance when McDonald's opened in Moscow and Beijing, respectively. They were unprepared to be smiled at by employees, and they had no idea what was inside a hamburger or how it should be eaten. The vast majority of McDonald's customers accepted the queue, which was not a common practice in many other countries. The physical setting of fast-food restaurants encourages discipline, and both customers and employees are standing, which establishes an egalitarian relationship.

Fast-food operations were started by individual entrepreneurs who had ideas and were willing to experiment. Once good ideas were launched, entrepreneurs sold out to organizers and managers who took fast-food operations into larger arenas.

During the 1960s and 1970, large corporations began to purchase chains. The Pillsbury Company bought Burger King, the Heublein Company bought Kentucky Fried Chicken, PepsiCo bought Taco Bell and Pizza Hut, and Royal Crown bought Arby's. Many fast-food chains subsequently were sold to investor groups or have been spun off into large restaurant conglomerates, such as Yum! Brands.

Franchisers initially managed a single outlet. Today, most franchisees are large groups that manage numerous outlets. It is very difficult for an individual to acquire a franchise from many large fast-food chains.

There have been many criticisms of the fast-food industry, including health-related concerns about consumption of so much fat, calories, and salt. As a result, many chains developed lighter entrees such as fish, salads, and salad bars. Other critics have been concerned with the exploitation of workers, who are paid minimum wages without benefits. Still others proclaim that the fast-food industry culture is creating a homogeneous diet among Americans. Soft drinks, hamburgers, fries, iceberg lettuce, fried chicken, and ketchup have become mainstays of America's diet as traditional foods or foods not easily converted into fast foods have faded.

The fast-food industry has also been criticized for targeting children. Since the 1950s, fast-food chains have targeted a large proportion of their advertising dollars on children. Fast-food chains hand out coloring books or pages, entice children with brightly colored Happy Meals and mascots, give away or sell inexpensive toys and other merchandise, offer playgrounds, and have tie-ins with children's movies. In addition, fast-food and junk-food companies now advertise and promote their foods in schools. The American School Food Service Association estimates that 30 percent of public high schools offer branded fast food for sale in their cafeterias or vending machines.

As fast-food chains have moved abroad, a number of additional criticisms have been raised, such as the homogenization or Americanization of the culinary world, the loss of food-supply genetic diversity, the vast waste generated by fast-food establishments, and the destruction of the rainforests.

Despite these concerns, fast-food operations have continued to expand in the United States and worldwide. The analysis of food consumption in the United States is measured by the United States Department of Agriculture's (USDA's) Economic Research Service (ERS), whose primary data source is the U.S. Census. The ERS Food Expenditure Series was developed in 1987, and data are available from 1929 through 2005. Statistics are available from other sources, including the National Restaurant Association, which estimated that fast-food restaurants generated $134 billion in sales during 2005 (Schlosser & Wilson, 2006). What is clear from all the statistics is that those figures have continued to rise. The largest growth, however, has been abroad. McDonald's, for instance, now has more operations in other countries than it does in the United States.

We are what we eat, and Americans are eating fast food. Figures show that, as a nation, we spend more money on fast food than the dollars spent on computers, higher education, or new cars. It's easy to spend those dollars, because fast food is now on almost every corner. Today it takes hard work and planning ahead to eat healthy. Good nutrition does not mean giving up all fast food. Still, experts agree that the best diet is one low in fat and high in fruits, vegetables, and whole grains.

The USDA MyPlate contains specific recommendations for the quantities and types of foods to eat from the major food groups of grains, fruits, vegetables, dairy, and meat or protein. While fast-food menus have changed over the years to offer fruit and vegetable choices, consumers might not realize that the basic burgers for the major chains have about 10 to 15 grams of fat, which is relatively lean for a hamburger. The real fat traps to avoid are the big signature burgers such as Burger King's Double Whopper with cheese at a whopping 1,010 calories and 67 grams of fat. That is more than an entire day's fat allowance for an adult. The McDonald's Angus Bacon and Cheese weighs in with 790 calories and 39 grams of fat. Wendy's Baconator Triple takes the prize with 1,360 calories and 91 grams of fat (McIndoo, 2011).

Fat and calorie numbers like these play a role in why fast food chains face criticism from consumer groups, such as the Center for Science in the Public Interest. Writers like Eric Schlosser, whose best-selling book *Fast Food Nation: The Dark Side of the All-American Meal,* are also forcing the issue, providing details about the content and culture of fast food. All the while, obesity rates in the United States continue to soar. Statistics from the Centers for Disease Control and Prevention (CDC) show that, from 2007 to 2009, an additional 2.4 million adults fit the criteria for obesity, raising the figure to over 72 million obese adults (CDC, 2011). So, while governments address this national health threat by passing laws forcing the mandatory posting of calories on menus in chain restaurants, the final responsibility still falls to each individual. Americans must decide if they will continue to choose convenience, price, and taste over more nutritious, healthy food.

*Andrew F. Smith*

*See also* Cheeseburger Bill; Fats; MyPlate.

## References

Centers for Disease Control and Prevention. "Vital Signs: State Specific Obesity Prevalence among Adults-United States, 2009." *Morbidity and Mortality Weekly Report* (August 3, 2010), www.cdc.gov.

"Did You Know." *Tufts University Health and Nutrition Letter* 26, no. 6 (August 2008): 3.

Goldstein, Myrna Chandler, and Mark A Goldstein. *Controversies in Food and Nutrition.* Westport, CT: Greenwood Press, 2002.

Emerson, Robert L. *The New Economics of Fast Food.* New York: Van Nostrand Reinhold, 1990.

Emerson, Robert L. *Fast Food: The Endless Shakeout.* New York: Lebhar-Friedman Books, 1979.

Jacobson, Michael F. *Fast-Food Guide,* 2nd ed. New York: Workman, 1991.

Levenstein, Harvey. *Paradox of Plenty: A Social History of Eating in Modern America.* New York: Oxford University Press, 1993.

Love, John F. *McDonald's: Behind the Arches.* New York: Bantam Books, 1986.

Luxenberg, Stan. *Roadside Empires: How the Chains Franchised America.* New York: Viking, 1985.

McIndoo, Heidi. "Fast Food on a Bun: How Do They Stack Up?" *Environmental Nutrition* 34, no. 1 (January 2011): 5.

Mintz, Sidney. "Afterward." In *Golden Arches East: McDonald's in East Asia,* edited by James L. Watson. Stanford, CA: Stanford University Press, 1997.

Perl, Lila. *Junk Food, Fast Food, Health Food: What America Eats and Why.* New York: Houghton Mifflin/Clarion Books, 1980.

Schlosser, Eric. *Fast Food Nation: The Dark Side of the All-American Meal.* New York: Houghton Mifflin, 2001.

Schlosser, Eric, and Charles Wilson. *Chew on This: Everything You Don't Want to Know about Fast Food.* Boston: Houghton Mifflin, 2006.

USDA Economic Research Service. "Food CPI and Expenditures: Measuring the ERS Food Expenditure Series" (March 26, 2007), www.ers.usda.gov.

Volpe, Tina. *The Fast Food Craze: Wreaking Havoc on Our Bodies and Our Animals.* Kagel Canyon, CA: Canyon, 2005.

## FATS

Historically, fat was considered a valued food. Those who could include increased amounts of fat in their diets had greater protection from starvation during times of scarcity. Even today, while food is plentiful in the developed world, in many parts of the developing world, people are often unable to consume sufficient amounts of food. For those individuals, carrying a little extra weight is considered far more desirable than being too thin. Women with rounder figures are believed to be more attractive than those who are lean; women with extra poundage are also thought to be more fertile and more likely to give birth to a healthy child.

By the second half of the 20th century, Americans tended to lump all fats together—assigning them all negative labels. Americans were told to limit their consumption of all types of fat. Fats were thought to raise the risk for a host of medical problems, such as heart disease and cancer. Moreover, those who consumed larger amounts of fat tended to become heavier or even obese. After all, excess weight and obesity have become epidemic in the United States.

Yet, in recent years, many people have begun to realize that fats are an integral part of the human body. According to Rosemary Stanton, in *Good Fats Bad Fats,* a book published in 2002, without fat, it is impossible to achieve optimal health. People need fat to regulate body temperature; fat protects the body from extreme heat and cold. Fat provides cushioning for internal organs and padding for bones. Fat stores energy, which is especially important during time of illness. Fat is required to build and support nerve and brain cells, and fat is needed to produce hormones and absorb some nutrients (Stanton, 2002). "We need to stop thinking of all body fat as undesirable. Some is essential" (Stanton, 2002).

A 2007 article entitled "Oil is Well" in *Prevention* magazine notes that, "consuming less than 20% of your calories from fats and oils may actually increase your risk of heart disease. That's because a deficit can lower your intake of vitamin E (a powerful antioxidant), keep 'good' cholesterol from rising, and spike triglycerides (type of fat found in the body)" (Sass, 2007).

**Some Fats Are Healthy and Some Are Not**   (Courtesy of Mark A. Goldstein)

*Unsaturated Fats*   There are two types of unsaturated fats that help to lower blood cholesterol: polyunsaturated fats and monounsaturated fats. Unsaturated fats, which are liquid at room temperature, are derived from plant or animal sources.

*Polyunsaturated Fats*   When consuming fats, it is important to distinguish between those that support good health and those that don't. More than thirty years ago, researchers discovered a class of fats known as polyunsaturated fatty acids. The two main types of polyunsaturated fatty acids are omega-3 and omega-6. Both are essential fatty acids that the body requires but is unable to manufacture. A 2007 article in *Natural Health* explains that, in general, omega-3 fatty acids—which are contained in fish, nuts, and flaxseed—are considered good fats. Most omega-6s—which are found in corn, cottonseed, and soybean oils; margarine; and processed foods—as well as "the infamous trans fats that come from the partial hydrogenation of vegetable oil" have a negative effect on the body (Wallace, 2007). There does appear to be one member of the omega-6 fatty acids, conjugated linoleic acid (CLA), which is "found only in the meat and milk of ruminants such as cattle" (Wallace, 2007), that is beneficial. There is some evidence that it may help with weight loss, build lean mass, increase immunity, and stop the growth of cancer cells. "The word fat here is crucial: Because CLA is found only in the fat of ruminants and their milk, you won't find it in skim milk or nonfat yogurt" (Wallace, 2007). (But new evidence has found CLA in white button mushrooms.)

Omega-3s were once a plentiful part of the U.S. diet. A 2007 article in *Environmental Nutrition* notes, "that's because cattle and chickens used to graze on rich sources of omega-3s like grass, wild plants, and seeds, instead of grains with scant omega-3s, which is what agribusiness now typically uses as livestock feed" (Antinoro, 2007).

A 2006 article in *Women's Health* noted that it is generally agreed that people should consume about 3,000 milligrams per day of omega-6 and 1,000 milligrams of omega-3. "That 3:1 ratio is important: Some studies show that eating too many omega-6s and not enough omega-3s may negate the positive health effects" (Duncan, 2006). A 2005 article in the *Saturday Evening Post* says that the "typical American diet tends to contain up to 30 times more omega-6 fatty acids than omega-3 fatty acids" (SerVaas, 2005). It is this imbalance that is thought to contribute to a host of medical problems.

One such problem is major depression. A study published in 2007 in *Psychosomatic Medicine* found that the omega-6 to omega-3 ratio in subjects with major depression to be 18 to 1. In subjects without depression, the ratio was 13 to 1. As the ratio rose, so did the degree of severity of the depression (Kiecolt-Glaser et al., 2007). The researchers also found an association between higher levels of omega-6 and inflammation-causing compounds that have been linked to arthritis, Type 2 diabetes, and heart disease.

Research published a year earlier in *Brown University Psychopharmacology Update* noted a possible link between suicide and higher omega-6/omega-3 ratios. Researchers studied 33 subjects with major depressive disorder. During a two-year follow-up, seven attempted suicide at least once. Two of these attempts were fatal. All of the subjects who attempted suicide had elevated ratios. Commenting on the study, David L. Katz, an associate professor of public health and director of the Prevention Research Center at Yale University School of Medicine, said, "While more research is needed before the use of omega-3 fatty acids can be considered among the routine therapies for depression, our knowledge is certainly sufficient to justify efforts to increase prevailing intake levels. We may hope that by doing so there might be less depression to treat" ("Omega-3 Fatty Acid Levels," 2006).

In a 2004 population study published in *Lipids,* researchers examined the association between consumption of omega-6 fatty acids and the murder rates in Argentina, Australia, Canada, the United Kingdom, and the United States. It is of interest that the researchers found that in areas where there was higher-than-average consumption of omega-6 fatty acids, there were also higher-than-average rates of murder. The rates of homicide appeared to correlate directly with increases in consumption of omega-6 fatty acids. The researchers concluded that, "these dietary interventions merit exploration as relatively cost-effective measures for reducing the pandemic of violence in Western societies, just as dietary interventions are reducing cardiovascular mortality" (Hibbeln, Nieminen, & Lands, 2004).

A culture stimulated tumor growth laboratory study published in 2005 in *Carcinogenesis* found that reducing the intake of omega-6 lowers the risk for cancer. It is believed that people who have higher intakes of omega-6 increase their risk for prostate cancer (Hughes-Fulford, Tjandrawinata, & Sayyah, 2005). In another article, published in 2005 in *GP,* the lead researcher of the study, Millie Hughes-Fulford, said that people who consume higher amounts of omega-6 are also at increased risk for colorectal and some breast cancers ("Omega-6 Link to Prostate Cancer." 2005).

A 2004 article in *Women's Health Weekly* describes Spanish researchers at the Universitat Autonoma de Barcelona who induced breast cancer tumors in rats. When the rats were fed excess amounts of omega-6, the tumors grew faster. While omega-6 fatty acids do not cause cancer, they clearly have the potential to "accelerate the clinical development of the disease" ("Excess Dietary Omega-6," 2004).

In her book, *The Ultimate Omega-3 Diet,* registered dietician Evelyn Tribole lists the omega-6 content of nuts. (Remember, nuts also contain omega-3 fatty acids.) While nuts are generally believed to be healthful, it may be wise to limit or avoid those with the highest levels of omega-6 (Tribole, 2007).

Tribole also offers a number of food substitutions that may help reduce the amount of omega-6 in the diet. Some of these are as follows (Tribole, 2007):

**Table 1. Nuts and Omega-6 Fat Measurements**

| Type of Nut (One Ounce or Two Tablespoons) | Omega-6 Fat Content (in Milligrams) |
| --- | --- |
| Walnuts | 10,800 |
| Sunflower seeds, roasted | 9,700 |
| Pine nuts | 9,400 |
| Hemp nut seeds | 9,400 |
| Pumpkin and squash seeds | 5,870 |
| Hickory nuts | 5,850 |
| Pecans | 5,850 |
| Brazil nuts | 5,820 |
| Peanuts | 4,450 |
| Pistachio nuts | 3,740 |
| Hazelnuts | 2,220 |
| Cashews | 2,170 |
| Chestnuts | 450 |
| Macadamia nuts | 370 |

*Source:* Evelyn Tribole. *The Ultimate Omega-3 Diet.* McGraw-Hill, 2007.

**Table 2. Healthy Substitutions**

| Instead of | Use |
| --- | --- |
| Granola | Flax-based or canola oil–based granola |
| Peanut butter | Almond butter, cashew butter, macadamia nut butter |
| Margarine | Canola oil margarine |
| Eggs | Omega-3 eggs |
| Potato chips | Baked chips; chips made with olive oil and high-oleic oils |
| Tuna in oil | Light tuna in water |

*Source:* Evelyn Tribole. *The Ultimate Omega-3 Diet.* McGraw-Hill, 2007.

**Monounsaturated Fats**   Monounsaturated fats, such as olive oil, canola oil, and peanut oil, have long been recognized as excellent for heart health. A 2007 article in *Food & Fitness Advisor* notes that "Monounsaturated fat is the best for heart health, because it decreases the LDL, or 'bad' cholesterol as well as total cholesterol but increases the HDL, or 'good' cholesterol" ("Cooking Oil Comparison," 2007).

Probably the best known monounsaturated fat is olive oil, the fat that is part of the Mediterranean diet. The positive role that the Mediterranean diet may play in cardiovascular health has been well documented by many studies. For instance, research presented before the spring 2007 annual meeting of the American College of Cardiology described a study of 202 individuals who had suffered a heart attack within the previous six weeks. Fifty of these subjects were placed on the American Heart Association low-fat diet, which required an intake of no more than 30 percent fat; 51 participants were placed on the Mediterranean diet, which allowed an intake of 40 percent fat. One hundred participants were not placed on any special diet. "After four years, 83 percent of those on the low-fat or Mediterranean diets hadn't suffered another heart attack, stroke, or other heart problems, compared to only 53 percent of the others "("'Healthy' Fats Just as Beneficial," 2007).

In recent years, researchers have determined that olive oil has the potential to do more than protect against cardiovascular disease. For example, a 2006 article published in *Archives of Neurology* examined the association between the Mediterranean diet and Alzheimer's disease. Researchers found that people who adhere to the Mediterranean diet have a reduced risk for developing Alzheimer's disease (Scarmeas, Stern, Mayeux, & Luchsinger, 2006). In fact, people who followed the diet quite strictly "had a 68 percent lower risk of Alzheimer's compared with those who had the lowest adherence" ("Eating a Mediterranean Diet," 2007).

In 2007 the *Journal of Agricultural and Food Chemistry* reported on a laboratory study that examined the role that olive oil may play in the prevention of peptic ulcers and some gastric cancers caused by *Helicobacter pylori* bacterium. Apparently, olive oil contains abundant amounts of polyphenols, powerful antioxidants that help make fruits and vegetables so healthful. Researchers found that, in the stomach, the polyphenols exerted a strong antibacterial activity. "These results open the possibility of considering virgin olive oil a chemopreventive agent for peptic ulcer or gastric cancer" (Romero, Medina, Vargas, Brenes, & De Castro, 2007).

A 2005 article in *Nature* notes that newly pressed extra-virgin olive oil contains oleocanthal, a compound that acts "as a natural anti-inflammatory compound that has a potency and profile similar to that of ibuprofen" (Beauchamp et al., 2005). Still another study, published in 2006 in *Current Pharmaceutical Biotechnology*, notes that researchers found that oleic acid, the primary monounsaturated fat in olive oil, may "suppress the overexpression and HER2 (erbB-2), a well-characterized oncogene playing a key role in the etiology, invasive progression and metastasis in several human cancers" (Menendez & Lupu, 2006). Heating olive oil breaks down some of its antioxidants. But unless a cook heats the oil until it begins to smoke, it should retain most of the benefits.

Nuts are another source of monounsaturated fats. A study published in a 2007 issue of *Lipids* added four weeks of 40 to 90 grams per day consumption of macadamia nuts to the diets of 17 men with high levels of blood cholesterol. Researchers found that the consumption of the nuts "modifies favorably the biomarkers of oxidative stress, thrombosis, and inflammation, the risk factors for coronary artery disease, despite the increase in dietary fat intake" (Garg, Blake, Wills, & Clayton, 2007).

The researchers conclude that macadamia nuts may play a role in preventing coronary artery disease. Almonds are also a wonderful source of monounsaturated fat. For those worried about weight gain from consuming nuts, which are high in fat content, there is an interesting study published in 2007 in the *British Journal of Nutrition*. Researchers found that even after eating a daily 344-calorie serving of almonds for 10 weeks, there was no change in body weight. The subjects simply ate smaller amounts of other foods (Hollis & Mattes, 2007).

**Bad Fats**   A few fats are known to be unhealthful. These include saturated fats, which are most often found in animal products such as whole milk and red meat. At room temperature, saturated fats are solid or waxy. Coconut oil, palm oil, and other tropical oils are also high in saturated fat.

Trans fats, which are also known as trans-fatty acids, are formed when hydrogen is added to vegetable oil, a process known as hydrogenation. This makes the fat harder and less likely to spoil. Many foods contain trans fats, including commercial bakery products, shortenings, and some margarines. The human body does not make trans fats and does not need them. It is of interest that a number of cities throughout the United States are prohibiting their use in restaurants. A 2007 issue of the *Harvard Health Letter* notes that trans fats are "now seen as the really bad fat. Beyond its effect on cholesterol, trans fat seems to make platelets 'stickier' (making blood clots more likely), stir up inflammation, and promote the production of extra-small LDL particles that are especially damaging to arteries" ("Time to Fatten Up Our Diets," 2007). However, it is important to realize that food labels may indicate that products contain "zero trans fats" when they actually contain no more than one-half gram of trans fat per serving ("When Zero Isn't Nothing," 2007).

A number of studies have shown a direct association between intake of bad fats and increased risk for certain medical problems. Thus, an article published in 2007 in *Cancer Causes and Control* reported that there is "some evidence" that the consumption of beef, lamb, eggs, dairy, fat, or cholesterol "may increase the risk of pancreatic cancer" (Chan, Wang, & Holly, 2007). Another study, published in the *American Journal of Clinical Nutrition* in 2008, determined that people who frequently eat saturated and trans fats have increased rates of subclinical atherosclerosis (Merchant et al., 2008). And still another study published in 2007 in *Circulation* concluded that, after covariates were adjusted, "high trans fat consumption remains a significant risk factor for coronary heart disease" (Sun et al., 2007). Those with the highest levels of trans fatty acids in their blood had three times the risk of developing coronary heart disease as those with the lowest levels (Sun et al., 2007).

For women having trouble conceiving, a 2007 study published in the *American Journal of Clinical Nutrition* has important information. Using data from the Nurses' Health Study, Harvard Medical School researchers found that even small amounts of trans fats have the potential to cause increases in infertility. Hence, a woman who consumes 2,000 calories per day and who obtains only 2 percent of her calories from trans fats, eats about four grams per day of trans fat or about the amount of trans fats in one doughnut. So, very small amounts of trans fats are able to have a dramatic effect on fertility. "Obtaining two percent of energy from trans fats rather than from monounsaturated fats was associated with a more than doubled risk of ovulatory infertility" (Chavarro, Rich-Edwards, Rosner, & Willett, 2007).

In the past, all fats were usually clumped together and considered bad for one's health. More recently, it has become quite evident that, while some fats are indeed unhealthful and should play a very limited role in the diet, there are fats that should be part of the daily diet. Just about everyone would benefit from more monounsaturated fats, and most people should be adding increased amounts of foods with omega-3s. On the other hand, trans fats should be avoided and saturated fats should be avoided or seriously limited.

*Myrna Chandler Goldstein and Mark A. Goldstein*

*See also* Calories; Carbohydrates; Cholesterol; Obesity.

### References

Allport, Susan. *The Queen of Fats*. Berkeley: University of California Press, 2006.

Antinoro, Linda. "Omega-3-Fortified Foods: Fish Out of Water or Healthful Addition to Diet?" *Environmental Nutrition* (July 2007) 30: 1.

Beauchamp, Gary K., Russell S.J. Keast, Diane Morel, Jianming Lin, et al. "Phytochemistry: Ibuprofen-Like Activity in Extra-Virgin Olive Oil." *Nature* 437 (September 1, 2005): 45–46.

Chan, June M., Furong Wang, and Elizabeth A. Holly. "Pancreatic Cancer, Animal Protein, and Dietary Fat in a Population-Based Study." *Cancer Causes and Control* 18 (December 2007): 1153–67.

Chavarro, Jorge E., Janet W. Rich-Edwards, Bernard A. Rosner, and Walter C. Willett. "Dietary Fatty Acid Intakes and the Risk of Ovulatory Infertility." *American Journal of Clinical Nutrition* 85 (January 2007): 231.

Colbert, Brandy. "Trans Fat Forestalls Fertility." *Vegetarian Times* 350 (May–June 2007): 16.

"Cooking Oil Comparison: What's Healthiest for You Heart? Olive, Canola, and Peanut Oils Get the Highest Marks in Terms of Healthy Fats, Versatility, and Flavor." *Food and Fitness Advisor* 10 (July 2007): 8–9.

Duncan, Nancy. "Mighty Omegas." *Women's Health* 3 (December 2006): 47.

"Eating a Mediterranean Diet Might Ward Off Alzheimer's." *Focus on Healthy Aging* 10 (January 2007): 2.

"Excess Dietary Omega-6 Speeds Breast Cancer by Altering Gene Activity." *Women's Health Weekly* (November 11, 2004): 4.

Garg, Manohar L., Robert J. Blake, Ron B.H. Wills, and Edward H. Clayton. "Macadamia Nut Consumption Modulates Favorably Risk Factors for Coronary Artery Disease in Hypercholesterolemic Subjects." *Lipids* 42 (June 2007): 583–87.

"'Healthy' Fats Just as Beneficial as Low-Fat Diet." *Heart Advisor* 10 (June 2007): 2.

Hibbeln, Joseph, Levi R.G. Nieminen, and William E.M. Lands. "Increasing Homicide Rates and Linoleic Acid Consumption among Five Western Countries, 1961–2000." *Lipids* 39 (December 2004): 1207–13.

Hollis, James, and Richard Mattes. "Effects of Chronic Consumption of Almonds on Body Weight in Healthy Humans." *British Journal of Nutrition* 98 (September 2007): 651–56.

Hughes-Fulford, Millie, Raymond R. Tjandrawinata, Chai-Fei Li, and Sina Sayyah. "Arachidonic Acid, An Omega-6 Fatty Acid, Induces Cytoplasmic Phospholipase A2 in Prostate Carcinoma Cells." *Carcinogenesis* 26 (September 2005): 1520–26.

Kiecolt-Glaser, Janice K., Martha A. Belury, Kyle Porter, David Q. Beversdorf, Stanley Lemeshow, and Ronald Glaser. "Depressive Symptoms, Omega-6: Omega-3 Fatty Acids, and Inflammation in Older Adults." *Psychosomatic Medicine* 69 (April 2007): 217–24.

Machowetz, Anja, Henrik E. Poulsen, Sindy Gruendel, Allan Weimann, et al. "Effects of Olive Oils on Biomarkers of Oxidative DNA Stress in Northern and Southern Europeans." *FASEB Journal* 21 (January 2007): 45–52.

Menendez, Javier A., and Ruth Lupu. "Mediterranean Dietary Traditions for the Molecular Treatment of Human Cancer: Anti-Oncogenic Actions of the Main Olive Oil's Monounsaturated Fatty Acid Oleic Acid." *Current Pharmaceutical Biotechnology* 7 (December 2006): 495–502.

Merchant, Anwar T., Linda E. Kelemen, Lawrence de Koning, Eva Lonn, et al. "Interrelation of Saturated Fat, Trans Fat, Alcohol Intake, and Subclinical Atherosclerosis." *American Journal of Clinical Nutrition* 87 (January 2008): 168.

Mihm, Stephen. "Does Eating Salmon Lower the Murder Rate?" *New York Times Magazine* (April 16, 2006): 18.

"Omega-6 Link to Prostate Cancer." *GP* (August 12, 2005): 2.

"Omega-6 Fatty Acids Linked to Depression and Inflammation." *Food and Fitness Advisor* 10 (July 2007): 2.

"Omega-3 Fatty Acid Levels as a Predictor of Future Suicide Risk." *Brown University Psychopharmacology Update* 17 (September 2006): 1–4.

Romero, Concepción, Edwardo Medina, Julio Vargas, Manuel Brenes, and Antonio De Castro. "In Vitro Activity of Olive Oil Polyphenols Against *Helicobacter pylori*." *Journal of Agricultural and Food Chemistry* 55 (February 7, 2007): 680–86.

Sass, Cynthia. "Oil Is Well!" *Prevention* 59 (December 2007): 75.

Scarmeas, Nikolaos, Yaakov Stern, Richard Mayeux, and Jose A. Luchsinger. "Mediterranean Diet, Alzheimer Disease, and Vascular Mediation." *Archives of Neurology* 63 (December 2006): 1709–17.

SerVaas, Cory. "How Do You Do the Omega Balance?" *Saturday Evening Post* 277 (July–August 2005): 99.

Sinn, Natalie, and Janet Bryan. "Effect of Supplementation with Polyunsaturated Fatty Acids and Micronutrients on Learning and Behavior Problems Associated with Child ADHD." *Journal of Developmental and Behavioral Pediatrics* 28 (August 2007): 82–91.

Stanton, Rosemary. *Good Fats Bad Fats.* New York: Marlowe, 2002.

Sun, Qi, Jing Ma, Hannia Campos, Susan E. Hankinson, et al. "A Prospective Study of Trans Fatty Acids in Erythrocytes and Risk of Coronary Heart Disease." *Circulation* 115 (April 10, 2007): 1858–65.

"Time to Fatten Up Our Diets." *Harvard Health Letter* (September 2007).

Tribole, Evelyn. *The Ultimate Omega-3 Diet.* New York: McGraw-Hill, 2007.

Wallace, Hannah. "The New Good Fat: Omega-3s. Omega-6s: Bad. Except for CLA, a Member of the Omega-6 Family That May Help Fight Weight Gain, Allergies, and More." *Natural Health* 37 (July–August 2007): 89–92.

"When Zero Isn't Nothing." *Harvard Reviews of Health News* (August 21, 2007).

Yost, Debora. "Powerful Protection against Heart Disease, Cancer, and Inflammation." *Life Extension* (September 2007).

## FIBER

Fiber in the diet is a bulky part of various plants that is not broken down by digestion. While fiber has little real nutritional value, it does have a host of health benefits and may help with everything from lowering cancer rates, the risk for diabetes, and levels of cholesterol and triglycerides to preventing constipation and heart disease; at the same time, it can help dieters feel full with fewer calories.

Also known as roughage or bulk, fiber is in the skins, seeds, leaves, and roots of various fruits and vegetables as well as in the bran and germ layers of popular grains. Since people lack the digestive enzymes to break down fiber, it moves through the digestive system largely unchanged and depending on the type of fiber, it may either speed up or slow down the passages of the food as waste.

Dietary fiber often is listed on food labels as soluble fiber, fiber that dissolves in water or fluids, and insoluble fiber, which does not dissolve in fluids. Soluble fiber is easily identified in oatmeal, nuts or seeds, lots of fruits, oat bran, and dried beans and peas. Insoluble fiber is found in brown rice, wheat bran, whole wheat bread, barley, and many vegetables and fruits. The soluble fiber, once eaten, dissolves in the fluids secreted by the digestive tract. As it is broken down by the fluids, the fiber forms a gel, which then passes slowly through the rest of the digestive area. Soluble fiber is known to slow the rate of digestion and absorption, which assists in stabilizing blood sugar levels in diabetics. The slow rate of digestion also helps reduce levels of low-density lipoproteins (LDL) or the "bad" cholesterol. LDL collects in the walls of blood vessels and can create blockages. Higher LDL levels also increase the risk of a heart attack or blood clot.

On the other hand, foods that contain insoluble fiber act to keep the digestive system running smoothly and on time, as the fiber goes through the system largely unchanged. Foods containing lots of insoluble fiber include fruits and vegetables with an edible skin or seeds. Each type of fiber plays a role in wellness, and nutritionists encourage a diet with a variety of both kinds of fiber. The government recommendation for daily intake of dietary fiber is 14 grams for every 1,000 calories consumed. That means that someone who routinely eats 2,000 calories each day should include at least 28 to 35 grams of dietary fiber in his or her food choices (United States Department of Agriculture, 2011).

Studies increasing show that a fiber rich diet improves an individual's health. Researchers from Northwestern University concluded that middle-age adults who consume large amounts of fiber are less likely to develop heart disease in their lifetime ("Fiber May Lessen Lifetime Risk," 2011). In fact, a study by

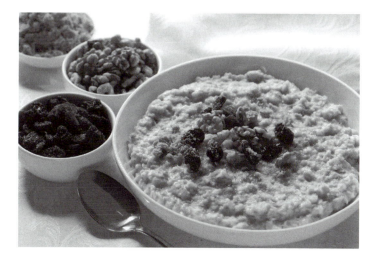

Oatmeal served with dried fruit and nuts is a high fiber meal. (Robyn Mackenzie/Dreamstime.com)

the National Cancer Institute in conjunction with the American Association for Retired Persons released in 2011 found that overall health substantially improved for men and women who eat the highest levels of dietary fiber. The nine-year study showed that men and women who ate from 25 to 29 grams of fiber per day were 22 percent less likely to die than those eating the least, from 10 to 12 grams of fiber per day (Park, Subar, Hollenbeck, & Schatzkin, 2011).

As baby boomers age, they are paying attention to the message a about fiber. According to market research firm Datamonitor, the variety of fiber-rich foods is growing dramatically. According to statistics from Datamonitor, 890 new products reached supermarket shelves in 2007, and more growth is expected (Raymond, 2007). Still, Americans have a long way to go to improve their fiber intake. According to the National Fiber Council, the average Americans eats about half of the recommended amount of dietary fiber (Raymond, 2007).

Scientists and food manufacturers are working to create a new type of fiber known as digestion-resistant starch. The starches are produced by heating or chemically adjusting existing starches as well as by genetically engineering plants to produce a more fiber-rich grain such as wheat and rice.

For grains, the refining process removes the bran, or outer coat of the grain, and this lowers its fiber content. That is why brown rice has more fiber than white rice, which has had the hull removed. It stands to reason that removing the skin from fruits and vegetables also lowers their fiber content. Refined and processed foods, including canned fruits and vegetables, are lower in fiber content than their fresh counterparts. The fiber content is shown on the label, and, as of 2011, manufacturers were required to list the total amount of fiber and the amount of fiber in each serving of food. Legislators are also considering a requirement that soluble fiber be listed separately from total fiber on nutrition labels since the soluble fiber contains the largest health benefit for consumers. Fiber supplements, while helpful, still lack the vitamins, minerals, and other nutrients found in fresh foods.

*Sharon Zoumbaris*

*See also* Cancer; Heart Health; Vegetables.

### References

"Dietary Fiber: Essential for a Healthy Diet." Mayo Clinic (November 19, 2009), www.mayoclinic.com/health/fiber/NU00033.

"Fiber May Lessen Lifetime Risk for Heart Problems: Study Finds That Odds of Disease Were Lowest for Those Who Consumed the Most Fiber." *Consumer Health News* (March 22, 2011), http://consumer.healthday.com/Article.asp?AID=651052.

"New Forms of Dietary Fiber to Boost Health." *Science Letter* (December 21, 2010): 166.

Park, Yikyung, Amy F. Subar, Albert Hollenbeck, and Arthur Schatzkin. "Dietary Fiber Intake and Mortality in the NIH-AARP Diet and Health Study." *Archives of Internal Medicine* (February 14, 2011), http://archinter.ama-assn.org.

Raymond, Joan. "Is Fiber the New Protein?" *Newsweek,* April 16, 2007, www.newsweek.com/2007/04/15/is-fiber-the-new-protein.html.

United States Department of Agriculture. "Dietary Reference Intakes: Macronutrients." *Food and Nutrition Information Center* (May 10, 2011), www.fnic.nal.usda.gov.

## FIBROMYALGIA

The hallmark of fibromyalgia (FM) includes the presence of multiple tender points at specific locations over the body combined with the report of widespread musculoskeletal pain. A good analogy is to consider pain as a radio signal. If the volume control on the receiver is broken and broadcasts only at a greatly amplified sound level, an otherwise normal listening experience will become difficult to tolerate. It is the same type of experience with pain in FM; even typically nonpainful stimuli like a gentle hug can cause discomfort because of pain amplification. This phenomenon is caused in large part by central sensitization, and, in fact, many researchers believe the central nervous system is the key factor in the pathology of FM. Like most chronic illnesses, the symptoms of FM extend far beyond the defining criteria. In addition to pain, many patients also report the following comorbidities (overlapping but separate disorders or symptoms):

- Fatigue
- Muscle and joint stiffness
- Insomnia
- Restless legs syndrome
- Balance issues, including orthostatic hypotension and dysautonomia
- Headaches, including migraine headaches

## Cognitive Lapses

- Raynaud's phenomenon
- Autoimmune disorders such as Sjögren's syndrome and rheumatoid arthritis
- Visual, auditory, tactile, and olfactory hypersensitivities
- Irritable bowel and irritable bladder
- Pelvic pain, endometriosis, vulvodynia
- Depression and anxiety disorders
- Temporomandibular joint dysfunction

The symptoms of FM may improve, may worsen, or may be continual, but the disorder is extremely unlikely to completely go away. Periods when symptoms worsen are termed *flares* and are often brought on by physical overexertion or stress. Many people with FM find that, at least some of the time, their illness prevents them from engaging in common everyday activities, such as traveling in a car for prolonged periods and climbing stairs. The disorder can be debilitating and often has a serious impact on family relationships, social friendships, and the ability to stay employed. It is understandable that life satisfaction levels suffer when someone cannot participate in what is considered a normal lifestyle. As is true with most chronic pain conditions, depression and anxiety are a common response to FM symptoms. Unfortunately, some medical providers continue to treat FM as only a psychosomatic disorder despite more and more research confirming that FM is, in fact, physical.

There are some further points to remember about this disorder. First, FM is not limited to the musculoskeletal system; research has shown brain and spinal cord involvement. Second, although some persons with FM may first experience primary immune system disorders such as rheumatoid arthritis, systemic lupus erythematosus, or Sjögren's syndrome, FM is not in itself an autoimmune disease. Third, we know this disorder is not the same as chronic fatigue immune dysfunction syndrome (CFIDS), because people with FM have chemical hallmarks in their spinal column fluid that are not present in CFIDS. Fourth, FM is not a mental illness. Studies have shown there is no higher incidence of mental illness in FM than in many other chronic pain populations. Overall, it is important to remember that FM is not a catchall diagnosis; it is a chronic, nondegenerative, noninflammatory disorder with an accepted diagnostic criteria.

The differences between rheumatic conditions involving joint deformity, termed *articular rheumatism,* and painful but nondeforming muscular rheumatism was recorded in the early to mid-1800s. A surgeon named William Balfour from Edinburgh, Scotland, and later the physician François Valleix in Paris, independently described unusually painful areas in patients with muscular rheumatism that produced shooting pain when palpated. *Fibrositis* was the term that preceded fibromyalgia. It first came into use in 1904, when English neurologist Sir William Gowers wrote a medical paper on low back pain. He speculated that low back tenderness was due to inflammatory changes in muscle fiber tissue and discussed for the first time the concept of pain amplification, as well as the possible contribution of disrupted sleep and fatigue to diffuse rheumatic muscle pain.

However, subsequent studies of muscle biopsies failed to find traditional indications of inflammation, and the term *fibrositis* was then considered a misnomer. At the turn of the 20th century, physician Sir William Osler coined the term *myalgia* and speculated that the pain of muscular rheumatism involved "neuralgia of the sensory nerves of the muscles." World War II saw an increase in the diagnosis of fibrositis in British soldiers, with 70 percent of all rheumatic patients in British army hospitals diagnosed with the condition.

Over time, the terms *fibrositis, fibromyositis, muscular rheumatism,* and even "tender lady syndrome" have all been used to describe this disorder. In 1973 the researcher Philip Hench first introduced the term *fibromyalgia,* which more accurately describes the symptoms. This current term is referenced by the following medical root words: *fibra* (Latin for fiber), *myo* (Greek for muscle), and *algos* (Greek for pain). Researchers such as Muhammad B. Yunus, Robert M. Bennett, I. Jon Russell, and others, seeking to clearly define FM in the 1980s, proposed the need for a unified classification system. In 1990, following a rigorous multisite research study, the American College of Rheumatology published a formal "Criteria for the Classification of Fibromyalgia." The American Medical Association recognized FM as a true illness and as a major cause of disability in 1987; the World Health Organization followed with the same recognition in 1992.

In most chronic illnesses a single lead cause eludes researchers, and FM is no different. However, scientists continue to develop a number of hypotheses about who may develop this disorder and why based on good objective evidence. Along with demographic studies and recorded clinical observations that highlight known risk factors, causation hypotheses are helpful in indicating further possible risk. Both known and suspected risk factors include gender, age, genetics, viral infection, stress, nervous system malfunctioning, sleep disturbances, and hormonal discrepancies.

**Gender, Age, and Genetics**  The two greatest known risk factors for FM appear to be a family history of the disease and being female. In fact, two recent studies have revealed that FM in a first-degree female relative is the greatest predictor of developing FM. No one knows why more women are diagnosed with FM than men. Various studies based on prevalence data show that women are seven to nine times more likely to have fibromyalgia than men and that the peak age for diagnosis in women is during the childbearing years. This has led researchers to suspect that either childbirth or menopause might be triggers for some women. However, there are no data to support the idea that gender-specific hormones such as estrogen, progesterone, or testosterone are linked to the development of the disorder.

FM is found in all age ranges, from children to the frail elderly. Research funded by the National Institutes of Health has begun to find out more about FM in both of these age spans. One study found that one-quarter of adult FM patients report their symptoms started before 15 years of age. Other studies have shown that the disorder's principal symptoms are the same for children as for adults, although children have more commonly reported nighttime growing pains, pain in extremities, poor sleep, and difficulty keeping up with their peers in athletic endeavors. In contrast, children have reported less low back pain, hand pain, or symptom changes associated with mood or weather. Indeed, pain is not one of the primary complaints in children with FM. This is likely because young children have a hard time knowing their pain isn't normal. Claudia Marek, author of *The First Year—Fibromyalgia,* interviewed a group of children and was amazed to discover 50 percent of her interviewees thought everyone they knew had pain but that other children were simply braver and better at coping with it than they were. Consequently, they were unwilling to verbalize their distress to others.

In fact, for many children with FM, the pain they experience is normal to them. Since they have not experienced life without the disorder, they cannot distinguish their symptoms as unusual. FM can be quite severe in childhood. Similar steps to those used for diagnosing FM in adults are used by pediatric providers: a medical history is taken, other possible causes for the symptoms are ruled out, and a tender point survey is performed. Children and adolescents with FM may report as few as five tender points. As discussed earlier, this can be because their experience of normal pain is skewed and leads to an underestimation of pressure pain severity during the test.

Children with FM are often misdiagnosed at first with mood disorders or other conditions, and it is not unusual for families seeking help for their children to have difficult experiences before receiving the correct diagnosis. Beyond the same discounting of symptoms adults with FM have received from the medical community in the past, some parents report they were unjustly accused of poor parenting by encouraging their child toward an imaginary disability, or even of inventing illness in a bid for the parents to receive heightened attention. Sometimes it is the cognitive problems experienced with FM that will first alert parents to seek medical help for their child. When this happens, the more recognized learning disorders such as dyslexia or attention deficit disorder are often explored and ruled out before finding the correct diagnosis. One discernable difference between children with dyslexia or other learning difficulties and those with FM is that those with learning difficulties will have a consistent struggle to perform certain tasks, whereas a young student who has no difficulty concentrating on schoolwork one day but struggles on other days may be displaying the "fibro-fog" of FM.

On the other end of the age spectrum, older adults bear the greatest burden of FM. One study found that only 9 percent of consecutively enrolled older adults tested for FM had previously received the diagnosis. Other painful conditions that come with aging may be the culprit. As an example, multiple surgeries, especially back and pelvic or abdominal surgeries, are associated as triggers for FM, and so age itself may also be a trigger for FM.

Alternately, one of the greatest risks for elderly patients who have been diagnosed with FM is that other diseases may be blamed on FM and thereby overlooked. For example, cardiac chest pain can be misdiagnosed as tender-point chest pain by either the patient or the clinician, while widespread pain from metastatic (spreading) cancer or the typical fatigue of undetected hypothyroidism (low thyroid disease) or anemia may be misinterpreted as the pain and fatigue of FM. Back pain with numbness, tingling, or radiating to the hips and legs may be neurologic in nature and not due to FM. Severe hip osteoarthritis (degenerating joint inflammation) is often overlooked in FM because of an older patient's longstanding pain, or may be attributed to the lessening mobility and deconditioning associated with normal aging. Autoimmune diseases such as polymyalgia rheumatica (PMR, an inflammatory condition) in persons older than 50 can also be misdiagnosed as FM despite a simple blood test called a sedimentation rate that could easily differentiate the two. This type of searching beyond the explanation of FM pain is critical; for example, undiagnosed PMR can sometimes progress to irreversible blindness.

By definition, no single surgery or round of medications will cure a chronic illness. Since that is the case, treatments for chronic illnesses are ongoing and lifelong. A biopsychosocial treatment schedule has proven to be the best approach for regaining good quality of life when living with FM.

The ultimate goal of health treatment is to reduce symptoms, promote physical fitness, and optimize the ability to perform activities of daily living. One health care provider alone cannot hope to accomplish this breadth of goals. An interdisciplinary team of providers is generally required for the best treatment outcome. The most important player on the team, however, is the person with FM. A patient who is active in the management of his or her FM is critical. A passive person with FM who expects a doctor's cure will be disappointed.

The FM patient who is proactive in his or her own health will need to assemble a treatment team and, further, become well educated about the disorder. This will mean staying informed about any current medication and its possible side effects, learning about common FM comorbidity symptoms, exploring cognitive behavioral strategies along with complementary and alternative therapies, exercising, and maintaining a nutritional diet. A good treatment team can provide the necessary knowledge.

### Treatment Team

*Primary Provider*   A single primary provider who can prescribe medications is the cornerstone of the treatment team. This might be a primary care physician, nurse practitioner, physician's assistant, internist, osteopathic physician (a holistic provider also called a doctor of osteopathy), or perhaps a physiatrist (a physician specializing in physical rehabilitation). The primary provider will be responsible for making the diagnosis, prescribing medications, and managing recommendations from other specialists.

*Physical Therapist*   A physical therapist (PT) can evaluate and treat regional pain, balance issues, and discuss energy conservation to manage fatigue. Treatments employed by PTs may include rehabilitation exercise, manual therapies, neurosensory balance analyses (measuring nerve transmission information to and from peripheral extremities to the CNS), gait analyses with corrective orthotics fitting, and a multitude of management strategies for long-term self-care. PTs can also teach patients to use spray-and-stretch, a treatment that requires a prescription from the provider for fluoromethasone cooling spray (a skin refrigerant). The PT can teach patients to spray the medication on selected muscles, which allows painfully tight muscles to be stretched with less discomfort. Patients can then use spray-and-stretch at home whenever needed. PTs may fit patients for prescription orthotics for foot pain and work in concert with an orthotist to ensure proper fitting. Finally, PTs may administer ultrasound therapies to reduce pain from regional syndromes, including temporomandibular joint dysfunction (also called TMD, a cause of jaw pain) and chronic back pain.

*Occupational Therapist* An occupational therapist (OT) can provide many of the same services as a physical therapist but commonly will focus more on physical modifications to workplace, home, or activities of daily living. Some PTs and OTs will divide the care of FM patients so that large muscles and joints are evaluated and managed by the PT, while smaller muscles and joints are evaluated by the OT. An example of this could include management of wrist pain or carpal tunnel syndrome by the OT and management of knee pain by the PT. In addition to providing individually fitted wrist splints and rehabilitative exercises, the OT might train the patient in such things as how to keep the body aligned in a neutral position during normal activity. The OT also has ergonomic expertise and can recommend a variety of equipment to ease pain and promote optimal posture.

OTs are usually well versed in creating an optimal work environment. They can help patients ask employers for special accommodations such as avoidance of bright or flashing lights, strong smells, cold environments, or loud noises. They can help clarify whether an employee can physically tolerate standing for prolonged periods of time; can perform repetitive tasks; and has a fast, unobstructed path to the restroom; and they can explain the need for that employee to take short, frequent stretch breaks. At home, they can help patients think twice about where they store commonly used items in the kitchen, how to hang pictures, and how to do housework, and they can remind patients of the need to pace themselves to avoid triggering a symptom flare. They are often the providers who suggest modifications such as vocational rehabilitation or suggest that patients consider disability.

*Speech Therapist* The speech therapist (ST) is a communications expert who can evaluate cognitive difficulties such as fibro-fog and differentiate them from cognitive deficits related to dementia, post-stroke, or head trauma. FM patients often report great distress about their perceived cognitive decline, so the ability to improve cognitive function is typically welcomed as life-enhancing. The ST will recommend a variety of nonpharmacologic strategies to maximize cognitive abilities and provide mental exercises to help enhance memory. Some of these strategies include establishing easily recalled routines, placing reminder notes, forming memory associations, decreasing multitasking, and reducing distractions.

*Clinical Exercise Specialist* The clinical exercise specialist (CES) is a fitness professional who has advanced training in working with special populations, including those with chronic illnesses. In this developing field, the CES works as a bridge between the medical clinic and a home or public exercise setting where ongoing postrehabilitative workouts can take place. The CES provides guidance that takes into account the recommendations of the primary provider, the PT, the OT, and the ST. The CES may work as a specialized in-home personal trainer or lead special population classes in a general exercise setting. CESs also work as medical research study team members, providing physical function testing or leading strictly defined study-based group exercise. In their close association with an FM client, they are often the first to hear about side effects or adverse events that might be related to a prescription drug, a developing comorbidity, or a change in disease course. They are an important link in knowledge and communication, encouraging a client with FM to seek direction and further treatment planning from the primary provider or other members of the treatment team.

*Psychologist*    The psychologist is one of many health care providers who can help maximize quality of life in someone with a chronic illness. Similarly, psychiatric mental health nurse practitioners (PMHNPs) and medical social workers possess some of the same skills. All can generally offer counseling related to cognitive-behavioral strategies. These strategies are often beyond the scope of the primary health care provider. Cognitive-behavioral strategies are formed by talk therapy and are individualized for each patient. For many with FM, these therapies can include fatigue control, decreasing catastrophic thinking, and boundary setting. There are numerous other types of counseling as well that these professionals can employ, depending on the needs of the patient or family they are treating. The PMHNP can also prescribe medication to augment therapy.

*Registered Dietitian*    The registered dietician (RD) is helpful in FM because many people's quality of life will improve through dietary change. The RD can help people learn not only what foods to avoid or minimize but how to introduce new foods into the diet and how to really enjoy new foods. In FM, obesity is often a problem, especially due to the sporadic nature of FM flare cycles and the resulting disruption of an exercise routine. The RD can individualize an eating plan based on each patient's food preferences. In general, they discourage diets and emphasize healthier eating for the long run. They also try to strip away moral value from food by discouraging naming certain foods "good" or "bad." Instead, they focus on which foods to eat often and which foods to enjoy less frequently or in smaller amounts. Another role of the RD is to help people with concurrent celiac disease, since gluten and its related products are so prevalent in the food supply. Lactose intolerance is a bit easier to negotiate, but an RD will have tips to minimize symptoms stemming from that problem as well.

The future of RDs in FM can involve helping patients remove or reduce dietary excitotoxins, including agents such as unbound glutamate. Similarly, as evidence mounts regarding agents such as aspartame and its influence on N-methyl D-aspartate (NMDA) receptor activity, those foods may need to be modified as well. These last two are particularly tricky, because dietary excitotoxins are common in our food supply but are not generally listed on food labels. When they are listed, they come in a variety of names and chemical compounds. The term *nutritionist* is not protected by law; therefore, anyone can claim the title of nutritionist, including many diet authors. The title of RD or LD (licensed dietitian) guarantees qualification by license and legal standards.

Others who can bring optimal care are the medical providers who specialize in the common comorbidities of FM. It is critical for the primary provider to seek evaluation and treatment recommendations for any diagnosed or undiagnosed symptom within the specialist's area of expertise. The primary provider does not ask the specialist to manage the patient's overall FM; he or she only refers the patient for treatment of the comorbidity. Specialists include a gastroenterologist, urologist, sleep specialist, endocrinologist, neurologist, rheumatologist, orthopedic surgeon, andpsychiatrist.

**Patient Education**   After assembling the FM treatment team, education about FM is invaluable. Education can occur individually between the provider and patient; in support groups; or through carefully selected books, media, and Internet sites. The primary provider is tasked with providing education regarding the validity of the FM diagnosis and the nondestructive nature of the condition on muscle. The provider outlines a rational treatment plan focusing on minimizing symptoms and restoring functionality. It is disheartening to learn that it is generally not possible to return to the state of health experienced before the onset of FM; most symptoms can never be totally eradicated. Having realistic expectations about the amount of relief possible from medications (generally 30 to 50 percent) is important for learning to cope with a new lifestyle reality. The primary provider will be supportive but realistic in terms of the lifelong nature of FM. Together patient and provider can review evidence-based educational materials. Touted cures can be discussed between the primary provider and the patient, but ultimately treatment choices and financial decisions belong to the patient.

*Kim D. Jones and Janice H. Hoffman*

*See also* Chronic Fatigue Syndrome (CFS); Depression; Immune System/Lymphatic System; Lupus.

## References

Blehm, R. "Physical Therapy and Other Nonpharmacologic Approaches to Fibromyalgia Management." *Current Pain and Headache Reports* 10, no. 5 (2006): 333–38.

Buskila, D., P. Sarzi-Puttini, and J.N. Ablin. "The Genetics of Fibromyalgia Syndrome." *Pharmacogenomics* 8, no. 1 (2007): 67–74.

Crooks, V.A. "Exploring the Altered Daily Geographies and Lifeworlds of Women Living with Fibromyalgia Syndrome: A Mixed-Method Approach." *Social Science and Medicine* 64, no. 3 (2007): 577–88.

Jones, C.J., K.D. Jones, D.N. Rutledge, L. Matallana, and D. Rooks. "Self-assessed Physical Function Levels of Women with Fibromyalgia: A National Survey." *Women's Health Issues* 18, no. 5 (2008): 406–12.

Jones, K.D., J.H. Hoffman, and D.G. Adams. "Exercise and Fibromyalgia." In *Understanding Fitness: How Exercise Fuels Health and Fight Disease,* edited by Julie K. Silver and Christopher Morin, 170–81.Westport, CT: Praeger, 2008.

Marek, Claudia C. *The First Year—Fibromyalgia: An Essential Guide for the Newly Diagnosed.* New York: Marlowe, 2003.

Otis, John. *Managing Chronic Pain: A Cognitive-Behavioral Therapy Approach Workbook.* New York: Oxford University Press, 2007.

Russell, I.J. "Fibromyalgia Syndrome: New Developments in Pathophysiology and Management. Introduction." *CNS Spectrums* 3, no. S5 (2008): 4–5.

Trock, David H., and Francis Chamberlain. *Healing Fibromyalgia. The Three Step Solution.* Hoboken, NJ: John Wiley, 2007.

Williams, D.A., and R.H. Gracely. "Biology and Therapy of Fibromyalgia: Functional Magnetic Resonance Imaging Findings in Fibromyalgia." *Arthritis Research and Therapy* 8, no. 6 (2007): 224.

Wood, P.B., J.C. Patterson, J.J. Sunderland, K.H. Tainter, M.F. Glabus, and D.L. Lilien. "Reduced Presynaptic Dopamine Activity in Fibromyalgia Syndrome Demonstrated with Positron Emission Tomography: A Pilot Study." *Clinical Journal of Pain* 8, no. 1 (2007): 51–58.

# FLAXSEEDS

The flax plant has a truly ancient history. During the Stone Age, it grew in Mesopotamia, which is now the southern portion of Iraq. There are recordings of the use of flaxseeds in the preparation of food in ancient Greece. In both ancient Greece and ancient Rome, flaxseeds were believed to have a number of healthful benefits. But after the decline of the Roman Empire, interest in flaxseeds waned.

That changed in the eighth and ninth centuries. The emperor Charlemagne reintroduced flaxseeds to the European palate. Centuries later, colonists planted flax in the United States. In the 17th century, flaxseeds arrived in Canada. Today, Canada is the world's largest producer of flaxseeds (George Mateljan Foundation, 2010). (Flaxseeds have also been used to make products such as rope, linen, linseed oil, and linoleum.)

Flaxseeds contain very good amounts of manganese and dietary fiber. They have good amounts of magnesium, folate, copper, phosphorus, and vitamin B6 (George Mateljan Foundation, 2010). Additionally, flaxseeds have alpha-linolenic acid (ALA), an omega fat that is a precursor to eicosapentaenoic acid, the type of omega-3 that is found in fish oil. Furthermore, they have lignans, phytochemicals (plant-based substances) that have estrogenic and anticancer effects (Turner, 2009). But it is important to review the research.

## Cancer

***Breast Cancer*** In a study published in 2004 in the *American Journal of Clinical Nutrition,* Canadian researchers supplemented the diet of 46 postmenopausal women with a daily muffin. For 16 weeks, the women ate muffins with a placebo or soy (25 grams of soy flour) or flaxseed (25 grams of ground flaxseed). At the end of the study, the researchers determined that the estrogen metabolism of those eating the flaxseed muffins, but not the soy or placebo muffins, had undergone a few changes. The levels of 2-hydroxyestrone, which is believed to be protective against breast cancer, had increased significantly. Second, the ratio of 2-hydroxyestrone to 16-alpha-hydroxyestrone (a metabolite that is thought to promote cancer) increased dramatically. This is also indicative of cancer prevention. So, flaxseeds appeared to have anticancer properties while the blood levels of the estrogen fractions (estradiol, estrone, and estrone sulfate) remained the same, which is important for bone health (Brooks et al., 2004).

***Prostate Cancer*** In a study published in 2008 in *Cancer Epidemiology, Biomarkers and Prevention,* researchers placed 161 men with prostate cancer on one of four diets at least 21 days before their scheduled prostatectomy: a flaxseed-supplemented diet (30 grams per day), a low-fat diet (less than 20 percent total energy), a flaxseed supplement low-fat diet, or a control (usual) diet. The men, who had a mean age of 59 years, remained on the diet for an average of 30 days.

Following surgery, the tumors were analyzed. Researchers found that tumors in the men who followed the diets that contained flaxseeds grew 40 to 50 percent more slowly than in the men who ate the low-fat or control diets. The researchers concluded that "flaxseed is safe and associated with biological alterations that may be preventive for prostate cancer" (Demark-Wahnefried et al., 2008).

**Hot Flashes** In a small study published in 2007 in the *Journal of the Society for Integrative Oncology,* Mayo Clinic researchers examined the use of flaxseeds to help women who did not want to take hormonal therapy manage their hot flashes. To be included in the study, women had to experience 14 hot flashes per week for at least one month.

For six weeks, every day, the women took 40 grams of crushed flaxseeds. At the conclusion of the study, the researchers found that the frequency of hot flashes had decreased by 50 percent—from 7.3 hot flashes to 3.6. However, a significant number of the women experienced gastrointestinal problems, a side effect that is not uncommon with flaxseed supplementation. Nevertheless, the researchers noted that flaxseed dietary therapy "decreases hot flash activity in women not taking estrogen therapy" (Pruthi et al., 2007).

On the other hand, a study published in 2006 in *Menopause* compared the effects of the 16-week consumption of daily muffins containing either 25 grams of soy flour, 25 grams of ground flaxseed, or wheat flour (control) on the frequency and severity of hot flashes in 99 postmenopausal women. Eighty-seven women completed the study. Of these, 31 ate the soy flour muffins; 28 ate the ground flaxseed muffins; and 28 ate wheat flour muffins. Although the researchers conducted extensive analysis of the results, they found that "neither dietary flaxseed nor soy flour significantly affected menopause-specific quality of life or hot flash symptoms in this study" (Lewis et al., 2006).

**Reduce Symptoms of Attention Deficit Hyperactivity Disorder** In a study published in 2006 in *Prostaglandins, Leukotrienes and Essential Fatty Acids,* researchers reviewed the effect that flaxseed oil had on 30 children with attention deficit hyperactivity disorder (ADHD) in Pune, India. The average age of the boys was seven years; the average age of the girls was eight and a half years. Boys outnumbered girls by three to one. The control group consisted of 30 healthy children without ADHD.

For three months, the children with ADHD were given daily flaxseed oil supplementation "corresponding to 200 mg [milligrams] ALA content along with 25 mg vitamin C twice a day." All of the children completed the study; no one had any side effects.

The researchers observed dramatic improvements in the symptoms of children with ADHD. "All the symptoms like impulsivity, restlessness, inattention, self-control, psychosomatic problems and learning problems showed highly significant improvement."

Social and learning problems, so often seen with ADHD, also improved. The researchers noted that "flax oil-based emulsion could be a useful adjunct for effective therapy of ADHD" (Joshi et al., 2006).

**Lower Blood Pressure**   In a 12-week study published in 2007 in the *European Journal of Clinical Nutrition,* Greek researchers supplemented the diets of 59 middle-aged men who had dyslipoidemia (abnormal fats in the blood) with flaxseed oil. The diet of a control group of 28 men was supplemented with safflower oil. The goal was to determine the effect that flaxseed oil had on the blood pressure.

The researchers found that when compared to supplementation with safflower oil, supplementation with flaxseed oil resulted in significant reductions in both systolic and diastolic blood pressure levels. By lowering blood pressure levels, flaxseed oil helps to maintain cardiovascular health (Paschos et al., 2007).

**Improved Cognition**   In a study published in 2005 in the *Journal of Nutrition,* Dutch researchers examined the association between dietary intake of phytoestrogens—specifically lignans, such as those contained in flaxseeds—and cognitive function in 394 healthy postmenopausal women who consume a Western diet. The researchers found that the women who included higher amounts of lignans in their diets had significantly better cognitive performance. This was particularly apparent in the women who were 20 to 30 years postmenopausal. The researchers wrote, "From our results, we conclude that higher dietary intake of lignans is associated with better cognitive function in postmenopausal women." Even so, the researchers noted that the results are far from conclusive. "Data on the relation between phytoestrogens and cognitive function are still sparse and far from sufficient to become conclusive" (Franco et al., 2005).

**Two Caveats**   Since the body is unable to break down whole flaxseeds, the seeds must be ground before consumed or added to another food such as yogurt or oatmeal. Small grinding machines, such as those used to grind coffee, are useful for grinding flaxseed.

It is generally recommended that people add one to two tablespoons of flaxseeds to their daily diets. However, as has previously been noted, flaxseeds may cause gastrointestinal problems. So, it is best to begin with a relatively small amount of flaxseeds, and slowly increase the amount.

*Myrna Chandler Goldstein and Mark A. Goldstein*

*See also* Attention Deficit Hyperactivity Disorder (ADHD); Cancer; Fiber; Hypertension.

## References

Brooks, Jennifer D., Wendy E. Ward, Jacqueline E. Lewis, et al. "Supplementation with Flaxseed Alters Estrogen Metabolism in Postmenopausal Women to a Greater Extent Than Does Supplementation with an Equal Amount of Soy." *American Journal of Clinical Nutrition* 79, no. 2 (February 2004): 318–25.

Demark-Wahnefried, Wendy, Thomas J. Polascik, Stephen I. George, et al. "Flaxseed Supplementation (Not Dietary Fat Restriction) Reduces Prostate Cancer Proliferation in Men Presurgery." *Cancer Epidemiology, Biomarkers and Prevention* 17, no. 12 (2008): 3577–87.

Franco, Oscar H., Huibert Burger, Corinne E.I. Lebrun, et al. "Higher Dietary Intake of Lignans Is Associated with Better Cognitive Performance in Postmenopausal Women." *Journal of Nutrition* 135 (May 2005): 1190–95.

George Mateljan Foundation. "Flaxseeds," http://whfoods.org/genpage.php?tname=food spice&dbid=81.

Joshi, Kalpana, Sagar Lad, Mrudula Kale, et al. "Supplementation with Flax Oil and Vitamin C Improves the Outcome of Attention Deficit Hyperactivity Disorder (ADHA)." *Prostaglandins, Leukotrienes and Essential Fatty Acids* 74, no. 1 (January 2006): 17–21.

Lewis, Jacqueline E., Leslie A. Nickell, Lilian U. Thompson, et al. "A Randomized Controlled Trial of the Effect of Dietary Soy and Flaxseed Muffins on Quality of Life and Hot Flashes during Menopause." *Menopause* 13, no. 4 (July–August 2006): 631–42.

Paschos, G.K., F. Magkos, D.B. Panagiotakos, et al. "Dietary Supplementation with Flaxseed Oil Lowers Blood Pressure in Dyslipidaemic Patients." *European Journal of Clinical Nutrition* 61 (2007): 1201–6.

Pruthi, S., S.L. Thompson, P.J. Novotny, et al. "Pilot Evaluation of Flaxseed for the Management of Hot Flashes." *Journal of the Society for Integrative Oncology* 5, no. 3 (Summer 2007): 106–12.

Turner, Lisa. "Just the Flax: Discover Delicious Flax Products—And Get the Most from Flaxseeds and Oils." *Better Nutrition* 71, no. 6 (June 2009): 60.

## FLEXIBLE SPENDING ACCOUNT (FSA)

Flexible spending accounts have been around for a while and are available to consumers through their employer-offered health insurance. Similar to a dependent care flexible spending account, these accounts allow individuals to pay predictable health care expenses with tax-free income.

Health care FSAs require an accurate assessment of health care costs for the upcoming year. Employees who enroll are allowed to set aside a certain amount of money from their pretaxed salary. The money is deducted from the employee's pay and placed into an account that can be used to pay for authorized medical expenses not covered by insurance. These expenses may include doctor's visits or copays, prescription medications, glasses or contact lenses, even braces or other dental procedures. This type of an account works well for planned expenses such as a monthly orthodontia bill or blood pressure medication, birth control pills, any expense that happens on an ongoing, monthly basis.

The fund can be used to pay medical bills even before the money is deducted from the employee's pay. However, an important fact for someone with a health care FSA to be aware of is that this is a use-it-or-lose-it account—any money left at the end of the year is forfeited by the employee.

Once the figure is determined at the beginning of the employer's plan year, the employee cannot alter the amount of money to be set aside even if the planned expenses change, such as a child getting his or her braces off early. Still, the money can be used for any other qualified expenses, and many people use left-over money to stock up on contacts or get a filling or crown they had been putting off because of the cost.

Another positive feature of flexible spending accounts is their ability to provide dollars for expenses that a basic health insurance plan may not cover. Services such as acupuncture, smoking cessation programs, chiropractors, and psychiatric care may be allowed. Plus, an employee can use the money as reimbursement for children's health care expenses as well as his or her own health care expenses. For these reasons, FSAs are growing in popularity due to the increasing use of nonconventional treatment plans and alternative medicine by many Americans. According to statistics from the National Center for Complementary and Alternative Medicine, a branch of the National Institutes of Health, At least 38 percent of adults in the United States and some 12 percent of children are currently using some form of complementary or alternative medicine. The most widely used complementary or alternative medicine therapies include acupuncture, biofeedback, hypnosis, massage, and meditation. In addition, employees are beginning to recognize that FSAs offer more flexibility and greater opportunity to use the money they would normally pay for vision and dental care insurance premiums.

To illustrate the savings, if a salary is taxed at 25 percent, only 75 cents per dollar is left to pay uncovered medical expenses. For an employee who decides to set aside $2,000 per year in a health care FSA, each full dollar of the $2,000 is available to reimburse qualified expenses. If employee used the full $2,000 deferred to his or her health care account, he or she would save approximately $500 in taxes. This, in turn reduces taxable income, similar to the way a 401(k) contribution works, because the money contributed to the FSA is transferred out before income taxes are applied.

**Changes in the Law**   Unfortunately for many employees, 2011 marks the start of significant changes to FSAs due to the 2010 Patient Protection and Affordable Care Act. There are two main changes that have the potential to raise health care costs. First, beginning in January 2011, qualified deductible items no longer include over-the-counter medicines unless they are prescribed by a doctor. This change may be felt most by people with chronic illnesses who depend on drugs that have changed from being available by prescription only to being available over the counter in recent years. Consumers and retailers have criticized this change, especially for loratadine (Claritin) and other allergy medicines, heartburn pills like famotidine (Pepcid), or even for pain relief drugs like acetaminophen (Tylenol). A few drugs, including insulin, are exempt.

Another big change to FSA rules will take effect in 2013, when the annual limit that employees may contribute to their plan will be restricted to $2,500. Employers had allowed larger deductions, often setting the figure between $2,500 and $5,000. However, according to insurance industry estimates, the average amount contributed to employee-sponsored FSAs in 2009 was just over $1,500—well below the $2,500 limit, meaning the cap may not have that much impact on middle-class Americans.

*Sharon Zoumbaris*

*See also* Acupuncture; Health Insurance; Health Savings Account (HSA); Managed Care.

### References

Fingar, Melissa. "FSAs, HSAs, and HRAs: Maximizing Available Health Care Options to Achieve Health Care Savings." *Journal of Compensation and Benefits* 21, no. 3 (May–June 2005): 21.

Geisel, Jerry. "IRS Limits FSA Reimbursements of OTC Medications." *Business Insurance* 44, no. 36 (September 13, 2010): 3.

Konrad, Walecia. "Flexible Spending, a Little Less So." *New York Times* (April 16, 2010), www.nytimes.com/2010/04/17/health/17patient.html.

Long, Emily. "Bill Caps Flexible Spending Account Contributions." Government Executive (December 4, 2009), www.govexec.com./story_page.cfm?filepath=/dailyfed/1209/120409/1.htm&oref=search.

## FOOD ALLERGIES. *See* ALLERGIES, FOOD

## FOOD AND DRUG ADMINISTRATION (FDA)

The Pure Food and Drug Act of 1906 marked the beginning of a series of reform legislation that laid the foundation for the consumer protection movement of the 20th century. The act protected consumers from false labeling of food and drugs and the sale of adulterated food.

It was a great expansion of the powers created by the Commerce Clause of the U.S. Constitution. This law began to have teeth, allowed offending products to be confiscated and destroyed, and allowed individuals and companies to be fined and individuals to be sentenced to jail. This act contained the seeds of the current U.S. Food and Drug Administration (FDA), an agency that monitors, regulates, and oversees food, drugs, biologics, medical and radiologic devices, diagnostic agents, and cosmetics.

Currently the FDA exists under the umbrellas of the U.S. Department of Health and Human Services headquartered in Rockville, Maryland. The headquarters is supported by field offices and laboratories across the United States and its territories. Within the FDA are offices that carry out the day-to-day activities of the various missions assigned to the FDA by law. The Office of the Commissioner supports the head of the agency. The offices that are most related to food are the Center for Food Safety and Applied Nutrition, the Office of Regulatory Affairs (ORA), and the Office of Criminal Investigations (OCI).

The ORA operates primarily through the field offices located around the country. It serves as an information-gathering arm of the agency. Inspections are conducted by investigators or consumer safety officers, who are also spread through the country in the field. These offices are divided into five basic geographic regions, which are subdivided into 13 districts. The support laboratories are also under the ORA.

In 2002 the OCI was established from the ORA to concentrate the enforcement powers and investigations of the FDA. The OCI agents are not involved with the day-to-day inspections, which make up the bulk of the ORA's work. The OCI agents uncover, investigate, and develop cases in criminal matters such as fraudulent labeling, intentional adulteration, intentional tampering, and other criminal acts. OCI agents are armed agents, not inspectors. Food Emergency Response Network, Strategic Partnership Program—Agroterrorism—and other programs are administered in cooperation with other federal agencies such as the Federal Bureau of Investigation.

The FDA has jurisdiction over a large portion of the food in distribution and vitamin supplements in the United States. The Center for Food Safety and Applied Nutrition monitors ingredients, packaging, food safety, and dietary supplements, and it coordinates packaging laws with the European Union and many other food-related activities.

The FDA, the oldest consumer protection agency of the U.S. government, has become more important and more varied as the needs of the public have changed with increased technology. As more was learned about the toxicity of preservatives in food, for example, the FDA was tasked to protect the public. This required a marriage of science and administration that continues today to be the center of the agency's operation. The FDA maintains a recall website for the benefit of consumers.

**Food and Drug Administration Modernization Act of 1997**   The Food and Drug Administration Modernization Act (FDAMA) of 1997 amends the Federal Food, Drug, and Cosmetic Act regarding the monitoring of food and drugs, devices, and biological products. By passing FDAMA, Congress expanded the power and purpose of the FDA in ways that recognized new complexities created by new technological, trade, and public health issues. The highlights of the FDAMA are discussed in the following sections.

*Prescription Drug User Fees*   The law extends the authorization of the Prescription Drug User Fee Act of 1992 for five additional years. The pharmaceutical industry gains from the extension of this program, because, through the expansion of the number of people working in the drugs and biologics sections (approximately 700 additional people), the FDA has substantially decreased the time that it takes for a new drug to be reviewed

*FDA Initiatives and Programs*   This part of the new law affords patients with increased access to experimental and innovative medications and devices. This makes it possible for promising drugs and devices to reach more patients in a more timely manner. It also takes advantage of computer databases to track side effects and increases patient access to information about the new drugs and devices.

An additional portion of the law allows patients using certain life-sustaining drugs or drugs that treat certain debilitating and serious diseases to be notified when a company intends to stop manufacturing that drug. The new law also applies the rules and regulations applicable to drugs to biological products, thus streamlining many processes.

*Information on Off-Label Use and Drug Economics*   Sometimes a drug that has been approved for one purpose turns out to also have other applications. Sometimes the second inadvertent application is more significant than the original. Before this law, dissemination of information regarding unapproved applications of the drug and even medical devices was prohibited. The current law allows the dissemination of peer-reviewed articles in medical journals that discuss other implications of drugs and devices, if the company agrees to file another application for that use of the drug.

Another change is the ability of drug companies to disseminate information about the economics of drug decisions to organizations that purchase drugs and devices in quantity because they treat many people. The purpose of this portion of the law is to allow managed care organizations and formulary committees and the like to make informed decisions about the economic implications of their purchasing decisions. Currently such information may not be provided to individual health care providers.

*Pharmacy Compounding*   Certain drug therapies are not manufactured in commercial quantities. In such cases, drugs must be compounded by hand by pharmacists. These drugs are exempted from the provisions of the law to ensure that pharmacists will continue to compound drugs needed by certain patients. To keep commercial manufacturers from avoiding the law by calling their activities compounding, the law states the definitions and quantities involved to minimize cheating.

*Risk-Based Regulation of Medical Devices*   The FDA, in an effort to place its resources where they are most needed, has created classes of medical devices. Those devices in Class I—that is, those that do not pose a large potential threat to public health if they fail or because they are not used in life-threatening cases—are exempted from premarket notification. The law requires that the FDA focuses on monitoring those devices in the marketplace that present the highest risk to human health and safety. The FDA has put a reporting system in place and can give most of its attention to larger-scale facilities that use the devices regularly and in very diverse conditions.

The act also allows the FDA to contact with outside agencies (which it approves) to review risks and performance of Class I and some Class II devices. There are limitations to the work that may be done by third parties under contract with the FDA.

*Food Safety and Labeling*   The act does away with previous provisions that required that the FDA approve any substances that came into contact with food prior to its use. The current law allows the manufacturer to notify the FDA of the intent to use certain packaging materials. If the manufacturer does not hear that such an action is objectionable within 120 days of the notification, it may go forward with the use of the packaging. The new rules have not yet been implemented as the agency awaits new appropriations. There is also provision in the law allowing the FDA more flexibility in approving and reviewing health claims and nutrient contents claims.

***Standards for Medical Products***   The act provides for new efficiencies and allows for the setting of priorities in use of resources; however, the act does not lower previously determined minimum standards. This also applies to medical products and drugs. Certain regulations are codified into the law, including certain presumptions about safety.

The law allows intervention by Congress to prevent certain medical devices that have been approved by the FDA from entering the marketplace, when standards are grossly deficient and would thereby present a serious health hazard.

*William C. Smith and Elizabeth M. Williams*

*See also* Food Safety; U.S. Department of Health and Human Services (HHS).

### References

Buchanan, Robert L. "Microbial Food Safety Risk Assessment at the FDA Center for Food Safety and Applied Nutrition: From Concept to Reality." U.S. Food and Drug Administration (2000), www.access.data.fad.gov/ScienceForums/forums00/SA-BUC.HTM.
U.S. Food and Drug Administration, "FDA Strategic Priorities 2011–2015," www.fda.gov.

## FOOD-BORNE ILLNESS

Food poisoning is produced by toxins released from bacteria and other organisms when these toxins are eaten. In most cases, this causes stomach cramping, vomiting, diarrhea, and fever, and dehydration when the body loses water faster than it can be replenished. The Centers for Disease Control and Prevention (CDC) tracks many of the over 250 food-borne diseases, including infections with the bacteria *Salmonella, Escherichia coli, Campylobacter jejuni, Shigella, Listeria,* and *Clostridium botulinum,* and with the Norwalk virus (*Norovirus*). The CDC has declared that the most common diseases in the United States are infections with *Campylobacter, Salmonella, E. coli,* and Norwalk.

Symptoms of *C. jejuni* infection include diarrhea, cramps, fever, and vomiting. Foods most likely to cause outbreaks include undercooked poultry, unpasteurized or raw milk, and contaminated water. Symptoms usually strike from 2 to 5 days after the infected food is eaten, and can last up to 10 days. Researchers suspect that the illness can lead to Guillain-Barre syndrome, a disorder in which the immune system attacks the body's nerves. Early symptoms of Guillain-Barre syndrome include weakness or tingling in the legs that can spread to the arms and upper body. Symptoms can increase in intensity, paralyzing certain muscles. In severe cases, the disorder can be life-threatening. *Campylobacter* has become increasingly resistant to a type of antibiotic used to treat it, and some scientists argue that the overuse of antibiotics in poultry feed has contributed to this development.

*Escherichia coli* 0157:H7 is one of the several strains of *E. coli* that causes illness. The bacteria brings with it severe diarrhea and often bloody stools along with stomach pain and vomiting, but little or no fever. It can strike anywhere from 1 day to 1 week after the bacteria is eaten, and lasts up to 10 days. People with weakened immune systems or children should get medical treatment immediately if they develop symptoms after eating undercooked beef, unpasteurized milk or juice, raw produce, salami, cold cuts, or other deli-style meat and poultry.

Infections with *Salmonella* bacteria mimic influenza, with symptoms that include fever, cramps, muscle aches, vomiting, and diarrhea. Foods suspected of carrying *Salmonella* include eggs, poultry, cheese, raw vegetables and fruit, and unpasteurized milk or juices. The symptoms appear after two or three days, and can last for a week. Severe illness can result if the infection spreads from the intestines to the bloodstream. Some cases have led to organ failure and death.

*Listeria monocytogenes* can grow slowly at refrigerator temperatures. Symptoms include fever, muscle aches, nausea, and diarrhea. These flulike symptoms can lead to premature delivery in pregnant women. *Listeria* is often found in fresh soft cheeses, unpasteurized or inadequately pasteurized milk, and deli meats and hot dogs. Gastrointestinal symptoms of may not appear until up to two days after infection, and infections in the blood, brain, or uterus may not appear for two to six weeks. Illness can require immediate medical treatment and can last for months. Of the 2,500 people a year who get seriously sick from *Listeria,* an estimated 500 die. According to the CDC, during 2008 most cases of *Listeria* occurred among people aged 65 years or older.

*Shigella* bacteria cause the disease shigellosis. Symptoms include diarrhea, fever, and stomach cramps starting a day or two after exposure. A severe infection

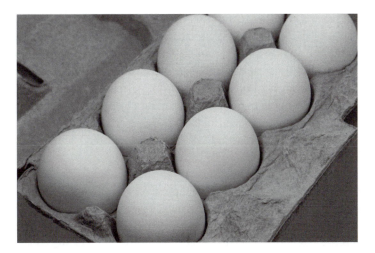

Chicken eggs, in addition to poultry, cheese, raw vegetables and fruit, and unpasteurized milk and juice, have been suspected of carrying salmonella. (Jennifer Pitiquen/Dreamstime.com)

with high fever may be associated with seizures in children younger than two years old. The illness lasts up to a week. People who are infected may not have visible symptoms but may still pass the bacteria on to others if they do not wash their hands after using the bathroom. Vegetables can be contaminated if they are grown in a field with sewage in it, and flies can breed in infected feces and then contaminate food.

The Norwalk virus (*Norovirus*) differs from other agents of food-borne illness because it is a virus rather than a bacterium. It is often associated with poorly cooked shellfish such as clams and oysters, or with fresh salad ingredients contaminated by infected food handlers. Symptoms include nausea, vomiting, and diarrhea, as well as headache and low-grade fever. The CDC estimates that Norwalk virus accounts for up to one-third of the food poisoning cases in the United States. A mild and brief illness usually develops one to two days after the contaminated food or water is consumed, and lasts for 24 to 60 hours. Severe illness or hospitalization is very rare.

*Clostridium botulinum* is the name of a group of bacteria found in soil that, when exposed to the right conditions, form spores and develop toxins. There are seven types of *botulinum* toxin designated by the letters A through G; only A, B, E, and F cause illness in humans. Food-borne botulism is often caused by eating home-canned foods with a low acid content, such as asparagus, green beans, beets, or corn. However, there have been reported outbreaks of botulism from unusual sources, such as homemade infused oils or improperly handled baked potatoes wrapped in aluminum foil.

The classic symptoms of botulism include double vision, blurred vision, drooping eyelids, slurred speech, difficulty swallowing, dry mouth, and muscle weakness. To prevent botulism, persons who practice home canning should follow strict hygiene rules; infused oils should be refrigerated; and potatoes baked while wrapped in foil should be kept hot until served or refrigerated. The toxins are destroyed by high temperatures, so boiling food for 10 minutes before eating is a way to ensure the safety of home-canned foods. People who survive an incident of botulism food poisoning can suffer from fatigue or other problems for months to years, and physical therapy may be needed for a full recovery.

Although botulism food poisoning is a rare form of food-borne illness, even more unusual and deadly is mad cow disease. Bovine spongiform encephalopathy (BSE) is a progressive neurological disorder found in cattle. An outbreak of BSE in the 1990s in England was blamed on the practice of feeding British cattle food that contained brains and other parts of infected sheep. To stop the spread of the disease, hundreds of thousands of cows had to be slaughtered. Scientists suspect that the infectious agent is an aberrant protein called a prion, which passes through infected meat and bone meal to young cattle. There is no known cure. Scientific studies have linked variant Creutzfeldt-Jakob disease in humans to BSE. There have been three verified cases of BSE in the United States, the most recent in March 2006.

**New Threats**   The infectious and parasitic diseases emerging as new threats to populations all over the world are spread thanks to the increased mobility of people. The *Cyclospora* parasite is among the almost 30 new disease-causing microbes and infectious diseases now recognized by the World Health Organization. According to the CDC, *Cyclospora* appeared in the United States in 1996, linked to Guatemalan raspberries. In 2005, health officials blamed *Cyclospora*-contaminated basil for 300 Florida illnesses.

New strains of bacteria, such as *Salmonella DT104,* have also appeared, and, according to epidemiologists, many of these strains now have a resistance to the drugs most commonly used to treat them. A 1994 outbreak of *Salmonella DT104* in the United Kingdom killed 10 people. The United States experienced its first outbreak of *Salmonella DT104* in October 1996, and since that time, there have been at least five reported outbreaks—one in Vermont, two in Washington State, and two in California.

Even familiar strains of *Salmonella* have global significance. *Salmonella enteritidis* infections have increased in 24 of the 35 countries that report outbreaks to the World Health Organization. In the United States, where the infections are linked to the internal contamination of commercial eggs, *S. enteritidis* had accounted for 6 percent of reported human infections in 1980; this figure had jumped to 26 percent by 1994. However, according to the latest CDC figures released in 2009, there was a decline in incident rates for *Campylobacter, Listeria, Salmonella,* and *E. coli* 0157:H7 in comparison to the rates recorded in the 1996–1998 period.

Although *E. coli* 0157:H7 was unknown before 1982, it gained prominence because of several tragic outbreaks around the world in countries including Canada, Japan, Africa, the United Kingdom, and the United States. The CDC estimates that there may be about 70,000 infections with *E. coli* 0157 in the United States each year. In addition to the bloody diarrhea and other familiar symptoms, *E. coli* 0157 has been identified by the CDC as the cause of hemolytic uremic syndrome, a life-threatening complication and a leading cause of kidney failure, especially in children.

*Sharon Zoumbaris*

*See also* Antibiotics; Bacteria; *E. Coli* Infection; Influenza; Salmonella; World Health Organization (WHO).

## Resources

Akkina J.E., et al. "Epidemiologic Aspects, Control and Importance of Multiple-Drug Resistant *Salmonella typhimurium* DT104 in the United States." *Journal of American Veterinary Medical Association* 214 (1999): 790–98.

Callaway, T.R., T.S. Edrington, R.C. Anderson, J.A. Byrd, and D.J. Nisbet, "Gastrointestinal Microbial Ecology and the Safety of Our Food Supply as Related to Salmonella." *Journal of Animal Science* 86, no. 14 (April 2008): E163–E172.

Centers for Disease Control and Prevention. "Preliminary FoodNet Data on the Incidence of Infection with Pathogens Transmitted Commonly through Food-10 States, 2009." *Morbidity and Mortality Weekly Report (MMWR)* (July 26, 2010), www.cdc.gov/mmwr.

Centers for Disease Control and Prevention. *Salmonella Surveillance Summary, 2006.* Atlanta: U.S. Department of Health and Human Services, 2008, www.cdc.gov/nationalsurveillance/ salmonella_surveillance.html.

"E. coli Outbreak: Questions Loom on Food Safety." *Tulsa World* (September 4, 2008): A14.

Hume, Scott. "Bush Boosts Food-Safety Budgets: Impact of Mad Cow Disease Incident Is Clear in Research and Testing Funds." *Restaurants and Institutions* (March 15, 2004): 60.

Martin, Andrew, and Griff Palmer. "China Not Sole Source of Dubious Food." *New York Times* (July 12, 2007): C1.

Neergaard, Lauran. "The COOL Law: Country-of-Origin Labeling of Foods." *Virginian-Pilot* (September 30, 2008): 3.

Nestle, Marion. *What to Eat.* New York: North Point Press, 2006.

Serrano, Alfonso, "How Safe Is Imported Food?" CBSnews.com (April 16, 2007).

U.S. Food and Drug Administration Center for Food Safety and Applied Nutrition. "Overview" (February 2001), www.cfsan.fad.gov/~lrd/cfsan4.html.

## FOOD RECALLS

Food recalls are voluntary actions taken by a manufacturer or distributor to protect U.S. consumers by removing a food or food product from the market if there is a belief that the products may cause health problems or death. Recalls are classified into several categories by the two main government agencies that are responsible for keeping food safe. The Food Safety and Inspection Service (FSIS) within the U.S. Department of Agriculture is the chief agency that inspects and regulates meat, poultry, and processed egg products, while the Food and Drug Administration (FDA) is responsible for the regulation and safety of all other food products.

Recalls may be initiated by the manufacturer or the distributor of a food product, and sometimes they are also requested by the FSIS. However, due to food safety laws that date back to the early 1900s, all recalls of food products are voluntary. The FSIS can legally detain any products in question if the company refuses to recall them. As soon as the FSIS learns of a potentially unsafe product, it conducts a preliminary investigation and weighs the need for a recall. The investigation includes contacting federal, state, and local health departments if necessary; collecting and analyzing food samples; interviewing consumers who allegedly became ill from the suspect food; creating a time line of incidents relating to the product; and contacting the manufacturer or distributor for more information.

**Classes of Recalls**   There are several official classes of recalls, from Class I to a market withdrawal. The Class I recall occurs in a situation where there is a reasonable chance that using the product or exposure to the product will cause serious health problems or death. A Class II recall is slightly less serious, and is called when use of the product may cause temporary or medically reversible adverse health problems or where the probability of serious health consequences is less likely. A Class III recall is initiated when use of or exposure to a product is not likely to cause any negative health consequences. Finally, a market withdrawal occurs when a product has a minor violation that would not be subject to legal action and the firm removes the product or corrects the problems. Examples of this situation might include product removal due to tampering without evidence that the tampering would cause health problems for consumers.

If or when a recall is initiated U.S. consumers are notified by the FSIS through a press release given to major media organizations in the case of a Class I and Class II recall. The press release is also posted on the FSIS website and usually includes a picture, if possible, of the recalled product. If and when the FSIS decided through further investigation that the company performing the recall has contacted all necessary parties or has made a reasonable effort to do so, the agency will then consider the recall complete.

For additional information on U.S. recalls of food and other products, the government has established several websites and hotlines. They include the USDA Meat and Poultry Hotline at 1-888-MPHotline (1-888-674-6854) or via e-mail at mphotline.fsis@usda.gov; via e-mail subscription on the FSIS home page or from www.govdocs.com/service/multi_subscribe.html?code=SFSIS; and for all government recalls, www.recalls.gov.

**Recalls**  Food recalls have included a wide variety of products from eggs to sausage, ground beef, and chicken nugget products, some produced in the United States and others imported from other countries. According to the FSIS website, in the summer months of 2010 recalls included 1 million pounds of frozen ground beef patties from a California company due to concerns about *E. coli* 0157:H7 contamination. Another recall was of 91,000 pounds of chicken nugget products from a Georgia chicken processing plant when consumers complained about finding small pieces of blue plastic mixed in with the frozen nuggets. Earlier in the summer, some 61,000 pounds of cooked canned and frozen beef products were recalled by a Chicago company when it was discovered they may have contained the animal drug ivermectin. The drug is an antiparasitic used to de-worm animals, and earlier FSIS testing had discovered samples that exceeded the levels established by the FDA. In just six weeks, there were approximately 21 major recalls listed on the FDA website that provides recalls and safety alerts to the public.

Nonmeat recalls during those same months included a broccoli raisin salad recalled by a large grocery store chain in Oregon and Washington, because the products had the potential to contain walnuts not listed on the label; romaine lettuce salad distributed in 20 states from Arkansas to Wyoming and Washington due to possible *E. coli* contamination; frozen, diced zucchini recalled from several states and Canada due to the possible contamination with *Listeria;* and black pepper recalled by an Ohio firm when it was believed the spice could have been contaminated with *Salmonella.*

*Sharon Zoumbaris*

*See also E. Coli* Infection; Food and Drug Administration (FDA); Food-borne Illness; Food Safety; U.S. Department of Agriculture (USDA).

### References

Centers for Disease Control and Prevention National Center for Infectious Diseases. "Avoiding Illnesses You Get through Food: Food Safety" (August 16, 2010), www.cdc.gov/ncidod/diseases/food/safety.htm.

"Food Product Recalls Reported." *Food Institute Report* 83, no. 30 (July 26, 2010): 12.

Kirby, David. *Animal Factory: The Looming Threat of Industrial Pig, Dairy, and Poultry Farms to Humans and the Environment.* New York: St. Martin's Press, 2010.

U.S. Food and Drug Administration. "Recalls, Market Withdrawals, and Safety Alerts" (August 16, 2010), www.fda.gov/Safety/recalls/default.htm.

## FOOD SAFETY

The term *food safety* is a relative one, and in the 21st-century United States, it is no longer just about potato salad left out in the sun or hamburgers not cooked enough on the grill. Today, U.S. consumers must contend with nationwide outbreaks of food-borne illness and tainted foods from countries such as China and Mexico, and at the same time weigh the effects of pesticides, poisonous metals, growth hormones, genetically modified foods, and irradiation.

Until recent years, Americans had shown only modest concerns about food-borne illness and even less interest in related safety issues such as pesticides or the overuse of antibiotics in livestock feed. However, that laid-back attitude is changing, according to a national survey that showed that three-quarters of Americans polled were more concerned about the food they eat today than they were five years ago, and 57 percent said they had stopped eating certain foods following a food scare ("*E. Coli* Outbreak," 2008).

As the U.S. food industry works overtime to influence what and how much people eat to preserve the economic health of their industry, Americans struggle to practice healthy nutrition by eating more fresh fruits and vegetables. Unfortunately, industry profits and food safety don't always work well together. Consumers have every right to be worried about the safety of their food. Statistics from the Centers for Disease Control and Prevention (CDC) show that some 76 million Americans are stricken with food-borne diseases each year.

The CDC serves as the lead federal agency for conducting disease surveillance and outbreak investigation. It estimates that, of those millions of food-borne disease cases each year, approximately 325,000 Americans require hospitalization, and 5,000 die (Eskin, Donley, Rosenbaum, & Mitchell, 2003). Sadly, many other victims—of all ages, races, and economic levels—suffer bouts of vomiting and diarrhea, never realizing they have a food-borne illness. The CDC estimates that 20 illnesses caused by *E. coli* 0157:H7 and 38 cases of salmonellosis occur for every case that is officially reported to federal public health authorities (Eskin et al., 2003).

Politicians and government officials call the U.S. food supply one of the safest in the world. Yet many Americans are getting sick from peanut butter, beef, raw spinach, strawberries, cantaloupe, ice cream, fruit juice, peppers, and many other foods. The summer of 2008 will be remembered for an outbreak of *Salmonella* that sickened at least 1,440 people across the United States and at that time was called the worst food-borne outbreak in at least a decade. Although the early evidence suggested that the bacteria traced to fresh tomatoes from Florida, the CDC and Food and Drug Administration (FDA) ultimately placed the blame on serrano and jalapeño peppers grown in Mexico.

A *Salmonella* outbreak of that size is not cheap. The Economic Research Service (ERS) of the U.S. Department of Agriculture (USDA) estimates that the economic cost of salmonellosis alone in 2007 was over $2 billion dollars. In calculating this figure, the ERS measured medical expenses, lost work, and premature death (USDA, 2011). The figure did not include associated costs, such as care for extended medical complications or pain and suffering. In other words, food-borne illnesses significantly costs the United States every year in both lives and dollars.

*Salmonella* is one culprit; however, it is far from the only food safety issue. The United States imports about 40 percent of its fresh produce, and this is a figure that continues to go up. The globalization of the nation's food supply means the average American eats about 260 pounds of imported foods each year (Serrano, 2007). Even though many of the outbreaks of food-borne illness come from meat, vegetables, and fruit produced in the United States, China's melamine scandal raised serious concerns about the safety of imports.

In 2008, dairy products from China were recalled around the world after they were found to contain melamine, a dangerous industrial chemical that artificially inflates protein content when added to a food. In China, the melamine-tainted milk killed 4 babies and sickened 54,000 children. Later that year, Wal-Mart pulled a brand of eggs from all its stores in China after tests discovered they were tainted with the same toxic chemical blamed for sickening the babies. The discovery of melamine in eggs raised a serious question about how deeply the chemical had penetrated China's food supply chain.

The outbreak of food poisoning from peppers in the summer of 2008 was not an isolated U.S. incident. In 1992, the fast food restaurant Jack in the Box was another canary in the coal mine, forcing federal agencies to recognize the need for improvements in

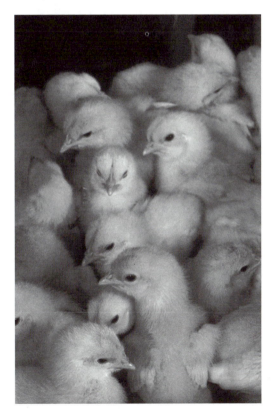

Food safety problems can develop anywhere from the farm to the table. (U.S. Department of Agriculture)

commercial food safety regulations. In the case of Jack in the Box, 732 people became ill and 4 children died due to deadly *E. coli* 0157:H7 in the meat. Public health officials eventually traced the contaminated beef patties back to their supplier, but not before hundreds of people were hospitalized and dozens of children suffered kidney failure. Their kidneys stopped working due to a serious urinary tract infection known as hemolyric uremic syndrome, caused by *E. coli.*

**History of Regulations**  As early as the 1860s, the safety of the nation's food supply was a growing public health concern. In response to the problem, President Abraham Lincoln signed legislation in 1862 to create the U.S. Department of Agriculture. Later, as the country continued its westward expansion, President Chester Arthur recognized the need to work with ranchers and meat packers to eradicate livestock diseases. He signed the Bureau of Animal Industry Act in 1884, which created the USDA's Bureau of Animal Industry, the forerunner of the Food Safety and Inspection Service (FSIS). Today, the FSIS has a leading role in the nation's food safety system.

By the end of the 19th century, the nation's slaughterhouses were the target of muckraking journalists whose stories of filth and disease terrified U.S. consumers as well as European trade partners. To quiet criticism of the nation's meat handling practices, Congress passed the Meat Inspection Act in 1890. That legislation authorized inspection of salt pork, bacon, and pigs for export. However, the law, and others that followed, did not calm overseas worries about the safety of U.S. meat exports. This unease about the quality of U.S. meat has been a recurrent theme in U.S. exports for decades. For example, in the summer of 2008, thousands of South Koreans rioted in the streets of Seoul to stop the import of U.S. beef into their country.

Things went from bad to worse in 1905, when the government faced an avalanche of U.S. consumer protests following the publication of Upton Sinclair's novel, *The Jungle.* In his book, Sinclair awakened the nation to real dangers in the food supply. He wrote in excruciating detail about the filthy conditions in Chicago meatpacking plants. The story focused on an immigrant who at one point described how, after the government inspectors left for the day, the "downers"—the sick, diseased, and injured cattle—were butchered: "It took a couple of hours to get them out of the way, and in the end Jurgis saw them go into the chilling rooms with the rest of the meat, being carefully scattered here and there so that they could not be identified" (Sinclair, 1984).

The book, combined with the efforts of the FDA and its director, Harvey Washington Wiley, pushed food safety to center stage. Wiley made national headlines in 1902 when he recruited young men to act as guinea pigs and test different food additives. The "poison squad" ate meals made with ingredients such as borax, salicylic acid, formaldehyde, sulfuric acid, sodium benzoate, and copper salts. Drawn into the debates over food safety, President Theodore Roosevelt and the Congress brought the 1906 Pure Food and Drug Act and the Federal Meat Inspection Act (FMIA) into law.

The FMIA called for the USDA to inspect meat largely by looking, touching, or poking and smelling the meat. The law was designed by Congress to prevent sick animals from getting into U.S. food; no one imagined a time when they would need to check for microscopic pathogens. The act also called for the USDA to appoint government inspectors, with some trained as veterinarians, to work in every U.S. slaughterhouse in operation at that time. However, the law kept inspectors from looking at the entire livestock operation from field to table. Instead, the government could only examine the animals in the slaughterhouse; they were not allowed to check livestock at any other point.

The law also left the USDA with no ability to recall tainted food once it left the plant. Those omissions continue to frustrate consumer advocates as well as government agencies. The USDA and FDA lack the specific recall authority available to other government agencies responsible for the safety of products such as toys, heart pacemakers, and automobiles. Those agencies may order a recall and impose monetary penalties if a company violates recall requirements. Neither the USDA nor FDA can order a company to recall potentially unsafe food. They also cannot fine a company that is slow to conduct a food recall or provides inaccurate customer lists.

Surprisingly, the 1906 FMIA did not address chicken slaughterhouses, because at the time Americans were buying what few chickens they ate directly from farms. Consumer demand for poultry did not increase until after World War II. One factor that kept U.S. chicken consumption low was a 1920 outbreak of avian influenza in New York City, which had been the hub of poultry distribution for the United States. By 1957, when the demand for chicken picked up, the USDA recommended that poultry processing plants only buy chickens from producers who voluntarily met USDA sanitation requirements. It wasn't long before Congress passed the Poultry Products Inspection Act of 1957. The new inspection requirements for poultry mirrored those for cattle and pigs—rules such as sanitary standards for processing facilities, and before-and-after inspections. Once again, inspection methods included using sight, touch, and smell but paid no attention to microscopic bacteria.

Decades earlier, typhoid fever, cholera, botulism, and trichinosis were common. However, they had disappeared in the United States thanks to pasteurization and improved canning and food preservation techniques. On the other hand, increasingly large livestock production practices created new problems. The Food Safety and Inspection Service (FSIS) was established in 1981 to monitor the handling of all U.S. meat, poultry, and egg products as critics began to call for tougher inspection methods that tested for invisible pathogens. Eggs were a perfect example: by the 1980s, disease-causing microbes had developed inside chickens and passed into the eggs.

The connection between *Salmonella* and poultry intensified, and in the 1990s U.S. scientists publicly acknowledged that laying hens were carrying *Salmonella enteritidis* internally. The increase in contaminated eggs was linked to U.S. industrial farming practices and to the crowded conditions of laying hens. With so many birds in such close quarters, the bacteria were easily passed from one hen to another. Many chickens had infected ovaries even though they showed no signs of sickness, and the infected birds shed the bacteria into the egg white. Once the shell was secreted around the egg white, the bacteria were invisibly sealed inside the egg. This situation was extremely rare in the 1960s and 1970s, but by the 1990s the number of cases of *Salmonella enteritidis* infection from transovarian transfer had increased dramatically.

The situation made headlines in 1994, when more than 200,000 people got food poisoning from contaminated ice cream (USDA, 2006). It was a massive job for the government to track down the common factor among hundreds of thousands of people, but officials finally pinpointed a specific brand of ice cream as the cause. The product was recalled. Researchers discovered that the ice cream had been transported by tanker trucks that previously carried unpasteurized eggs. Those eggs were infected with *Salmonella*. Today, the USDA estimates that more than 70 billion eggs are sold each year in U.S. stores, and that 19 percent contain *Salmonella* bacteria (Nestle, 2006). This means that U.S. consumers are buying millions of *Salmonella*-infected eggs each year. In 2006, the FSIS implemented a "*Salmonella* attack plan" to try to lower the rate of infection in U.S. eggs.

**A Federal Maze**   A look at current federal food safety responsibilities reveals a mishmash of agencies and laws. There are as many as 12 government agencies with at least a small regulatory role in the foods Americans eat. However, the two main agencies responsible for food safety are the USDA and the FDA. The USDA, through the FSIS, regulates meat, poultry, and processed egg products along with foods that contain them. It also oversees pasteurized egg products.

The FDA, which works on food safety chiefly through its Center for Food Safety and Applied Nutrition, has the lead responsibility for administering food safety regulations. The agency addresses the safety of all other foods, including fresh fruits and vegetables, milk, eggs, and any processed foods that do not contain meat, poultry, or processed egg products. It also oversees canned and imported foods, some 80 percent of the nation's food supply. This creates a complicated system of checks and balances. For example, the USDA regulates spaghetti sauce with meat stock, but the FDA regulates spaghetti sauce without meat stock. The USDA oversees pizza with meat toppings; the FDA inspects the safety of cheese pizza. The USDA performs daily slaughterhouse inspections, whereas the FDA only inspects plants in its jurisdiction once every five years.

At the same time, in recent years, the FDA office in charge of food safety has had its workload increased, its budget cut, and its number of employees reduced. According to the Government Accountability Office, the FDA's Center for Food Safety and Applied Nutrition saw its budget drop 14 percent from 2003 to 2006 (Sylvester, 2008). The FDA is now conducting half the food-safety inspections it did 10 years ago, with fewer inspectors in the field. The number of food-import inspectors has also dropped about 20 percent, while food imports have climbed. Figures show that just over 1 percent of fish, vegetables, fruit, and other imported foods were inspected by the FDA in the spring of 2007 (Schmidt, 2007). This spells trouble for U.S. consumers: as problems with melamine in Chinese dairy products and *Salmonella* in Mexican peppers illustrated, imports are a growing food safety concern for the nation.

In recent years, FDA inspections discovered a number of problems with other products from China, including frozen catfish tainted with veterinary drugs, fresh ginger polluted with pesticides, and melons contaminated with toxins. Federal records also suggest that China is not the only country with food export problems. In 2007, government inspectors seized more food shipments from India and Mexico than from China, according to the *New York Times* (Martin, 2007). To deal more effectively with the growing volume of imports, the FDA and the USDA have adopted an inspection philosophy that prioritizes foods, sources, or producers they suspect represent the biggest risk to public health. Basically, these agencies only have the resources to examine a fraction of the food products imported into the United States.

**Changes in Regulations**   Beginning in October 2008, a new federal rule took effect requiring retailers to identify the country of origin when labeling imported foods. Consumers who are worried about lax safety regulations can avoid imports from any country they want—sort of. The country-of-origin labeling (COOL) law designates where items originated, from Chile to the United States. However, labels are not required for processed foods or mixed foods. This means that cantaloupe slices from Guatemala or Mexico would have labels, but a frozen pea and carrot mix would not. Plain raw chicken would be labeled, but not breaded chicken tenders. Bagged lettuce could be labeled, but if radicchio was added, no label is required.

Jean Halloran of Consumers Union has said that the COOL law is "a very good thing because we'll have a lot more information," but she cautioned that consumers can still be fooled given all the exceptions (Neergaard, 2008). She suggested that the labels will help consumers who are worried about safety regulations in certain countries to avoid imported food from those areas. Another benefit is the additional information readily available for people who suspect they have food poisoning; they could potentially help investigators pinpoint the origin of suspicious foods thanks to the new labels. Stores that violate the law can be fined.

The COOL law is one of several food safety changes inspired by poisoning tragedies involving imported foods. On the domestic front, the government agreed with consumer advocates and put a new system using research and technology into place following the Jack in the Box outbreak of *E. coli*. Designed to be more than a scientific version of the poke-and-sniff method already used by inspectors, the Hazard Analysis and Critical Control Point (HACCP) program puts the responsibility for safety on food processors and producers, requiring them to identify points in their production line where there is an increased risk of contamination. The HACCP system also requires the use of steam and acid carcass washes to protect against invisible pathogens. Although the fundamental principles of the HACCP program offer a sound tool for companies to improve food safety, consumer advocates say that, in practice, the program is often used as a substitute for government inspection rather than the two systems working in tandem.

The HACCP concept was developed in the 1960s, when the U.S. National Aeronautics and Space Administration (NASA) needed safe food for space flights.

Today, meat and poultry HACCP systems are regulated by the USDA, and seafood and juice HACCP systems are regulated by the FDA. The seafood rules were finalized in 1995, the final rule for the juice industry took effect in 2002, and the USDA rules for meat and poultry processing were finalized in 1999. There are two overall types of procedures in the HACCP program: carcass inspection and verification inspection. Government and industry experts agree that identifying and preventing hazards that could cause food-borne illness has improved overall food safety.

Carcass inspection requires inspectors, stationed on the slaughter line at a fixed location, to view the meat postmortem. Meanwhile, the verification inspector examines plant records as well as microbial samples of the meat for testing and analysis. Since the HACCP system has been initiated in the United States, the severity of food poisoning incidents remains a problem, but the overall number of cases of listeriosis and salmonellosis is on the decline.

However, beginning in 2007, scientists noted an increase in the prevalence of *E. coli* in beef products. By mid-October of 2008, USDA meat inspectors had recorded a 50 percent increase in contaminated beef samples over the number from the same time in the previous year (Shin, 2008). Although their findings are not conclusive, researchers are testing whether the use of an ethanol product called distillers grain in cattle feed may be connected with the increase in contaminated beef. Scientists say there is still a lot they do not understand about the bacteria, and federal efforts to improve slaughterhouse safety will continue.

**Additional Food Safety Issues**   One area where consumer advocates want more government oversight is in the use of antibiotics in livestock feed, which in turn could improve the nation's growing problem of antibiotic resistance. Antibiotics were first given to livestock to accelerate growth, but as more and more animals were crowded into smaller areas, the antibiotics were also used to hold at bay diseases that would cut into producer's profits. A sick cow cannot legally be slaughtered in a U.S. slaughter house. Some estimates show that the volume of antibiotics used in animal feed equals or exceeds that used in human medicine.

U.S. livestock feed holds another potentially fatal food safety hazard. In April 2008, the FDA issued a final regulation to keep certain cattle parts from all animal feed in an effort to protect U.S. consumers from bovine spongiform encephalopathy (BSE), also known as mad cow disease. BSE spread in Great Britain in the 1990s when cattle were fed bone meal and meat from other animals that had the disease.

The new FDA measure restricts the addition of cattle brains and spinal cords to U.S. animal feed if the parts are from cattle older than 30 months of age. Carcasses of cattle not inspected by the FDA are also prohibited from being ground up and put into cattle feed if the animals are older than 30 months of age. The FDA maintains that the risk of BSE in cattle less than 30 months of age is low, and that their parts can be used in feed with minimal risk of infection. The United States is one of the few countries in the world that allows any animal parts in livestock feed, a fact that for years prompted South Korea to ban imports of U.S. beef. The South Korean government decided to allow American beef after U.S.

government officials increased funding for several aspects of BSE control. Specifically, the USDA, through the Food Safety and Inspection Service, received an extra $4 million in the 2005 federal budget to improve how it monitored BSE regulations, and the Agricultural Research Service was awarded another $5 million to develop better BSE-testing technologies (Hume, 2004).

**Technological Innovations** Irradiation of food to kill pathogens, genetically modified crops whose genes are altered to improve resistance to insects and pesticides, and growth hormones used to increase milk production in dairy cows are technological innovations considered important food safety issues by U.S. consumer advocates. Whether these and other developments represent a danger depends on one's viewpoint. In general, government agencies and scientists support these technologies as tools to promote food safety and combat world hunger, whereas critics oppose them as untested and potentially dangerous.

*Irradiation* Right from the start, U.S. consumers were skeptical of the idea of treating food with radiation. In 1963 the FDA approved irradiation to kill insects in wheat and flour. The FDA then approved irradiation to kill growth sprouts in potatoes in 1964. Controversy arose in 1968, when the FDA rejected a petition to use radiation to sterilize canned bacon, reporting noticeable problems in animal studies that raised doubts about the safety of the bacon. The FDA continues to approve irradiation of various foods. For example, in 2008 it increased permissible irradiation levels for fresh iceberg lettuce and fresh spinach.

Opponents of food irradiation technology call it one more threat to food safety and suggest that it takes attention away from the root causes of the food hygiene problem. They argue that huge farms and industrialized animal agriculture, as well as antibiotics and hormones in animal feed, have contributed to the growing presence of dangerous pathogens in livestock.

*Genetically Modified Organisms* Genetically modified organisms, or GMOs, are considered a food safety issue by some Americans. Supporters see no health risk in genetically modified corn or canola, or their use in U.S. agriculture. Opponents of GMOs point to a lack of research and suggest they could have hidden dangers for consumers. All known food allergens are proteins, and since genes code for proteins, genetically modified crops end up with a new protein when a foreign gene is inserted. Critics say this could cause unexpected allergic reactions: for example, anyone allergic to fish who eats a tomato that has been genetically modified to include a fish gene could have an allergic reaction to the tomato. Opponents also suggest that, during the process of genetic engineering, the newly inserted gene could damage the plant's own genes or increase the levels of toxins the plant produces.

*Recombinant Bovine Growth Hormone* Another controversial technology that has resulted from genetic engineering is the use of bovine growth hormone in dairy cows. Also known as recombinant bovine growth hormone (rBGH) or recombinant bovine somatotropin (rBST), its use in U.S. dairy cows was approved by the FDA in 1993 after years of testing and studies. The hormone, a genetic replica of the hormone the animals produce naturally, was one of the first applications of genetic engineering used in U.S. food production. The hormone is injected into the cows after they give birth to boost their milk production by up to a gallon per day and keep them making milk longer. The FDA ruled that milk and meat from cows given rBGH were the same as those from other cows and safe for U.S. consumers.

Critics dispute those findings and warn that rBGH is bad for the health of the cows and may even pose a cancer risk for people. In a 2000 study in the *Journal of Reproductive Medicine,* research showed that women who drank milk with rBGH were three times more likely to have twins than women who did not. The reason appears to be the substance IGF-1 (insulinlike growth factor), which is found in cows' milk and encourages cells to divide. Milk from cows treated with rBGH has three times more IGF-1 than milk from untreated cows. According to the study's author, Gary Steinman, an assistant clinical professor of obstetrics, his research showed a relationship between bovine growth hormone in the food supply and the fact that the U.S. rate of twin births has almost tripled in the last 30 years (Barone, 2007). Steinman says the use of assisted reproductive technologies in the United States doesn't fully account for the increase in multiple births in this country. He added that "[t]he rate has gone up twice as fast here in the U.S. as in Britain, where there's been a moratorium on synthetic BGH" (Bakalar, 2006).

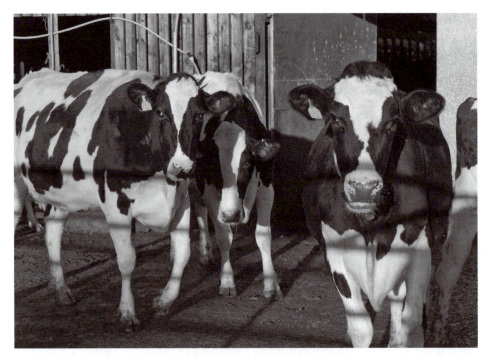

Genetically engineered bovine growth hormone (rBGH or rBST) is a genetically modified organism (GMO) and is controversial because it has been injected into dairy cows in the United States to increase milk production. (Eileen Groome/Dreamstime.com)

Scientific studies have found that high levels of IGF-1 in the blood have been associated with prostate and breast cancer, although no studies have shown that milk from cows treated with rBGH directly causes cancer. Use of the artificial hormone is banned in Canada and in the European Union.

**Consumer Groups** Following the *Salmonella* outbreak in the summer of 2008, a number of consumer advocates, scientists, and public health officials called on Congress to reform the FDA via new food safety legislation. With one voice, they asked for a large increase in resources and funding for the FDA, for mandatory recall authority for the FDA and USDA so they could act quickly in public health situations, for traceability in the form of mandated detailed records as a way to follow food all the way back to its origin, and for increased inspections and civil penalties for manufacturers and producers who violate food safety laws. The letter was signed by the Consumers Union, the Consumer Federation of America, the Center for Science in the Public Interest (CSPI), Public Citizen's Global Trade Watch, the Center for Foodborne Illness Research and Prevention, and Safe Tables Our Priority, now known as Stop Food Borne Illness.

The Consumer Federation of America is a nonprofit association of some 300 consumer groups using research, education, and advocacy to advance the interests of average Americans. The Consumers Union is the nonprofit publisher of *Consumer Reports* magazine; the group's mission, as stated on its website, is to advocate a fair, just, and safe marketplace for all U.S. consumers.

The Center for Science in the Public Interest was founded by a small group of scientists during the ecology boom of the early 1970s as an advocate for nutrition, health, and food safety. Characterized as an independent science-based organization, it seeks to educate the public on food and nutrition findings and to counterbalance the influence of the food industry on government regulations. The organization publishes the award-winning *Nutrition Action Healthletter;* according to the CSPI website, this newsletter is considered the largest health publication in North America, with a circulation of 900,000 subscribers. The CSPI is funded by subscriptions to the newsletter and by individual donors. It accepts no advertising, corporate funding, or government grants.

Like the CSPI, Public Citizen was founded in the early 1970s as a nonprofit consumer advocacy organization with the specific mission of representing U.S. consumers. Started by Ralph Nader, Public Citizen emphasizes its role as a government watchdog.

The Center for Foodborne Illness Research and Prevention is a national nonprofit health organization, started in 2006 by two women whose lives were tragically touched by food poisoning. Executive director Patricia Buck and her daughter, director Barbara Kowalcyk, founded the organization after Kowalcyk's son and Buck's grandson, Kevin Kowalcyk, died from complications due to an *E. coli* infection. The organization is dedicated to working with other organizations, the government, and industry to develop better food protections and to prevent food-borne illness through research, education, and advocacy. It is funded through individual contributions, corporate sponsorships, and government grants.

Safe Tables Our Priority is another nonprofit organization, which recently changed its name to Stop Food Borne Illness. It brings attention to the problem of food safety in the United States, and describes itself on its website as devoted to victim assistance, public education, and policy advocacy for safe food at the grass-roots level. The organization started after the 1993 *E. coli* tragedy associated with Jack in the Box hamburgers. Members include scientists, doctors, and people with direct links to the Jack in the Box victims.

**Food Safety ABCs** Food-borne pathogens are invisible to the naked eye. They don't smell bad or taste funny, but they can make you very sick or even kill you. The FSIS education program, the Fight BAC Campaign, was designed to educate consumers on basic food safety. The FSIS lists four cornerstones of food safety: ensure that hands and work surfaces are clean, keep foods separate to prevent cross-contamination, cook to proper temperatures to kill bacteria, and refrigerate food promptly.

Bacteria can spread between countertops, cutting boards, and food, so it's important to wash hands and surfaces with hot, soapy water. Anyone handling food should wash his or her hands for at least 20 seconds with warm, soapy water, especially after using the bathroom, changing diapers, handling pets, or touching food. Cloth towels and sponges should be cleaned frequently; cloths should be run through the hot cycle of the washing machine, and sponges through the dishwasher. Produce should also be rinsed under running tap water and scrubbed with a vegetable brush.

Cross-contamination is a serious safety concern when handling raw meat, poultry, seafood, and eggs. The key is to keep these foods away from each other and from the already prepared foods. Cooked food should never be put on a serving plate or cutting board that previously held raw meat, chicken, or seafood without first washing that plate in hot, soapy water. When grocery shopping, consumers should keep meat products, seafood, chicken, and eggs separate from other foods.

When cooking food, it is difficult to tell by looking if it has reached a safe minimum internal temperature. Steaks, roasts, and fish need to reach an internal temperature of 145 degrees Fahrenheit; pork, ground beef, and egg dishes must reach 160 degrees; and chicken breasts and whole chickens and turkeys all need to reach 165 degrees, according to USDA food safety recommendations. Hot dogs, cold cuts, bologna, and other deli meats need to reach a temperature of 165 degrees when being reheated.

When it comes to leftover food, it is important to refrigerate or freeze meat, chicken, eggs, seafood, or any other perishables within two hours of cooking or purchasing. During the summer, one hour is a safer limit. It is safe to thaw frozen food in the refrigerator, in cold water, or in the microwave, but it is never safe to thaw food at room temperature. Once frozen food is thawed, it should be cooked immediately. The USDA also recommends dividing leftovers into shallow containers for quicker cooling if there is a lot of food to be stored.

There are accepted rules of storage for cooked as well as raw foods. To keep food safe to eat, refrigerator temperatures should not go above 40 degrees

Fahrenheit. Eggs can be kept for a maximum of five weeks when fresh and for one week when hard-boiled. Deli meats that include egg, chicken, ham, and tuna should not be kept more than five days. A package of hot dogs may be refrigerated for a week once opened, and if unopened can be kept for a maximum of two weeks. Ground meats should never be kept in the refrigerator uncooked for more than a day or two, and the same is true for seafood and for chicken or turkey.

Beyond home preparation, shoppers should be careful when buying fresh meat, poultry, and seafood. For example, when buying fresh, whole fish, examine the fish's eyes to be sure they are clear and bulge a little. Only a few fish, such as walleye, have naturally cloudy eyes. Whole fish or fillets should be firm with shiny flesh. Dull flesh or dark spots around the edges of the fish mean that it is old. The flesh should spring back when pressed and should have bright red gills free from slime. Any fresh seafood should be used within two days of purchase and should be kept in the coldest part of the refrigerator or in a special meat-keeper section.

Consumers may be confused by the various types of date labels on food. They include a sell-by date that tells the store how long to display the product for sale; consumers should buy these foods only before the sell-by date. A best-if-used-by date is only a recommendation; it does not address the safety of the food. A use-by date records the last day recommended for the peak quality of the product, as determined by the manufacturer.

**The Future**   The occurrence, transmission, and control of food safety in the United States are a serious battleground in a rapidly changing world of pathogens and bacteria. There are as many opinions on how to combat these threats and improve food safety as there are pathogens to make people ill—everything from more regulation to less regulation, from added import fees to no import fees. Unfortunately, the current food safety strategy from both government and industry still puts much of the responsibility on consumer behavior. Their overemphasis on education gives the impression that if people get sick, it is their own fault for not making sure their food was safe. Consumers do have a role to play, but they are only one partner. Government and industry must recognize the importance of safety, even if it affects profits.

If all parties commit to improve agricultural practices, apply food technologies to reduce or eliminate pathogens, and educate persons who handle food, it may be possible to limit the spread of food-borne diseases before they take on larger or more deadly proportions. Also troubling is the shift in the focus of health education in U.S. secondary schools. Health classes now deal primarily with the prevention of alcohol and other drug use, giving little or no attention to food safety education.

Advocates say the best solution must include regulations and changes in the laws that would keep the pathogens out of the food supply in the first place. Treatments such as irradiation, added antibiotics, or the use of GMOs will not substitute for real changes in how government and industry deal with recognized problems. In the end, Americans looking for a reminder of how serious food safety problems can be need only read Upton Sinclair's *The Jungle* or watch the 1978 cult film, *Attack of the Killer Tomatoes*.

*Sharon Zoumbaris*

*See also E. Coli* Infection; Food and Drug Administration (FDA); Food-borne Illness; Food Recalls; Genetically Modified Organisms (GMOs); Irradiation.

### References

Bakalar, Nicholas. "Rise in Rate of Twin Births May Be Tied to Dairy Case." *New York Times* (May 30, 2006), www.nytimes.com/2006/05/30/health/30twin.html.

Barone, Jennifer. "Milk Drinkers More Likely to Have Twins." *Discover* 28, no. 1 (January 2007): 48.

Callaway, T.R., T.S. Edrington, R.C. Anderson, J.A. Byrd, and D.J. Nisbet. "Gastrointestinal Microbial Ecology and the Safety of Our Food Supply as Related to *Salmonella*." *Journal of Animal Science* 86, no. 14 (April 2008): E163–E172.

"*E. coli* Outbreak: Questions Loom on Food Safety." *Tulsa World* (September 4, 2008): A14.

Eskin, Sandra B., Nancy Donley, Donna Rosenbaum, and Karen Taylor Mitchell. "Ten Years after the Jack-in-the-Box Outbreak Why Are People Still Dying from Contaminated Food?" Stop Foodborne Illness (2003), www.stopfoodborneillness.org.

Hume, Scott. "Bush Boosts Food-Safety Budgets: Impact of Mad Cow Disease Incident Is Clear in Research and Testing Funds." *Restaurants and Institutions* (March 15, 2004): 60.

Martin, Andrew, and Griff Palmer. "China Not Sole Source of Dubious Food." *New York Times* (July 12, 2007): C1.

Neergaard, Lauran. "The COOL Law: Country-of-Origin Labeling of Foods." *Virginian-Pilot* (September 30, 2008): 3.

Nestle, Marion. *What to Eat.* New York: North Point Press, 2006.

Schmit, Julie. "U.S. Food Imports Outrun FDA Resources." *USA Today* (March 19, 2007): B1.

Serrano, Alfonso. "How Safe Is Imported Food?" CBSnews.com (April 16, 2007).

Shin, Annys. "Does Ethanol Raise Risks?" *Washington Post* (November 4, 2008): H1.

Sinclair, Upton. *The Jungle.* New York: Buccaneer Books, 1984.

Sylvester, Lisa, interview by Lou Dobbs. *Lou Dobbs Tonight.* CNN, June 20, 2008.

U.S. Department of Agriculture Economic Research Service. "Foodborne Illness Cost Calculator: *Salmonella*," June 24, 2011. www.ers.usda.gov/data/foodborneillness/salm_Intro.asp.

U.S. Department of Agriculture Food Safety and Inspection Service. "Celebrating 100 Years of the Federal Meat Inspection Act (FMIA)" (May 15, 2006), www.fsis.usda.gov/About_FSIS/100_Years_FMIA/index.asp.

U.S. Food and Drug Administration Center for Food Safety and Applied Nutrition. "Overview" (February 2001), www.cfsan.fad.gov/~lrd/cfsan4.html.

## FREE RADICALS

Free radicals are among the newest villains Americans face in their pursuit of good health. Despite their reputation for trouble, free radicals are actually a natural by-product of oxygen metabolism in cells. Everyone, whether healthy or not, has them. They create problems for health when they outnumber the antioxidants whose job is to neutralize them. This imbalance often occurs in people who deal constantly with mental or physical stress, depression, or anxiety or have extensive exposure to environmental pollution or vitamin deficiency. When the free radicals outnumber their antioxidant counterparts, the end result is called oxidative stress, and it can lead to cell damage, disease, or even possible cognitive decline such as Alzheimer's disease.

The best way to combat the effects of oxidative stress is through a diet filled with antioxidant-rich foods such as berries, broccoli, legumes, nuts, fish, lean meats, and other fruits and vegetables. Other ways to combat free radicals is by getting plenty of sleep, taking part in regular, moderate exercise, and reducing exposure to pollution and toxic chemicals. Health professionals say it is also important to stop smoking and avoid excess alcohol. In other words, lead a healthy lifestyle.

Consumers, especially baby boomers, are looking at new, exotic superfruits to aid in their battle with free radical damage. Those superfruits include açaí, goji, and pomegranate. The fruits are being turned into juices and supplements and added to other foods because they contain the highest levels of antioxidants. A study presented at the American Chemical Society national meeting in 2010 suggested that berries rich in antioxidants may even help reverse age-related damage from oxidative stress and inflammation ("How to Protect Your Brain," 2010). Studies are also underway to test the effects of exercise on oxidative stress and the damage it can create.

Another study, the largest of its kind, put together antioxidant values for over 3,000 foods for use in other research. The eight-year effort led by researchers at the University of Oslo in Norway examined the antioxidant properties of plants, spices, herbs, berries, fruit and fruit juices, vegetables, nuts and seeds, and a number of dietary supplements ("More Reason to Eat," 2010). One of the most important results: scientists found no antioxidants in animal-based foods, emphasizing again the importance of fruits and vegetables as part of a healthy diet.

*Sharon Zoumbaris*

*See also* Açaí Berry; Antioxidants; Stress; Vegetables.

### References

Crawford, Mark. "Antioxidants: High Expectations for a High Qualify of Life." *Nutraceuticals World* 14, no. 2 (March 2011): 36 (5).

"Free Radicals: Where They Come from and What to Do about Them." *Mind, Mood and Memory* 6, no. 11 (November 2010): 1 (2).

"How to Protect Your Brain from Chronic Oxidative Stress: Avoiding Factors That Increase the Formation of Toxic Free Radicals Can Help Prevent Brain Aging and Disease." *Mind, Mood and Memory* 6, no. 2 (February 2010): 6.

"More Reason to Eat Your 5 to 9 Daily Servings of Fruits and Vegetables; Herbs, Spices, Berries and Traditional Plant Medicines Ranked Highest in Disease-Busting Antioxidants." *Duke Medicine Health News* 16, no. 4 (April 2010): 4 (2).

# G

## GARLIC

Garlic is a common ingredient in cooking, and it is also considered a familiar dietary supplement, used for high cholesterol, heart disease, and high blood pressure. Some people also believe garlic can prevent certain types of cancer, including stomach and colon cancers.

Garlic can be taken in tablets or capsules or can be eaten raw or cooked. Raw garlic cloves are often used to infuse oils or to make liquid extracts. While garlic appears to be safe for most adults, there are side effects, including increased body odor and bad breath, heartburn, allergic reactions, and upset stomach. These side effects are found to occur most commonly with raw garlic.

Garlic has also been found to thin the blood or reduce the clotting ability in blood in some people, similar to aspirin's effect on blood properties. This can create problems for individuals both before and during surgery. Garlic has also been found to interfere with the effectiveness of an HIV drug, saquinavir. The National Center for Complementary Alternative Medicine (NCCAM) has funded research to study whether garlic interacts with certain drugs and how it may thin the blood.

**Prized in Ancient Times**   Garlic has been prized as a culinary ingredient and a health remedy for thousands of years. Ancient Egyptians buried it with pharaohs and were said to have fed it to slaves building the pyramids to keep them healthy. It continues to play a major role in the food of that region, where it is added to many foods along with olive oil and garlic's cousin, the onion. The ancient Greeks and Romans were believed to have fed garlic to their athletes, soldiers, and slaves.

For years, China outproduced the rest of the world in garlic exports. However, garlic production was sharply curtailed in 2007 following several other publicized problems with Chinese food exports, including pet food. At that time, the Chinese government demanded that higher safety standards be instituted.

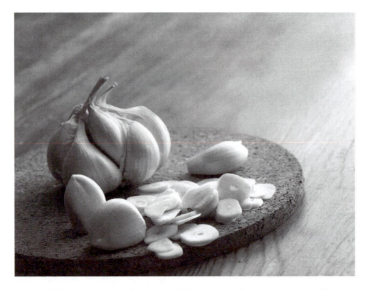

Garlic cloves are sliced for cooking. Scientists suggest garlic is a natural antibiotic and provides many positive health benefits. (Yap Kee Chan/Dreamstime.com)

Before the crackdown, China had been exporting at least $10 million worth of garlic to the United States every month. This crackdown created a black market for garlic, and shipments of smuggled garlic have been confiscated in Norway and Sweden.

**Special Properties**   What is it about garlic that leads people to turn to smuggling to get enough of it? Garlic is a member of the onion family, along with shallots, leeks, and chives. All contain the same bioactive sulfur compounds as well as flavonoids, B vitamins, and measurable amounts of manganese and selenium. Its sulfur-containing nutrients offer superior health benefits by increasing the level of hydrogen sulfide, which leads to relaxed arteries and improved blood flow. Sulfur is found in every cell of the human body and helps maintain healthy joints and boosts the immune system. Its anti-inflammatory properties have convinced scientists to study it as a possible anticancer agent.

However, an NCCAM-funded study on the safety and effectiveness of three garlic preparations (fresh garlic, dried powdered garlic tablets, and aged garlic extract tablets) for lowering blood cholesterol levels found no benefit (Gardner et al., 2007). And according to NCCAM, a clinical trial on the long-term use of garlic supplements to prevent stomach cancer found no effect (NCCAM, 2008).

Researchers agree they have a lot to learn about garlic and why, like many other herbs and plants, it is so beneficial. To achieve the greatest health benefits from garlic, the cloves should be crushed or chopped, which activates the enzyme allinase, which in turn stimulates allicin, which breaks down to a variety of healthful compounds. The dicing or crushing allows the allicin to begin working, even though the garlic is cooked.

*Sharon Zoumbaris*

*See also* Antioxidants; Blood Pressure; National Center for Complementary and Alternative Medicine (NCCAM).

## References

Challem, Jack. "Sulfur-Rich Nutrients: What Do Garlic, Glutathione, Glucosamine, NAC, Alpha-lipoic Acid, Chondroitin and MSM Have in Common?" *Better Nutrition* 71, no. 12 (December 2009): 18.

"Customs Intercepts Smuggled Garlic from China." *Morning Edition, NPR News* (July 8, 2010).

Gardner, Christopher D., et al. "Effect of Raw Garlic vs Commercial Garlic Supplements on Plasma Lipid Concentrations in Adults with Moderate Hypercholesterolemia." *Archives of Internal Medicine* 167, no. 4 (February 26, 2007): 346–53.

Marano, Daniel A. "The Gift of Garlic: As Ancient As Its Role in Cooking and Healing Is, Only now Are Scientists Starting to Capture Its Healthful Properties." *Psychology Today* 42, no. 2 (March–April 2009): 56.

National Cancer Institute. "Garlic and Cancer Prevention: Questions and Answers" (July 9, 2007), www.cancer.gov/newscenter/pressrelease/garlic.

National Center for Complementary and Alternative Medicine. "Herbs at a Glance: Garlic" (2008), www.nccam.nih.gov.

## GENDER IDENTITY AND SEXUAL ORIENTATION

Gender identity and sexual orientation are often misunderstood terms. Are they determined by genetics, hormones, or culture? It's an age-old question with complex answers and solutions. Adolescents who suffer from gender identity disorder (GID) may experience social isolation and are vulnerable to depression and suicide. However, when they are younger, girls with GID face less overall social rejection than boys; it remains more acceptable to be a tomboy than a sissy.

Childhood is usually a pretty simple time in a person's life. Boys are boys, and girls are girls. Adults sometimes help kids keep the distinctions clear by dressing boys and girls differently, by treating them in different ways, and by making sure they know that they are expected to act in different ways. Also, boys tend to hang out with boys, and to regard girls as icky or unappealing in other ways. Girls prefer to hang out with other girls, regarding boys as gross or not people one wants to spend time with.

But, at about age 10 or so, things change. Hormones become active in both boys' and girls' bodies, and childhood standards and norms no longer hold true. Boys—at least most of them—begin to feel that maybe girls are not so bad after all. It may be all right to spend some time with them—actually, to spend a lot of time with them in more intimate ways than they had ever imagined. And most girls are willing to give boys a second chance—and even a third and fourth chance to see if there might not be more to the male sex than they had ever imagined.

Some boys continue to like hanging out with other boys, and even begin to feel that they would like to do more than just play baseball and smoke cigarettes behind the barn with them. Even though they have received the message thousands of times that it's time to start going out with girls, somehow a date with a boy seems more appealing and more natural. And some girls feel the same way about other girls. And yet other boys and girls just are not sure to whom they are most strongly attracted, boys or girls—or both.

Finally, some boys and girls are no longer entirely sure they are really male or female at all. The hormones that begin to flow in a male's body may suddenly carry a strange and terrifying message: "Did you know that you are really a girl, and not a boy?" Or, on the other hand, "You have been brought up as a girl, but now is the time to admit that you feel more like a boy." It is no wonder that adolescence has often been called the period of Sturm und Drang, "storm and stress," as almost-men and almost-women for the first time in their lives begin to assess their own sexual nature.

**Terminology** No discussion of sexual orientation and gender identity can proceed without a clear understanding of the meaning of a number of essential terms. To begin with, *sexual orientation* means the sex to which a person is primarily attracted physically, emotionally, and sexually. To say that one is *heterosexually oriented* means that one is attracted primarily to someone of the opposite sex; someone who is *homosexually oriented* is attracted primarily to someone of

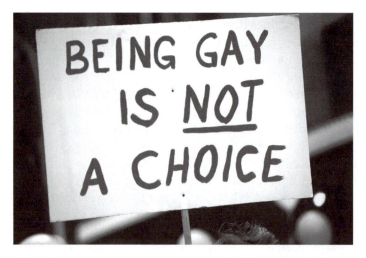

This sign presents an opinion on a much debated topic, "Being gay is not a choice." Many people in the gay liberation movement believe that sexual orientation is not a conscious choice, a view supported by the American Psychological Association. (Photo-Disc, Inc.)

the same sex. The terms *homosexual* and *heterosexual* are not very good as nouns, because they tend to define a person exclusively or primarily in terms of her or his sexual orientation. "That woman is a homosexual" suggests that her sexual orientation is the most important defining characteristic one can assign to her, which typically is not the case. Some people are attracted to both sexes, perhaps equally, but usually to some extent or another. They are said to have a *bisexual* orientation.

The issue of one's sexual orientation has long been a matter of considerable controversy in the United States and many other (but not all) parts of the world. As a result, a very large vocabulary of pejorative terms has developed to talk about anyone whose sexual orientation is outside the usual heterosexual norm recognized by society. Gay, lesbian, faggot, fairy, queer, and dyke are only a few of those terms, none of which is especially helpful in discussing the issues of sexual orientation.

The term *gender identity* means something very different from sexual orientation. Gender identity refers to the perception that one has of his or her own sexual status. A man may have been born with male genitalia and still feel deep down in his heart and soul that he is somehow a woman. Someone born with the reproductive system of a woman might feel that she is a man in a woman's body. Although these feelings are not typical of most men and women, they are not uncommon, and they are the basis of profound psychological and emotional struggles for people who experience them. Such individuals sometimes decide that they can no longer live a lie and commit to a series of medical procedures through which they change their physical gender, from male to female or female to male. Such individuals are known as *transgendered* individuals.

Gay men, lesbians, bisexuals, and transgendered individuals all experience a common reaction from general society, often a feeling of not belonging. It is small wonder, then, that a number of social and political organizations have been established to deal with issues common to those who belong to one of these categories. These groups often define themselves as gay, lesbian, bisexual, and transgendered (GLBT) groups and, in some cases, throw in the word *queer* (as in gay, lesbian, bisexual, queer, and transgendered) as an in-your-face political statement to the general community.

Groups interested in issues of sexual orientation and gender identity may add yet another term to their name: *questioning,* resulting in organizations that call themselves gay, lesbian, bisexual, transgendered, and questioning (GLBTQ). The term *questioning* refers to and emphasizes the fact that many adolescents are at a stage in their lives when they really do not know the category to which they belong—that is, whether they are more attracted to someone of the same sex, of the opposite sex, or to both sexes, or even how they feel about their own sexual identity.

A final category of individuals to be mentioned includes *transvestites,* sometimes the least understood of all nontypical groups. Transvestites are individuals who take pleasure in dressing and acting as members of the opposite sex: men dress as women, and women dress as men. Such individuals are almost without exception heterosexual. The term almost always applies to the former case—men who dress as women—because that condition is regarded as somehow abnormal or unnatural. On the contrary, many women dress and act in a manner not unlike that of men in everyday society, so the practice is generally not regarded as abnormal or unnatural. Instead, it is more likely to be regarded as a statement of status in (at least) U.S. society. That is, it is permissible for a woman to want to move up in the world by dressing like her superior, a man, while it is largely unthinkable that a man would want to move down in the world by dressing like a woman. But that analysis is for another time.

**Gay, Lesbian, Transgender**   One reason that adolescence is such a difficult time in a person's life is that so many questions have to be answered in the transition from childhood to adulthood. Does one want to simply adopt and accept the attitudes, beliefs, and lifestyle of one's parents, or should one break away and form a new and independent life? Should one be a Democrat, Orthodox Jew, and attorney because those are the choices one's parents made or want their children to make? Or does one's conscience push one toward the Republican Party, atheism, and a career as a concert pianist?

The matters of sexual orientation and gender identity are not so much matters of choice—evidence now suggests that both characteristics have strong genetic roots—but deciding how to act on one's innermost convictions about these issues *is* a decision one has to make. In a society in which homosexual behavior and transgenderism are still the subject of considerable disapproval, acknowledging to oneself and one's family and friends that one may be lesbian, gay, or a potentially transgendered individual can be far more difficult than announcing that one is no longer a Democrat or an Orthodox Jew.

Public opinion polls suggest that attitudes about homosexual behavior in the United States have undergone significant changes in the past few decades. In its most recent poll on the question (June 2008), the Gallup Poll organization found that the nation was evenly split on the question of whether homosexual relations are "morally acceptable" or "morally wrong," with 48 percent of respondents agreeing with each position. But that result represents a significant shift in less than a decade. When the same question was asked in 2001, the majority of respondents—53 percent—agreed that homosexual relations were "morally wrong," while only 40 percent thought they were "morally acceptable" (Gallup, 2009).

This trend is more apparent when viewed over a longer time span. In 1983, Gallup asked respondents whether they thought homosexuality was "an acceptable alternative lifestyle or not": 51 percent of respondents said no, while 34 percent said yes. Twenty-five years later, when Gallup asked the same question, these positions had been reversed: 57 percent of respondents agreed that homosexuality "was acceptable," while 40 percent said that it was not (Gallup, 2009).

These data send mixed messages to adolescents in the United States who are questioning their sexual orientation and gender identity. For one thing, they indicate that at least 4 out of 10 Americans still regard homosexual behavior as morally unacceptable. That means that something like 4 out of 10 parents, school teachers and counselors, religious leaders, neighbors, family friends, and others with whom one comes into contact on a daily basis regards the questioning teen-ager as morally repugnant. Many of the resources on which adolescents depend for support and guidance in dealing with difficult personal questions—such as one's religious beliefs, political commitments, sexual orientation, and gender identity—may not, therefore, be available in dealing with this issue.

The problems faced by adolescents dealing with issues of sexual orientation and gender identity have been documented in a number of surveys and studies. In 2001, for example, the Massachusetts Department of Public Health reported on a study it conducted of suicides and suicide attempts among high school stu-dents in the state. It found that about 40 gay, lesbian, and bisexual students had attempted suicide at least once, compared to a rate of 10 percent among hetero-sexual students (Healy, 2001). Similar results have been reported in a number of other studies on suicide rates among teenagers (Massachusetts Department of Elementary and Secondary Education, 2007, p. 50; Trevor Project, 2009).

In one of the most comprehensive (if somewhat dated) studies of the issues faced by GLBTQ students, more than 40 percent of respondents reported not feeling safe in school because of their sexual orientation or gender identity; more than 90 percent heard homophobic remarks from fellow students; 30 percent heard similar remarks from faculty and administrators; and 69 percent reported having experienced some form of verbal or physical harassment. Even among those respondents who said they felt safe at their schools, 46 percent reported verbal harassment, 36 percent reported sexual harassment, 12 percent reported physical harassment, and 6 percent reported some type of physical assault (The Body, 2001).

One consequence of the problems GLBTQ students face is their tendency to turn to alcohol and illegal drugs as a form of relief and compensation. A study by researchers at the University of Pittsburgh in 2008 found that the rate of alcohol and substance abuse among gay, lesbian, and bisexual students is about 190 per-cent that of heterosexual students, and, among some subgroups of GLB students, the rate may reach 400 percent that of their heterosexual counterparts. Lead re-searcher Michael P. Marshal explained that homophobia, discrimination, and vic-timization are largely responsible for these substance use disparities in young gay people. History shows that when marginalized groups are oppressed and do not have equal opportunities and equal rights, they suffer. Our results show that gay youth are clearly no exception (Addiction, 2008).

**Options for GLBTQ Youth**   Some adolescents are fortunate in that they can turn to trusted resources—parents, teachers, religious leaders, friends, neighbors, and relatives—when they have questions about their sexual orientation or gender identity. Somewhat strangely enough, the one group of individuals whom they may not be able to turn are older gay men, lesbians, bisexuals, and transgendered individuals. The problem has traditionally been that older GLBT individuals are hesitant to offer their help to younger men and women and boys and girls for fear of being labeled as predators. The connection between child molestation and ho-mosexual behavior has been emphasized for so long that concerns about one's legal safety may prompt many older GLBT individuals from associating with younger questioning youth under almost any circumstances. The abundance of evidence that refutes this connection has made this problem only slightly less of an issue (see, for example, Newton, 1978).

In any case, a number of resources have been developed over the past two decades to which GLBTQ youth can turn for assistance in dealing with their own questions about sexual orientation and gender identity. Without much doubt, the availability of the Internet has been a key factor in increasing the number of these resources to which young people can turn. For example, Youth Resource is a project of Advocates for Youth that provides information on a range of topics of interest and concern to GLBTQ youth. It provides a link to dozens of local organizations, such as school and campus groups, to which one can turn for direct advice and assistance. A search for the state of Alabama, for example, returns the names of 4 youth groups that deal with sexual orientation and gender identity issues among teenagers, 1 campus organization, and 13 peer-education groups. Another online resource is the National Youth Advocacy Coalition, whose primary objective is to "strengthen the role of young people in the LGBTQ rights movement" (National Youth Advocacy Coalition, 2009).

A number of nonelectronic resources are also available for GLBTQ youth. Perhaps the best known of these resources is the Gay, Lesbian, and Straight Education Network (GLSEN), founded in 1990 to work to "to assure that each member of every school community is valued and respected regardless of sexual orientation or gender identity/expression" and "to develop school climates where difference is valued for the positive contribution it makes in creating a more vibrant and diverse community" (Gay, Lesbian, and Straight Education Network, 2009).

Resources are also available for adults who want to learn more about ways in which they can act as a resource for GLBTQ youth. Probably the oldest and most widely respected of these organizations is Parents and Friends of Lesbians and Gays (PFLAG). PFLAG was founded in 1972 by Jeanne Manford after her son was beaten in a gay pride parade in New York City. Manford's goal was to provide a safe haven for parents of gays and lesbians and to provide information and support for mothers and fathers who were unsure how to deal with news that a son or daughter was gay or lesbian. Today PFLAG has more than 200,000 members in over 500 chapters in all 50 states and the District of Columbia. In addition to working with individual parents, the organization works on a local and national basis for equal rights for all individuals regardless of sexual orientation or gender identity.

**Progress?**    In some ways, dealing with issues of sexual orientation and gender identity are easier for young men and women today than it was a half century ago. In the 1950s, many GLBTQ youth probably knew little or nothing about homosexuality. One of the most common themes in the biographies of gay men and lesbians of the times was that "I thought I was the only person in the world like me." Today, stories of gay men, lesbians, bisexuals, and transgendered individuals appear everywhere in the public media. One consequence of this change has been that the age at which young men and women acknowledge being gay, lesbian, or bisexual has become younger and younger (Elias, 2007).

In that context, perhaps "coming out of the closet" (acknowledging one's sexual orientation) may be easier for teenagers in the 21st century than it ever was in the United States.

On the other hand, "being out" means that young men and women often have to deal with difficult issues at an earlier age than ever before. As with issues of sexually transmitted infections and contraception, questions about sexual orientation and gender identity are increasingly problems about which adolescents need more accurate information and guidance from adults.

Individuals seeking sex reassignment medical surgery and hormone therapy as treatment for gender identity disorder may consider deducting some of those medical expenses following a federal ruling in May 2010. Robert Donovan, born anatomically male, underwent a three-part treatment plan that included hormonal therapy, sex reassignment surgery, and breast augmentation. He legally changed his name and on his 2001 tax return claimed medical expense deductions. The IRS challenged his claim and also questioned whether he was properly diagnosed. However, the Tax Court rejected the IRS's arguments and ruled that GID is a well-recognized mental disorder, included in the American Psychiatric Association's *Diagnostic and Statistical Manual of Mental Disorders*. The court ruled that the costs of the surgery and hormone therapy were qualified medical deductibles but the breast augmentation was cosmetic surgery and was not deductible. It remains to be seen what effect, if any, this will have on insurance coverage in the future for those individuals seeking medical intervention for GID.

*David E. Newton*

*See also* Adolescence; Depression; Health Insurance; Suicide.

## References

American Social Health Association. "STD/STI Statistics > Fast Facts" (2009), www.ashastd.org/learn/learn_statistics.cfm.

The Body. "Fact Sheet: Lesbian, Gay, Bisexual and Transgender Youth Issues" (2001), www.thebody.com/content/whatis/art2449.html.

Elias, Marilyn. "Gay Teens Coming Out Earlier to Peers and Family." *USA Today* (February 7, 2007), www.usatoday.com/news/nation/2007-02-07-gay-teens-cover_x.htm.

Gallup. "Americans Evenly Divided on Morality of Homosexuality" (2009), www.gallup.com/poll/108115/americans-evenly-divided-morality-homosexuality.aspx.

Gay, Lesbian, and Straight Education Network. "Our Mission." www.glsen.org/cgi-bin/iowa/all/about/history/index.html.

"Gay Youth Report Higher Rates of Drug and Alcohol Use." *Addiction* (March 25, 2008), www.addictionjournal.org/viewpressrelease.asp?pr=74.

Goldman, Leon. "Syphilis in the Bible." *Archives of Dermatology* 103, no. 5 (May 1971): 535–36.

Healy, Patrick. "Massachusetts Study Shows High Suicide Rate for Gay Students" (2001), www.glsen.org/cgi-bin/iowa/all/news/record/399.html.

Herpes.com. "The Truth about HSV-1 and HSV-2" (2009), www.herpes.com/hsv1-2.html.

Massachusetts Department of Elementary and Secondary Education. *2005 Youth Risk Behavior Survey.* Boston: Massachusetts Department of Elementary and Secondary Education, December 2007.

National Youth Advocacy Coalition. "About the National Youth Advocacy Coalition" (2009), www.nyacyouth.org/about/index.php.

Newton, David E. "Homosexual Behavior and Child Molestation: A Review of the Evidence." *Adolescence* 13, no. 49 (Spring 1978): 29–43.

The Trevor Project. "Suicidal Signs" (2009), www.thetrevorproject.org/info.aspx.

Wells, Jean T., and Gwendolyn McFadden. "Sex-Change Surgery Deductible Medical Expense." *Journal of Accountancy* 209, no. 5 (May 2010): 70.

# GENETICALLY MODIFIED ORGANISMS (GMOs)

Genetically modified (GM) foods derive from genetically modified organisms (GMOs)—plants created for human or animal consumption using biotechnology instead of conventional plant breeding. The term most commonly used in the United States to describe the technology is genetic engineering (GE). Scientists and researchers describe the modified DNA produced in the process as recombinant DNA (rDNA). In Europe, genetic engineering is generally referred to as genetic modification, mainly because this term translates easily among different languages. The foods produced from genetic engineering are also called biotech foods, gene foods, bioengineered foods, gene-altered foods, transgenic foods, and, among the harshest critics of the technology, Frankenfoods.

Techniques for isolating and altering genes were first developed by U.S. geneticists during the early 1970s. In 1982, researchers succeeded in transferring genes between plant species. In conventional plant breeding, seeds and plants can be improved, but not chemically altered. In a GM food, DNA changes occur thanks to scientists who introduce specific traits into a plant by inserting one or more new genes into its genetic code. Unlike plants produced through conventional breeding, GM plants are given genes from vastly different organisms.

Scientists have mixed the genes of animals and vegetables as well as those of vegetables and bacteria. The most widely used gene transfer is the introduction of a Bt gene into corn, cotton, or soy. Bt, or *Bacillus thuringiensis*—a naturally occurring bacterium—produces proteins that poison insect larvae. The Bt bacterium is related to the common bacterium responsible for food poisoning and is a close relative of the organism that causes anthrax. Surprisingly, Bt toxin has been used for years by organic growers, who spray it on plants to kill pests. The toxin breaks down rapidly after killing the pests, and there is no evidence of health problems for people eating food sprayed properly with it. When the Bt toxin genes are inserted into corn, the plants generate their own pesticides, allowing them to kill insects such as the corn borer. The long-term effects of eating Bt corn have not been studied to date.

**Advantages and Disadvantages** Supporters of genetically modified foods say they offer several clear advantages, including pest resistance for crops, herbicide tolerance, disease resistance, and a better ability to withstand difficult growing conditions. The potential for improved nutrition, or for the development of new pharmaceuticals in foods such as tomatoes and potatoes, are expected to improve living conditions around the world.

Corporations such as Monsanto consider GM foods, especially Monsanto's Bt corn, a great success in protecting the environment by eliminating the overuse of chemical pesticides and herbicides. Thanks to the transfer of the Bt insect toxin genes, the plants do the work of the pesticides by easily killing the insects that feed on them. In addition to the Bt gene transfer, several crops (including Bt corn) have been genetically modified for resistance to weed-killing herbicide sprays. According to biotech companies, their statistics show that farmers who plant herbicide-tolerant plants reduce the amount of herbicide chemicals they spray on their crops. One prime example is the Monsanto strain of soybeans genetically modified to withstand the company's herbicide, Roundup. According to Monsanto, farmers who plant Monsanto soybeans use fewer applications of Roundup, thereby reducing costs and limiting dangerous chemical runoff.

Biotech companies also promote the eventual development of GM foods containing added vitamins and minerals, which they suggest will one day eliminate malnutrition around the world. Given these possibilities, corporate officials have little patience for critics, who they characterize as overzealous environmentalists with no scientific evidence to back up their charges.

The critics of GM foods are equally adamant about their concerns, which fall into three main categories: environmental hazards, human health risks, and economic effects. Red flags on GE food safety were raised due to research published in February 2009 and highlighted several potential problems, including the development of antibiotic-resistant genes, allergic responses, and some effects noted in short-term animal trials that scientists determined should require more investigation (Palmer & McCullum-Gomez, 2010).

Critics worry about unintended harm to other plants, insects, and animals when GM crops spread through natural pollination, are carried away on the wind, and fertilize other plants. Scientists call this phenomenon gene flow. It occurs when the plants fertilized by stray crop pollen reproduce, and their offspring take on the herbicide- and pest-resistant characteristics of the GM crops. Some critics of genetic engineering believe that genes introduced to GM plants could spread uncontrollably or create unstoppable superweeds. Gene flow would force farmers to use stronger herbicides or risk losing their crops. Biotech corporations have suggested that farmers should combat gene flow by planting non-GM crops around the GM fields, creating a buffer zone.

Critics also predict that, just as antibiotics have been overused—creating more antibiotic-resistant diseases—the overuse of pesticides on U.S. farms will mean chemical after chemical will become less effective—allowing superpests and superweeds to flourish. The Union of Concerned Scientists says there are signs that the most popular Bt crops will lose their effectiveness as weeds become resistant (Mellon & Rissler, 2003). Scientists also expect those plants to fall victim to Bt-resistant pests.

Another environmental fear is that GM crops with pest-killing genes will destroy helpful insects. Opponents of GM foods say the monarch butterfly symbolizes this risk. In the spring of 1999, a laboratory study published in *Nature* indicated that pollen from Bt corn could kill the larvae of monarch butterflies (Losey, Rayor, & Carter, 1999). At the time, Bt corn varieties had been planted on 20 million acres across the United States, including areas directly in the migratory path of the butterflies. Earlier tests on Bt crops by the Environmental Protection Agency (EPA) failed to consider the crops' potential effects on monarch butterflies or on other moths or butterflies not damaging to crops. They only tested the Bt toxin's ability to kill the larvae of pests such as the corn borer.

Following the study's release, a storm of protests forced the U.S. Department of Agriculture (USDA) to review just how real the threat was to the monarch population. The results of the USDA's 2001 study showed that only one Bt corn variety had high enough levels of Bt toxin to easily kill the monarch larvae. Luckily, that seed did not sell well and was not widely planted. But the crisis demonstrated a lack of government vigilance and bolstered critics' claims that many insects, as well as animals higher up in the food chain, were at risk from GM crops. The 2001 USDA study did not address whether GM crops had the potential to cause future abnormalities, such as delayed development, impaired reproduction, altered growth, or shortened life spans.

The monarch butterfly was again center stage in the debate over GM foods in November 2007, when environmental officials with the European Union (EU) announced study results showing that two varieties of GM corn harmed butterfly species, specifically the monarch. In a statement, EU environment commissioner Stavros Dimas called the "potential damage on the environment irreversible" and said the level of risk generated by cultivation was unacceptable (Kanter, 2007).

Farmers and environmentalists opposed to GM plants also argue that altered seeds threaten biodiversity. Farmers have saved their seeds through hundreds and thousands of seasons, using each generation of seeds to improve properties such as resistance to pests, drought, wind, and changing weather. But the use of GM seeds, controlled by a few large biotech corporations, could eliminate many varieties of plants. Modern consumers may not realize that only 1 percent of vegetable varieties grown a century ago are still available for purchase today. If, or when, a crop is attacked by a new disease, as occurred with U.S. corn in 1970, today's researchers must look to a rapidly shrinking pool of heirloom seeds for solutions. Critics worry that someday those seeds simply won't exist if GM crops continue to cross-pollinate conventional fields.

Cross-pollination from GM crops has also been an important legal issue. Monsanto and other companies have sued farmers for patent infringement; Monsanto claims that the farmers obtained their GM seeds without paying royalties to the company. The farmers argue that the crops were the result of cross-pollination they could not control. Monsanto has won the majority of its patent infringement claims. The company has also successfully sued farmers who saved and planted seeds from those cross-pollinated fields.

Opponents of GM foods fear that there are unstudied and potentially devastating health risks for humans who eat the foods as well. Changing the fundamental DNA of a food could cause new diseases or health problems. At a minimum, critics argue, these untested genetic combinations could create proteins that trigger severe allergic reactions. One example that critics cite involved deaths from L-tryptophan, an amino acid pill that killed 38 people and sickened thousands in 1989. The Japanese manufacturer of the pill used genetically engineered bacteria in its production, and, although it is not clear how the toxins developed in the drug, opponents of genetic engineering suspect the bacteria was a factor. Ultimately, no definite cause was pinpointed, but scientists agreed that some people were genetically more likely to react fatally to the amino acid in its pure form. L-tryptophan was banned, and opponents of genetic engineering continue to raise questions about the role GM bacteria played in the tragedy.

Finally, critics of GM foods concerned with their effects on humans warn that the food supply could quickly be contaminated by allergens unexpectedly created in GM crops, as happened with StarLink corn contamination. In April 1997, the biotech firm Aventis Crop Science applied to the EPA for a license to sell StarLink, a genetically engineered Bt corn. However, introduction of the Bt gene in StarLink produced a protein, called Cry9C, not present in other Bt corn crops. Scientists noticed that this particular protein did not digest well in people and did not break down in heat, two major characteristics common when food proteins trigger allergic reactions.

Based on this information, the EPA rejected StarLink for human consumption, but granted a split registration that allowed it to be used for animal feed. StarLink was also not licensed for export. In September 2000, StarLink was detected in Taco Bell taco shells, and the parent company, Kraft Foods, immediately issued a voluntary recall. In the months that followed, StarLink was discovered in more and more yellow corn products in the United States and in other countries.

To many critics of GM foods, this episode raised serious questions about the U.S. government's ability to keep such foods separate from conventional foods. Before the StarLink incident was over, U.S. companies were forced to recall over 300 contaminated food products in 2000 and 2001. The incident heightened fears among European consumers. Corn exports from the United States to Europe were halted, and companies were forced to buy back contaminated corn. In the United States, farmers filed class-action suits in Nebraska, Iowa, and Illinois to recoup big losses that had resulted when their corn was contaminated or commingled with StarLink. Aventis eventually reached an agreement in 17 states to compensate farmers for their losses.

Although StarLink represented only 1 percent of the total U.S. corn crop in 2000, when it accidentally mixed with other corn varieties, it may have contaminated up to 50 percent of the year's corn harvest. There were still more costs for Aventis. Following the discovery of StarLink contamination in foods, over two dozen people reported severe allergic reactions and filed a class-action suit. The U.S. Food and Drug Administration (FDA) and the Centers for Disease Control and Prevention (CDC) tested blood samples from a majority of those people, and, although it did appear that the claimants suffered severe allergic reactions to something, the CDC ruled that StarLink was not responsible.

Cost is a third area used by critics of GM foods, who argue that the foods are priced no more cheaply than their conventional counterparts and fail to benefit consumers nutritionally. Another economic downside of GM foods, according to critics, is that patents are placed on GM seeds and prices go up, meaning small farmers may not be able to afford the engineered seeds. Because growers are not allowed to save GM seeds from year to year, if their conventional seeds are altered by the GM plants, small farmers may be left with nothing to grow. Critics say that, one way or another, small farmers will ultimately be squeezed out, leaving giant biotech companies in control of the world's seed and food supply.

**Government's Role**   In the United States, three agencies have jurisdiction over genetically modified organisms: the U.S. Department of Agriculture, the Food and Drug Administration, and the Environmental Protection Agency. Over-all, the FDA has the bulk of the responsibilities for GMOs, because it is respon-sible for the safety and nutrition of food and food additives. In 1986, the Reagan administration formally published the *Coordinated Framework for Regulation of Bio-technology* that set up how the three agencies would divide their responsibilities.

The most striking aspect of the system is that it remains voluntary. The FDA does not require safety reviews on GM foods and only requires labeling if the composition of a GM food is radically different from that of its conventional counterpart. If a company voluntarily decides to submit a GM plant for evalua-tion, the end result is usually a statement from the FDA finding the engineered crop substantially equivalent to its nonengineered version. In other words, FDA policy begins with the premise that plants developed through biotechnology are not inherently unsafe or different in any significant way. They are evaluated on their physical characteristics rather than on how they were created. If it looks like a tomato, smells like a tomato, and tastes like a tomato, it must be a tomato, even if it contains genes from fish or bacteria.

The EPA has the strongest regulations of the three agencies but plays a much smaller role in the regulation of biotechnology. The agency oversees the manu-facture, sale, and use of plant pesticides and other toxic substances as well as ben-eficial insects and other living organisms. However, only two classes of GM plants fall under the EPA's control: plants containing Bt toxins with resistance to certain insects and GM plants with a resistance to viruses.

The third agency, the USDA, oversees plants and plant pests and controls the testing of GM crops in order to protect U.S. crops from pests. If agricultural cor-porations can demonstrate to the USDA that their GM crop is not a pest, they are free to plant and sell the crop on U.S. farmland. A smaller agency within the USDA, the Animal and Plant Health Inspection Service (APHIS), also oversees the safety of GM organisms and their overall impact on U.S. agriculture. The ser-vice focuses on new GM plants and evaluates potential problems with pests or weed escapes that could damage U.S. agriculture.

Although several guidelines influence field testing of genetically modified plants, the USDA rarely rejects new GM plants. Between 1987 and 2005, APHIS approved more than 10,000 field test requests out of the 11,000 it received (Becker & Cowan, 2006). Field test approval leaves deregulation as the only real hurdle facing biotech companies before they can market a new GM food in the United States. After they gather several years of data from regulated field trials, developers go back to APHIS and petition for deregulation. If the petition is accepted—and the vast majority are—then the GM product is treated as equivalent to the conventionally grown product and is sold to consumers without a label or any mention of genetic changes.

The FDA released a series of policy statements in 1992, including "Foods Derived from New Plant Varieties." This landmark statement said GM foods were presumed generally recognized as safe (GRAS) and marketable as such. It's important to remember that the FDA deals with food safety after a product is on the shelves. The agency first created and applied the idea of substantial equivalence in the case of the FlavrSavr tomato. The GRAS designation of GM foods cemented the policy that when the nutritional content of a GM food appears the same as its conventional version, the FDA will not require any testing or special labeling. In 2006, the FDA published new policies calling for voluntary consultation with GM companies in the early stages of development.

**Labeling**   The argument against labeling genetically modified food is largely economic. Basically, those who favor GM foods take a strong stand against labeling, calling it cost-prohibitive, unnecessary, misleading, and inefficient. In the United States, GM plants are routinely harvested and mixed with conventional crops. Advocates of GM foods say the cost to consumers of segregating bioengineered foods from conventional foods would raise food prices but provide no other real benefits.

Opponents of GM foods already distrust such foods. They describe a complete lack of studies to support the industry's position and argue that without scientific reassurance that GM foods are safe to eat, labels are vital for consumers who want to avoid the foods. Critics also point to legislation that exists outside the United States. They say it is in America's best interest to have internationally clear standards and labels rather than the current U.S. policy, which creates a distinct economic disadvantage for farmers due to large export losses.

**European Response to GM Foods**   Fear of genetically engineered food has flourished in Europe for decades and has effectively stopped efforts by U.S. biotech corporations to promote genetically modified crops in countries outside the United States. Despite scientific and industry reassurance that GM foods are safe for human consumption, and a ruling by the World Trade Organization against import bans in the European Union, genetic engineering technology continues to be rejected by an overwhelming majority of Europeans. Internationally, some 35 countries have restrictions on GM foods, ranging from mandatory labeling to outright bans (Rees, 2006).

**Corporations**   Profits were a driving force behind the early development of GMOs. In the 1990s, some big U.S. corporations faced a deadline when older pesticides were due to come off patent, releasing those chemical formulas into the public domain. New seed patents became the focus of corporations such as Cargill and Archer Daniels Midland, which together hold patents on 80 percent of the world's grain. The other major players—Syngenta, DuPont, Monsanto, and Aventis—control two-thirds of the world's agrochemical market. By 2006, almost 50 percent of the corn planted in the United States was Monsanto's Bt or Roundup Ready seeds (Lerner & Lerner, 2007).

The Monsanto Company has developed more genetically engineered seeds and plants than any other corporation. During the 1990s, it patented and sold GM varieties of rice, cotton, and soybeans. All these plants are engineered to resist the company's top-selling herbicide, Roundup, now the most profitable herbicide in the world. In 2002, the picture for Monsanto was not so positive; the company had suffered a 65 percent drop in sales of Roundup. But by 2008, thanks to the purchase of seed companies, advances in GMO technology, and the pairing of the seeds with its herbicide, the company posted huge earnings. In January 2008, Monsanto reported annual earnings of over $256 million in the fiscal first quarter, compared to $90 million for the same period in 2007 (Simpkins & Patalon, 2008).

Along with large biotech corporations, other organizations that strongly support GM technology include Sense About Science and the National Center for Food and Agriculture Policy (NCFAP). Sense About Science is a British lobby group that was launched in 2002. The website refers to a network of scientists who support an evidence-based approach to technological developments. The NCFAP is a private, nonprofit research organization formed in 1992. Consumer advocates have called the organization a pro-GM industry group whose funding for NCFAP biotechnology studies is linked to such donors as Monsanto, Grocery Manufacturers of America, DuPont, Aventis, and the Rockefeller Foundation.

**Environmentalists**    Opponents of genetically modified foods agree on several basic concepts, most importantly that the benefits of GMOs do not outweigh the risks. They wonder how the world's poor will find enough resources to buy genetically engineered seeds when they lack money to buy seeds now. Corporations such as Monsanto have shown no willingness to give away free seeds, and they have taken legal action against inadvertent cross-pollination.

The groups opposed to genetically engineered foods include Greenpeace, the Center for Food Safety (CFS), the Alliance for Bio-Integrity, GM Watch, and the Union of Concerned Scientists. Greenpeace has offices in 40 countries across Europe, the Americas, Asia, and the Pacific. The group started in 1971 and has grown into an international advocate for the environment. Greenpeace officially applauds scientific progress on molecular biology, but it criticizes the untested use of genetically modified organisms as a giant genetic experiment by corporate interests.

The Alliance for Bio-Integrity was founded by lawyer Stephen M. Druker, who played a key role in the 1998 lawsuit against the FDA. The CFS is a nonprofit, public interest environmental advocacy organization that began in 1997 for the direct purpose of challenging GM food technologies and promoting alternatives. The organization has offices in Washington, D.C., and San Francisco. The CFS joined the 1998 lawsuit against the FDA along with the Alliance for Bio-Integrity.

GM Watch was founded in 1998 in Norfolk, United Kingdom, in response to growing international concern about genetic engineering, and now has contacts in several European countries. A private, nonprofit organization, GM Watch specifically functions to publicly question the genetic engineering industry.

**The Future**   The controversy continues. On one side are those who demand the right to know what they are eating. They call genetically modified foods an experiment in progress with unknown consequences. On the other side are corporations, governments, and scientists who say no evidence of harm has come to light and argue that the use of biotechnology is imperative to feed a hungry world.

Consumers must ask themselves whether this technology is being pushed to the market before risks are understood and managed. Consumers who do not want to eat genetically modified foods have found ways to avoid them. The Organic Foods Production Act of 1990 (OFPA) is a uniform organic standard in place for farmers that is enforced by the USDA. Although the agency proposed rules over the years to permit irradiated foods and biotech foods, the organic standard ultimately adopted in 2002 explicitly excludes any GM foods. For now the label's net effect means no GM ingredients are used in organic products.

Consumers wishing to avoid GM products can also scan labels for common GM ingredients such as corn oil, corn syrup, cornstarch, soy protein, soy oil, soy sauce, lecithin, cottonseed oil, and canola oil. An FDA report published in 2000 listed those foods among many that tested positive for the presence of unlabeled genetically modified ingredients. The FDA list also included various well-known items: Duncan Hines cake mix, Jiffy corn muffin mix, Ultra Slim-Fast, Aunt Jemima pancake mix, and Kellogg's Corn Flakes to name a few. For shoppers who want information on GM-free foods, the "True Food Shopping List" from the Greenpeace website provides a list of foods without GM ingredients.

*Sharon Zoumbaris*

*See also* Environmental Protection Agency (EPA); Food and Drug Administration (FDA); L-Tryptophan; Organic Food; U.S. Department of Agriculture (USDA).

## References

Becker, Geoffrey S., and Tadlock Cowan. "Agricultural Biotechnology: Background and Recent Issues." *Congressional Research Service (CRS) Reports and Issue Briefs* (September 2006).

Center for Food Safety. "Genetically Engineered Food," www.centerforfoodsafety.org/geneticall7.cfm.

Druker, Steven M. "A Report on the Results of *Alliance for Bio-Integrity v. Shalala, et al.*" Alliance for Bio-Integrity (October 1, 2003), www.biointegrity.org/report-on-lawsuit.htm.

Hart, Kathleen. *Eating in the Dark: America's Experiment with Genetically Engineered Food.* New York: Pantheon Books, 2002.

Kanter, James. "EU Officials Propose Ban on Genetically Modified Corn Seeds." *International Herald Tribune* (November 21, 2007).

Lerner, K. Lee, and Brenda Wilmoth Lerner, eds. *Biotechnology: Changing Life through Science.* Farmington Hills, MI: Thomson Gale, 2007.

Losey, John E., Linda S. Rayor, and Maureen E. Carter. "Transgenic Pollen Harms Monarch Larvae." *Nature* 399, no. 6733 (May 20, 1999).

Mellon, Margaret, and Jane Rissler. "Environmental Effects of Genetically Modified Food Crops: Recent Experiences." Paper presented at Genetically Modified Foods—The American Experience, Copenhagen, June 12–13, 2003. Reproduced by Union of Concerned Scientists, www.ucusa.org/food_and_agriculture/science_and_impacts/impacts_genetic_engineering/environmental-effects-of.html.

Palmer, Sharon, and Chris McCullum-Gomez. "Genetically Engineered Foods Update." *Environmental Nutrition* 33, no. 7 (July 2010).

Rees, Andy. *Genetically Modified Food: A Short Guide for the Confused.* Ann Arbor, MI: Pluto Press, 2006.

Sample, Ian. "The Return of GM: Biotech Firm Mans Barricades as Campaigners Vow to Stop Trials: Small Field Near Cambridge the Latest Battleground in Fight to Prevent GM Trials." *Guardian* (February 16, 2008).

Simpkins, Jason, and William Patalon III. "Monsanto Reaps Huge Rewards from Its Blossoming Seed Business." Money Morning (January 7, 2008), www.moneymorning.com/2008/01/07/monsanto-reaps-huge-rewards-from-its-blossoming-seed-business/.

Thomson, Jennifer A. *Seeds for the Future.* Ithaca, NY: Cornell University Press, 2007.

## GHRELIN

Ghrelin is a new and promising discovery in the fight against obesity. Pronounced GRELL-in, research on this growth hormone has shown that it not only has an effect on whether a person is hungry, it may also help defend against symptoms of stress-induced depression and anxiety. Early research demonstrated that ghrelin plays a role in sending hunger signals to the brain. A study published in the May 23, 2002, issue of the *New England Journal of Medicine* first suggested that ghrelin may turn out to be an important reason people feel hungry and why it's so hard for dieters to keep weight off.

Later studies using mice found that fully sated mice that received ghrelin were drawn to high-fat food, suggesting it may work in the brain to cause continued eating of pleasurable foods. In 2009, a research group from the University of Texas in Dallas reported that blocking the body's response to ghrelin signals could potentially decrease food intake, once again raising hopes for a breakthrough in the treatment of obesity.

In a country where obesity is an epidemic, understanding how ghrelin works could lead to effective weight-loss drugs. Other potential uses include as a drug to promote weight gain in anorexics and cancer patients. Scientists know that part of the brain's hypothalamus controls food intake, but until recent years the only chemical substances known to turn it on had been found in the brain. New research now shows ghrelin's receptors are in the brain; however, more importantly, its primary site of production is in the stomach, which pumps it into the bloodstream.

From there hormone travels to the pituitary, a vastly different mechanism from other peptides that affect appetite. Those are made in the brain, do not travel into the bloodstream, and only work when injected directly into the appropriate brain regions.

Ghrelin, a peptide consisting of 28 amino acids, was first identified by Kenji Kangawa of the National Cardiovascular Center Research Institute in Osaka, Japan. The name uses the root *ghre,* which means growth in Hindi and related languages, and the name's initial letters also refer to ghrelin's role as a growth hormone–releasing factor. Following its identification in 1999, doctors have started looking at ghrelin in the treatment of obesity as well as in wasting syndromes stemming from AIDS, cancer, heart disease, and a variety of other illnesses.

Although the hormone's role in the body is not yet fully understood, recent studies show that people suffering from wasting illnesses manufacture more ghrelin than normal. In fact, the highest blood concentrations of ghrelin recorded are in people suffering from anorexia nervosa. Apparently while anorexics are starving themselves to death, blood analysis indicates large amounts of ghrelin are released as normal body mechanisms continually signal the need for food.

The report also found that after a group of 13 obese people dieted and lost some 17 percent of their body weight, their ghrelin levels were significantly higher throughout the day than before the weight loss, when ghrelin levels would rise before meals but fall afterward. Scientists suggest that this increase in ghrelin in people who have lost weight dieting may reflect the body's attempt to regain lost pounds, a mechanism that originally evolved to defend against starvation during humankind's early history, when food supplies fluctuated erratically. Today in developed nations such as the United States, with an abundance of high-calorie foods, scientists speculate this early survival advantage may now contribute to obesity.

On the other hand, low ghrelin levels were noted in people who underwent gastric-bypass surgery. They experienced a drop in their ghrelin levels but did not appear to suffer any side effects. According to a study, people who undergo this surgery describe a generalized disinterest in food with a noticeable drop in ghrelin production. Researchers say that following bypass surgery, stomach cells that produce ghrelin are no longer exposed to food and ghrelin production may no longer be stimulated. During gastric-bypass surgery, surgeons sew much of the stomach shut, leaving room for a dieter to eat only a small amount of food.

Still, researchers warn against high expectations about ghrelin's prospects. They say similar hopes were raised years ago for leptin, a hormone that acts as an appetite suppressant. Yet after years of research, no useful medication was developed, because researchers found that patients quickly developed a tolerance to leptin. Nonetheless, the discovery of ghrelin is a major advance in the understanding of what controls appetite, and this leaves researchers hungry to learn more.

*Marjolijn Bijlefeld and Sharon Zoumbaris*

*See also* Amino Acids; Obesity.

## References

Cummings, David E., D.S. Weigle, R.S. Frayo, P.A. Breen, M.K. Ma, E.P. Dellinger, and J.Q. Purnell. "Plasma Ghrelin Levels after Diet-Induced Weight Loss or Gastric Bypass Surgery." *New England Journal of Medicine* 346, no. 21 (May 23, 2002): 1623–30.

Fischman, Josh. "A Hungry Hormone." *U.S. News & World Report* (June 3, 2002): 53.

Flier, J.S., and E. Maratos-Flier. "The Stomach Speaks—Ghrelin and Weight Regulation." *New England Journal of Medicine* 346, no. 21 (May 23, 2002): 1662–63.

Lemonick, Michael D. "Lean and Hungrier: Is a Recently Discovered Hormone the Reason Why Folks Who Lose Weight Can't Keep It Off?" *Time,* June 3, 2002, 54.

Perello, Mario, Ichiro Sakata, Shari Birnbaum, Jen-Chieh Chuang, Sherri Osborne-Lawrence, Sherry A. Rovinsky, Jakub Woloszyn, Masashi Yanagisawa, Michael Lutter, and Jeffrey M. Zigman. "Ghrelin Increases the Rewarding Value of High-Fat in an Orexin-Dependent Manner." *Biological Psychiatry* 67, no. 9 (May 1, 2010): 880–86.

Pinkney, Jonathan, and Gareth Williams. "Ghrelin Gets Hungry." *Lancet* 359, no. 9315 (April 20, 2002): 1360.

Travis, John. "The Hunger Hormone? An Appetite Stimulant Produced by the Stomach May Lead to Treatments for Obesity and Wasting Syndromes." *Science News* 161, no. 7 (February 16, 2002): 107–9.

## GINGER

Ginger, which is mentioned in ancient writings from China, India, and the Middle East, has long been praised for its aromatic and culinary qualities. However, it is probably best known for having myriad medicinal properties. Of these, the first and foremost is ginger's ability to bring relief from gastrointestinal problems such as nausea. Ginger is also thought to be useful for anti-inflammatory illnesses such as osteoarthritis. And some people think that ginger may promote cardiovascular health (Klotter, 2009). Of course, it is important to review the research.

**Nausea** A study published in 2003 in the *Australian and New Zealand Journal of Obstetrics and Gynaecology* examined the effect ginger extract had on the morning sickness of 120 women, all of whom were less than 20 weeks pregnant. The study only included women who had daily bouts with morning sickness for at least one week and women for whom no relief was obtained from dietary modifications.

The women received either 125 milligrams of ginger extract (1.5 grams of dried ginger) or a placebo four times per day for four days. After the first day of treatment, the women consuming ginger extract had significantly less nausea than the women taking the placebo. While there were no significant differences in vomiting, the women on ginger experienced less retching. The researchers concluded that "Ginger can be considered a useful treatment for women suffering from morning sickness" (Willetts, Ekangaki, & Eden, 2003).

A second study on the use of ginger for morning sickness in Australian women was published in 2004 in *Obstetrics and Gynecology*. For three weeks, 291 women who were less than 16 weeks pregnant were given either 1.05 grams of ginger or 75 milligrams of vitamin B6 every day. In both groups, more than half of the

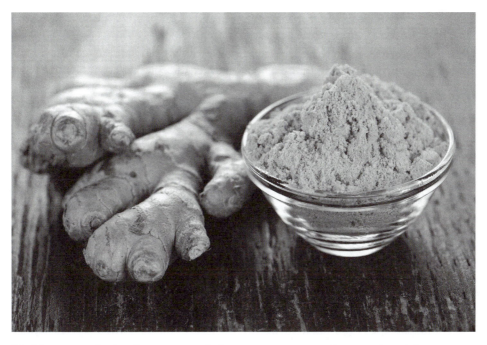

Health care professionals recommend ginger to ease nausea from motion sickness, pregnancy, and cancer chemotherapy. Here, fresh and powdered ginger root sit on a table. (Elena Elisseeva/Dreamstime.com)

women improved; there were no significant differences in outcomes. The researchers concluded that, for "women looking for relief from their nausea, dry retching, and vomiting, the use of ginger in early pregnancy will reduce their symptoms to an equivalent extent as vitamin B6" (Smith et al., 2004).

A third study, published in 2003 in the *American Journal of Obstetrics and Gynecology,* compared 187 pregnant women who took ginger for nausea and vomiting with a control group of 187 who did not take any treatments. The ginger appeared to "mildly" help the women with their nausea and vomiting, and it did not "appear to increase the rate of major malformations above the baseline rate" (Portnoi et al., 2003).

In a study conducted in Thailand and published in 2007 in *Alternative Medicine Review,* researchers attempted to determine whether ginger could reduce or prevent the nausea and vomiting that often follows major gynecologic surgery. Researchers studied a total of 120 women undergoing major gynecologic surgery. Before surgery, 60 women received two capsules of ginger; another 60 women received a placebo. The researchers indicated that the women who had presurgery ginger had statistically significantly less nausea and vomiting that the women who took the placebo. The researchers noted that "ginger has efficacy in prevention of nausea and vomiting after major gynecologic surgery" (Roxas, 2007).

Another study from Thailand, published in 2006 in the *American Journal of Obstetrics and Gynecology,* reviewed five randomized, double-blind, placebo-controlled trials with a total of 363 patients. All of the studies compared the use of a fixed dose of ginger to a placebo on 24-hour postoperative nausea and vomiting in patients having gynecological or lower extremity surgery. The incidence of postoperative nausea and vomiting in those who received at least one gram of ginger was more than a third less than those who received placebos. Still, the study has some limitations. For example, the majority of the patients were Asian with an average weight of only 50 kilograms (110 pounds). Dosage requirements may need to be increased for people who are larger. Nevertheless, the researchers concluded that "use of ginger is an effective means for reducing postoperative nausea and vomiting" (Chaiyakunapruk et al., 2006).

It is also well known that people receiving chemotherapy treatments frequently experience nausea. A study published in 2006 in *Neurogastroenterology and Motility* attempted to determine whether high-protein meals combined with ginger could help control the postchemotherapy nausea. For three days after chemotherapy treatments, 28 cancer patients were placed in one of three groups. The control group ate their normal diets. A second group ate a protein drink and one gram of ginger root twice each day. A third group ate a protein drink and additional protein power and one gram of ginger root twice a day. The researchers found that the "high protein meals with ginger reduced the delayed nausea of chemotherapy, and reduced the use of antiemetic [antinausea] medications. Anti-nausea effects of high protein meals with ginger were associated with enhancement of normal gastric myoelectrical [electricity generated by muscle] activity and decreased gastric dysrhythmias [abnormal stomach electrical activity]" (Levine et al., 2006).

**Cardiovascular and Diabetic Health**  Researchers at Kuwait University studied the role that ginger plays in rats that have been treated to develop diabetes. In a study published in 2006 in the *British Journal of Nutrition,* researchers noted that rats that developed diabetes tended to have high blood sugar and weight loss. The researchers fed these rats raw ginger—500 milligrams per kilogram of body weight per day—for seven weeks. A separate group of rats, which did not receive any ginger, served as the control group. At the end of the study, the rats that were fed ginger had considerably lower levels of blood sugar, cholesterol, and triglycerides than the rats in the control group. Ginger also appeared to lessen some of the complications associated with diabetes, such as protein in the urine, excessive urine output, and excess water intake. "Therefore, it can be concluded from these studies that raw ginger has significant potential in the treatment of diabetes" (Al-Amin et al., 2006).

**Osteoarthritis of the Knee**  In a study published in 2001 in *Arthritis and Rheumatism,* subjects with moderate to severe pain from osteoarthritis in their knees were divided into two groups. One group took 255 milligrams of concentrated ginger root twice daily for six weeks, while the other group had placebos. Following a washout period, the group that originally had ginger was given placebos, and the group that originally had placebos was given ginger. In the end, 247 patients were evaluated. The researchers found that the ginger markedly improved the pain from osteoarthritis. "A highly purified and standardized ginger extract had a statistically significant effect on reducing symptoms of OA [osteo-arthritis] of the knee." But some of the participants reported gastrointestinal side effects, such as belching, gas, nausea, and mild heartburn (Altman & Marcussen, 2001).

In an article published in 2005 in the *Journal of Medicinal Food,* researchers from the Department of Orthopedic Surgery at Johns Hopkins University School of Medicine noted that the anti-inflammatory properties of ginger have been known for centuries. More recently, many studies have been conducted on these properties, and it is now generally recognized that "ginger modulates biochemical pathways activated in chronic inflammation" (Grzanna, Lindmark, & Frondoza, 2005). But an article published in 2007 in *American Family Physician* appears to disagree. Commenting on the use of ginger for arthritis, Brett White wrote, "Mixed results have been found in limited studies of ginger for the treatment of arthritis symptoms" (White, 2007).

Though ginger allergies are uncommon, they are known to exist. And people taking blood-thinning medications, such as warfarin, should check with their health care provider before consuming even moderate amounts of ginger.

*Myrna Chandler Goldstein and Mark A. Goldstein*

*See also* Diabetes; Heart Health.

## References

Al-Amin, Zainab M., Martha Thomson, Khaled K. Al-Qattan, et al. "Anti-Diabetic and Hypolipidaemic Properties of Ginger (*Zingiber officinale*) in Streptozotocin-Induced Diabetic Rates." *British Journal of Nutrition* 96 (2006): 660–66.

Altman, R.D., and K.C. Marcussen. "Effects of a Ginger Extract on Knee Pain in Patients with Osteoarthritis." *Arthritis and Rheumatism* 44 (2001): 2531–38.

Chaiyakunapruk, Nathorn, Nantawarn Kitikannakorn, Surakit Nathisuwan, et al. "The Efficacy of Ginger for the Prevention of Postoperative Nausea and Vomiting: A Meta-Analysis." *American Journal of Obstetrics and Gynecology* 194, no. 1 (January 2006): 95–99.

Grzanna, Reinhard, Lars Lindmark, and Carmelita G. Frondoza. "Ginger—An Herbal Medicinal Product with Broad Anti-Inflammatory Actions." *Journal of Medicinal Food* 8, no. 2 (2005): 125–32.

Klotter, Jule. "The Many Benefits of Ginger." *Townsend Letter* (February–March 2009): 45–46.

Levine, M.E., M. Gillis, S. Yanchis, et al. "Protein and Ginger for the Treatment of Chemotherapy-Induced Delayed Nausea and Gastric Dysrhythmia. *Neurogastroenterology and Motility* 18, no. 6 (June 2006): 488.

Portnoi, G., L.A. Chng, L. Karimi-Tabesh, et al. "Prospective Comparative Study of the Safety and Effectiveness of Ginger for the Treatment of Nausea and Vomiting in Pregnancy." *American Journal of Obstetrics and Gynecology* 189, no. 5 (November 2003): 1374–77.

Roxas, Mario. "The Efficacy of Ginger in Prevention of Postoperative Nausea and Vomiting after Major Gynecologic Surgery." *Alternative Medicine Review* 12, no. 4 (December 2007): 373.

Smith, S., C. Crowther, K. Willson, et al. "A Randomized Controlled Trial of Ginger to Treat Nausea and Vomiting in Pregnancy." *Obstetrics and Gynecology* 103, no. 4 (April 2004): 639–45.

White, Brett. "Ginger: An Overview." *American Family Physician* 75 (2007): 1689–91.

Willets, Karen E., Abie Ekangaki, and John A. Eden. "Effect of a Ginger Extract on Pregnancy-Induced Nausea: A Randomised Controlled Trial." *Australian and New Zealand Journal of Obstetrics and Gynaecology* 43, no. 2 (March 2003): 139–44.

## GINSENG

Ginseng is the common name for a family of tropical herbs that have been used medicinally for centuries. The Asian form of ginseng or *Panax ginseng,* is very popular, especially in China and Korea. The Panax ginseng is now so popular in some areas that it is difficult to buy. The high demand led to the development of a North American ginseng, *Panax quinquefolius,* which is now used as a substitute for the Asian variety of the herb. However, both species are becoming difficult to find in the wild, which has opened up large commercial growth of the ginseng market.

Wild ginseng has become increasingly rare due to its increased popularity and worldwide overharvesting of the root. According to U.S. botanists, Chinese ginseng is now so difficult to acquire that the U.S.-grown roots have become increasingly sought after. A portion of the wild U.S. ginseng grows in national forests such as the Great Smoky Mountains National Park in North Carolina and Tennessee. In the Asian market, the twisted, tangled roots found only in the wild are considered more potent than the commercially grown herb.

The Panax ginseng is native to Korea and China and has been popular for many centuries. It has been used to improve immune system function, and it is used in the treatment of depression and anxiety, erectile dysfunction, symptoms related to menopause, and high blood sugar.

U.S. ginseng, like its Asian counterpart, is used as a tonic to boost the immune system and is also used to treat stress. There is anecdotal evidence that ginseng can fight infections such as the flu and that it might help prevent colds or make symptoms milder. U.S. ginseng has also been used to treat a variety of infections, including HIV/AIDS; however, any reports of its success are only anecdotal.

Ginseng grows wild in many U.S. old-growth forests including those in Wisconsin. Wild ginseng is prized, because commercial ginseng is difficult to grow. It takes four years for the plants to mature, and, once the plants are harvested, the land cannot be replanted with ginseng. Commercial growers of ginseng create canopies to protect the sensitive plants and keep them in the shade, which they need to survive. A pound of fresh ginseng sells for $135, and the dried roots are worth $460 a pound ("The Spice of Life," 2011). The sale of Wisconsin ginseng in 2010 was estimated to be over $30 million (NPR, 2010).

The root of the plant is dried and ground up so it can be taken internally through tablets, capsules, extracts, and teas, along with other applications for external use. The root contains chemical components known as ginsenosides, and this is where the medicinal properties are thought to be strongest.

While ginseng is believed to have some effect on lowering blood glucose, the National Center for Complementary and Alternative Medicine, part of the National Institutes of Health, has funded studies to examine just how ginseng affects insulin resistance. The organization is also looking at ginseng in relationship to Alzheimer's disease and cancer. Still, scientific evidence at this point is based on small clinical trials, and researchers say more evidence is necessary before they can conclusively support any of the health claims associated with ginseng.

Side effects have been reported from long-term ginseng use, while short-term doses appear to be safe in most cases. Common side effects include stomach upset, insomnia, and headaches. There have also been reports of allergic reactions in individuals. Scientists caution people with diabetes to consult their physician and to use extra caution with ginseng, especially if they are already taking medication to lower their blood sugar.

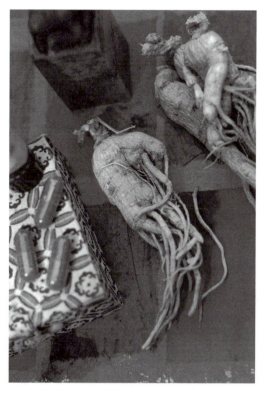

Ginseng root is used in Chinese herbal medicine to boost the immune system and is available in supplement capsules. (Antaratma Images/Dreamstime.com)

Other potential problems from ginseng include the possibility of adverse drug interactions. Studies showed that patients being treated for leukemia experienced liver toxicity when ginseng was taken in combination with another prescription (Bilgi, Bell, Ananthakrishnan, & Atallah, 2010).

*Sharon Zoumbaris*

*See also* Diabetes; Insomnia; Traditional Chinese Medicine.

### References

"Asian Ginseng." National Center for Complementary and Alternative Medicine (September 2005), www.nccam.nih.gov/health/asianginseng/ataglance.htm.

Bilgi, N., K. Bell, A. Ananthakrishnan, and E. Atallah. "Imatinib and Panax Ginseng: A Potential Interaction Resulting in Liver Toxicity." *Annals of Pharmacotherapy* 44, no. 926 (May 2010): 8.

Castleman, Michael. "75 Safe and Effective Herbal Remedies: Treat Dozens of Common Ailments Naturally." *Mother Earth News* (October–November 2010): 36.

Coates, P., et al., eds. "Asian Ginseng." *Encyclopedia of Dietary Supplements.* New York: Marcel Dekker, 2005.

"Wisconsin Ginseng Commands Premium Price," Morning Edition, November 2, 2010, NPR. http://www.npr.org/templates/story/story.php?storyId=130993658.

"The Spice of Life: Wild Ginseng Is Disappearing from Southeast Parks at an Alarming Rate." *National Parks* 85, no. 1 (Winter 2011).

## GLYCEMIC INDEX

The glycemic index (GI) is a measure of how quickly blood glucose levels rise in response to food. In other words, consuming a high-GI food will cause an individual's blood glucose to spike more dramatically than consuming the same amount of a low-GI food. Blood glucose, more commonly referred to as simply blood sugar, is critically important for normal bodily function. While fluctuations in blood glucose in response to meals are normal, frequent spikes in blood glucose (resulting from high-GI foods or otherwise) have been associated with an increased risk of numerous diseases, ranging from the development of Type 2 diabetes to cardiovascular disease (Ludwig, 2002). Thus, low-GI foods are generally considered healthier than their high-GI counterparts, although there are numerous caveats to this trend.

Originally developed in 1980 by Dr. David Jenkins, the glycemic index was intended as a way to help diabetic patients control their blood sugar. Jenkins identified foods' glycemic index values by measuring the area under the curve on a graph of blood glucose levels for two hours after a meal (of that food). This value was then divided by the area under the curve of some reference food and multiplied by 100 to yield a figure ranging from 0 to 100.

At first, a variety of reference foods were used, most commonly pure sugar or white bread. However, due to the culturally specific nature of foods such as white bread, glycemic index values today are more often reported relative to pure glucose in order to yield standardized glycemic index values for given foods (though comparisons to white bread are still in use). These foods are then typically divided loosely into categories of low (less than 55), medium (56 to 69), and high (70 to 100) GI, where 100 is pure glucose.

**Glycemic Index Foods** Although finding the precise GI of any given food requires a controlled test, there are general guidelines that can be followed in identifying low-, medium-, and high-GI foods. Fruits and vegetables tend to be low GI, while processed carbohydrates tend to be high GI. When comparing sources of carbohydrates, simple carbohydrates tend to be of lower GI. For instance, although bread has a relatively high GI, it is less than pure glucose, which has a GI of 100 by definition. Processed foods tend to have higher GI values. For instance, white bread and white pasta have higher GI values than whole-wheat bread and whole-wheat pasta. A few examples are given below.

Low-GI foods (less than 55): Raw carrots, apples, grapefruit, peanuts, peas, skim milk, lentils

Medium-GI foods (56 to 69): Bananas, pineapple, raisins, sweet corn

High-GI foods (70 to 100): Rice, white bread, white potatoes, watermelon (Mayo Clinic, 2009)

**Glycemic Index and Diabetes**   One of the primary uses for the glycemic index is to help diabetic individuals control their blood sugar. Normally, the pancreas releases insulin in response to the high blood glucose following a meal in order to bring blood glucose levels back down to normal by stimulating fat and muscle cells to uptake glucose from the blood. However, in people with Type 1 diabetes, the pancreas has lost its ability to produce insulin, and in people with Type 2 diabetes, the body has developed resistance to insulin. The resultant hyperglycemia can contribute to a plethora of complications ranging from diabetic retinopathy to heart attack and stroke. Thus, it is critical for diabetics to control their blood glucose artificially via insulin injections, other medications, exercise, and dietary control. It is with this last point—dietary control—that the glycemic index can be a factor. While carbohydrate counting is still the most important dietary control for diabetics, the type of carbohydrate (i.e., glycemic index) also has an influence on blood glucose. Thus, it is beneficial for diabetic patients to plan meals consisting primarily of foods from the low- and medium-GI categories and avoid high-GI foods. However, while planning low- and medium-GI meals, it is important not to neglect carbohydrate counting. The American Diabetes Association describes GI planning as useful in "fine-tuning blood glucose management" as an adjunct to everything else (American Diabetes Association, n.d.).

**Low–Glycemic Index Diets**   While the glycemic index was originally developed to help people with diabetes, it can also be a useful tool for helping nondiabetic patients eat healthier. Although there are several variations of the low-GI diet, the principle remains the same: restricting oneself to low- and medium-GI foods while avoiding high-GI foods. The reasoning is similar to that for diabetics—avoiding high-GI foods results in a smaller rise in blood glucose after eating. Promoters of the low-GI diet have touted numerous health benefits, including weight loss and a reduced risk of Type 2 diabetes, hypertension, cardiovascular disease, and even cancer.

While no high-quality long-term studies have been conducted to evaluate the health effects of the low-GI diet specifically, animal studies and short-term human studies have suggested that low-GI diets lead to some weight loss relative to high-GI diets (Ludwig, 2002). Since weight loss is generally associated with a decreased risk of developing diabetes, hypertension, and cardiovascular disease, it is reasonable that a low-GI diet is also protective against such chronic diseases. However, several small studies have suggested that a low-GI diet may have protective effects against diabetes and cardiovascular disease, independent of the weight loss (Ludwig, 2002). While the low-GI diet has occasionally been promoted as reducing the risk of cancer as well, the current scientific evidence does not support this claim (Mulholland, Murray, Cardwell, & Cantwell, 2009). The precise physiological mechanisms by which eating a low-GI diet leads to weight loss and its other health benefits are uncertain, but possible explanations include improved satiety from low-GI foods over high-GI foods (although whether this is true is currently the subject of debate among nutrition scientists) and reduced insulin resistance from avoiding the blood glucose spike associated with high-GI foods (Ludwig, 2002).

Regardless, one of the major benefits of the low-glycemic diet over other diets is that there are no known risks to the low-GI diet, unlike many other popular diets. Furthermore, the low-GI diet is easier to maintain long term than many other more extreme diets. For example, while many other diets may lead to greater short-term weight loss, the extreme impact on one's normal diet from such diets often causes people to abandon them and resume their previous eating habits, thereby counteracting any health benefits gained. Since the low-GI diet does not require calorie counting or extremely rigid attention to foods eaten (low- and medium-GI foods allow for a wide variety of foods), it is generally easier to maintain long term (Mayo Clinic, 2009).

**Criticisms**   While the glycemic index can certainly be a valuable tool in helping individuals eat healthier, there are several important criticisms to be aware of. A common criticism of the glycemic index system is that the real glycemic index of any given meal depends on many factors in addition to what types of food are consumed. Factors such as meals within the past several hours, the composition of food in previous meals, cooking methods, and even the specific variety of the food in question can all greatly impact the glycemic index. For example, white potatoes can range from moderate to high GI, depending on the particular variety. This makes it difficult to predict the true GI of a given meal, since foods are rarely eaten in isolation following an overnight fast (the conditions under which the standardized GI value is measured).

More specific criticisms relating to the use of low-GI diets tend to focus on the fact that GI measures neglect the total carbohydrate content in various foods, an idea captured in the concept of glycemic load. Glycemic load multiples a food's GI by its carbohydrate content. Thus, foods can have a high GI while still having a low glycemic load and vice versa. For example, despite having a high caloric count and high carbohydrate and fat content, ice cream actually has a low to medium glycemic index (Foster-Powell, Holt, & Brand-Miller, 2002). Blindly following the low-GI diet might lead one to erroneously conclude that ice cream and other high-calorie snack foods are healthful.

The glycemic index can be a useful tool to help diabetics control their blood glucose and to help others lose weight and reduce their risk of various chronic diseases. Still, due to its imitations, dieting according to the glycemic index must be done with consideration of other facets of healthy eating, such as avoiding very sugary or high-fat foods, even if they are low GI. Fortunately, most low-GI foods, such as fruits and vegetables, are considered healthy by almost any standard. Ultimately, the glycemic index can be a useful tool in conjunction with other nutritional tools to help keep a healthy weight and reduce the risk of developing diabetes and cardiovascular disease.

*David Chen*

*See also* Carbohydrates; Diabetes; Nutrition.

## References

American Diabetes Association. "Glycemic Index and Diabetes" (n.d.), www.diabetes.org/food-and-fitness/food/planning-meals/glycemic-index-and-diabetes.html#.

Foster-Powell, Kaye, Susanna H.A. Holt, and Janette C. Brand-Miller. "International Table of Glycemic Index and Glycemic Load Values: 2002." *American Journal of Clinical Nutrition* 76, no. 1 (2002): 5–56.

Ludwig, David S. "The Glycemic Index: Physiological Mechanisms Relating to Obesity, Diabetes, and Cardiovascular Disease." *Journal of American Medical Association* 287, no. 18 (2002): 2414–23.

Mayo Clinic. "Glycemic Index Diet: Losing Weight with Blood Sugar Control" (2009), www.mayoclinic.com/health/glycemic-index-diet/MY00770.

Mulholland H.G., L.J. Murray, C.R. Cardwell, and M.M. Cantwell. "Glycemic Index, Glycemic Load, and the Risk of Digestive Tract Neoplasms: A Systematic Review and Meta-Analysis." *American Journal of Nutrition* 89, no. 2 (2009): 568–76.

## GRAHAM, SYLVESTER

Sylvester Graham (b. July 4, 1794, in West Suffield, Connecticut; d. September 11, 1851, in Northampton, Massachusetts) is considered one of the United States' first food faddists and health reformers. Graham believed that a high-fiber, natural-food diet would remedy cholera, alcoholism, premature aging, violence, sexual abuses, and digestive ills. His early followers included the Kellogg brothers, John and Will, who were famous for their religious colony and health sanitarium at Battle Creek, Michigan. In 1897 John and Will produced their whole-grain cereal and formed the Battle Creek Food Company. Later, Will split with his brother and opened the Battle Creek Toasted Corn Flake Company, which eventually became the Kellogg Company. Graham's fanaticism and zeal for natural food attracted early followers, like the Kelloggs; those supporters became known as Grahamites. The graham cracker is one famous result today of Graham's health campaign in the early 19th century, although it is more like a cookie than the high-fiber bread he promoted.

Graham was also one of the nation's earliest vegetarians, a lifestyle choice based on his firm belief, long before the discovery of nutrition, that diet and health were directly connected. At that time, U.S. upper classes followed a diet of meat-eating gluttony, which led to overweight and the associated diseases of obesity. Graham was named president of the American Vegetarian Society, founded in 1849 in New York City. The society's membership included Harriet Beecher Stowe and journalist Horace Greeley.

Like many other health reformers, Graham had an early history of bad health. He was the youngest of 17 children born to Massachusetts minister John Graham, who died when Sylvester was just two years old. According to records, Graham's mother was "in a deranged state of mind" after her husband's death, so the court appointed a guardian for Sylvester and two older siblings. Sylvester's health and education suffered as he was passed from relative to relative, finally settling years later in Newark, New Jersey, where he was eventually reunited with his mother

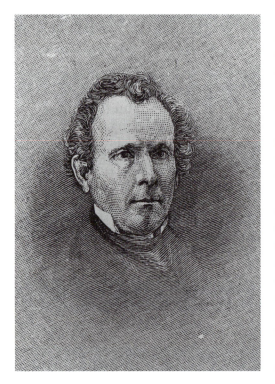

Sylvester Graham was an early advocate of dietary reform in the United States. He was known for his interest in vegetarianism and advocated radically different dietary habits. (Courtesy of the Library of Congress)

and an older brother. It was at this time that Graham began to prepare for the ministry. He studied at Amherst Academy but was expelled after one quarter. He then studied privately with a minister and was ordained in 1826, the year he married the woman who had previously nursed him through a nervous breakdown.

While Graham was primarily interested in saving souls, he also lectured on the evils of alcohol for the Pennsylvania Society for Discouraging the Use of Ardent Spirits. This temperance group worked to moderate the per capita consumption of alcohol, but Graham from the first advocated total abstinence. Soon he was also talking about diet and sex as well as alcohol. During this time, he studied human physiology and diet. The cholera epidemic of 1832, the first of three cholera epidemics in the United States during the 19th century, gave Graham a renewed platform when he suggested that greasy, spicy meat, combined with "excessive lewdness," caused the cholera outbreak.

His most famous advice was that thick, coarse bread, baked at home and eaten daily, should be the mainstay of every diet. He believed his bread, made from the whole of the wheat and coarsely ground, known as "dyspepsia bread" or "temperance bread," was best when eaten a day old. Although his bread was eventually nicknamed "the graham cracker," it bore no physical resemblance to today's modern cracker, which is made with refined flour and high-fructose corn syrup. Graham was convinced of the bread's healing powers.

Graham also recommended hard mattresses, open bedroom windows, cold baths, and a raw-food, vegetarian diet as best, because it was closest to nature. Even though he realized that people were devoted to white bakery bread, he continued to condemn it as a horrible food choice. Graham's book, *Treatise on Bread,* sold for four dollars per dozen and described the bread-making process as the province of the loving wife and mother. However, because he accused bakers of adulterating their products with additives, many people, including well-known author Ralph Waldo Emerson, publicly ridiculed Graham's diet.

The dietary world of the 1830s was filled with disease and bad health caused by consumption, chronic indigestion, and dyspepsia—a blanket term for constipation, stomachaches, headaches, and foul breath. Americans ate meat at every meal—some 180 pounds yearly per person—and foods were soaked in grease or gravy and washed down with whiskey. Long before the discovery of nutrition, fiber, vitamins, minerals, and cholesterol, Graham insisted that diet and health were directly connected. He believed that eating meat, particularly pork, led to sexual excess. Sexual excess then led to increased consumption of more rich foods and unhealthy meat, which, according to Graham, predisposed an individual to disease.

After the cholera epidemics subsided, Graham continued to lecture to mass audiences, traveling through Massachusetts, New York, New Jersey, Pennsylvania, Rhode Island, and Maine. In 1837, as his popularity faded, he moved to Northampton, Massachusetts, with his wife Sarah and their two children. He died there on September 11, 1851, at the age of 57.

In the United States, talk of Grahamism would continue for many years, as followers such as abolitionists William Lloyd Garrison, Horace Greeley, and Henry Stanton remained firm believers in his health ideals. Ellen Harmon White, spiritual leader and founder of the Seventh-day Adventist Church and founder of Battle Creek, Michigan's Western Health Reform Institute, also continued to recommend Graham's ideas and diet following his death. Slowly but surely, the U.S. medical and scientific communities would one day come to accept Graham's theory that diet and health were interrelated. Although he was ahead of his time, Graham's belief that eating too much salt, meat, and fat can cause health problems is now accepted nutritional wisdom.

*Marjolijn Bijlefeld and Sharon Zoumbaris*

*See also* Kellogg, John Harvey; Nutrition; Vegetarians.

## References

Armstrong, David, and Elizabeth Metzger Armstrong. *The Great American Medicine Show: Being an Illustrated History of Hucksters, Healers, Health Evangelists, and Heroes from Plymouth Rock to the Present.* New York: Prentice Hall, 1991.

DiBacco, Thomas V. "Behind the Graham Cracker, a Health Food Tale: One Man's Battle to Make Americans Think about Nutrition." *Washington Post* (July 25, 1989): 3.

*Dictionary of American Biography.* Farmington Hills, MI: Gale Group, 2001.

*Encyclopedia of World Biography,* 2nd ed. Farmington Hills, MI: Gale Group, 1998.

Farmer, Jean. "The Rev. Sylvester (Graham Cracker) Graham: America's Early Fiber Crusader." *Saturday Evening Post* (March 1985): 32–37.

Gordon, John Steele. "Sawdust Pudding." *American Heritage* (July–August 1996): 16–18.

Nissenbaum, Stephen. *Sex, Diet and Debility in Jacksonian America: Sylvester Graham and Health Reform.* Chicago: Dorsey Press, 1988.

## GRIEF

Grief occurs when a person experiences loss or affliction. It is an internal reaction, a deep sense that is wholly unique to each individual. The scope of the loss or affliction can be personal—such as the death of a loved one, unemployment, or diagnosis of a life-threatening condition—or public, as in the case of Hurricane Katrina, the terrorist attacks of September 11, 2001, or the death and funeral of President John F. Kennedy.

While the terms *grief, bereavement,* and *mourning* are often used interchangeably, they are not quite the same thing. Basically, grief is a collection of feelings such as sorrow, intense sadness, despair, anxiety, irritability, or guilt—all part of a reaction to bereavement, which is the loss or death of someone or something important to an individual. Mourning, however, is the social face of grief, the way in which society calls for individuals to honor the dead or to publicly deal with the aftermath of bereavement.

With any loss, something has been taken away, and the natural human instinct is to grieve. The intensity differs from person to person and depends on the nature of the grief trigger. Grieving affects a person physically, mentally, emotionally, and socially. There is no right or wrong way to grieve and no formal timetable for the process.

Although grief is not an illness, it can cause physical and emotional symptoms. A grieving person may experience disturbed sleep, stomach upset, headaches, crying spells, a weakened immune system, and a lack of concentration. Feelings of shock and disbelief, sadness, guilt, anger, and fear are common. Early in the grieving process, people have reported they thought they were in a bad dream or not in their right mind. If symptoms persist for an extended period of time, they may cause clinical depression and other serious health issues.

Grief stresses the body and can affect the immune system, which can exacerbate preexisting physical ailments. Studies, which began over 20 years ago, have shown that grieving people are less able to fight off disease and may have fewer natural killer cells than their nongrieving counterparts (Bower et al., 2003).

Sometimes medical or counseling assistance is needed to get through the grieving process. Medications are available to help with sleeplessness or anxiety, but a person should discuss this with his or her personal physician and should remember to eat right, exercise, and get enough rest. If the grief is overwhelming, the grieving individual should talk to a mental health professional trained in grief counseling or consider joining a support group. Practicing stress management techniques, learning new skills, and socializing can also help a grieving person.

When feelings or thoughts such as that life is not worth living or guilt and blame are prolonged, a person may be suffering from complicated grief. Among those who suffer the loss of someone significant, about 1 in 11 may experience complicated grief. Also known as protracted or chronic grief, it couples aspects of post-traumatic stress disorder with depression. Psychotherapy, interpersonal therapy, or psychodynamic therapy may offer help through exploration of one's emotions and feelings. Limited research has been conducted on the use of psychiatric drugs, but there has been some benefit shown from administering certain types of antidepressants. If a grieving person displays suicidal tendencies, a mental health professional or local emergency service should be contacted.

A family member or friend can help someone who is grieving by spending time with and listening to that person while encouraging him or her to work through the grief. Friends who offer statements such as, "with time, you'll get over this," may offer false comfort and not allow the person to fully mourn. Instead, offer to cook dinner or shop for food since it is often difficult for the grieving person to concentrate on everyday activities. If the grieving person is displaying extreme behavior or acting out of the ordinary, friends or family should recommend that the person seek professional help.

Psychiatrist Elisabeth Kubler-Ross wrote about five stages of grief in 1969: denial (This can't be happening to me); anger (Why is this happening? Who is to blame?); bargaining (Make this not happen, and in return I will ___); depression (I'm too sad to do anything); and acceptance (I'm at peace with what happened). Her frames of reference were the feelings of terminally ill patients, but her five-stage model became the basis for addressing a spectrum of loss experiences from divorce to the death of a pet.

A grieving person does not have to go through all of these stages or in any particular order. The Hospice Foundation of America characterizes grief as a roller coaster "full of ups and downs, highs and lows. Like many roller coasters, the ride tends to be rougher in the beginning; the lows may be deeper and longer. The difficult periods should become less intense and shorter as time goes by, but it takes time to work through a loss." Kubler-Ross noted in her final book that the five stages were not intended to match multifaceted emotions with singular categories and that the grief process is as individual as a person's life.

In *The Truth about Grief: The Myth of Its Five Stages and the New Science of Loss*, author Ruth Davis Konigsberg challenges the wisdom and validity of the five stages of grief. She describes how professional counseling became a burgeoning profession from the 1970s to the 1990s and how grief evolved into a journey-like process. She points to contemporary research to debunk the most common myths regarding grief including: "we grieve in stages," "express it; don't repress it," "grief is harder on women," "grief never ends," and "counseling helps." For the myth related to grieving in stages, she describes a Yale University study, reported in the *Journal of the American Medical Association* in 2007, which concluded that study participants (recently bereaved individuals) readily accepted the death of a loved one. This is contrary to the Kubler-Ross model, where acceptance is the final grief stage and is defined as recognizing that a loved one is gone. Konigsberg's bottom line is that "science is beginning to tell us that most people are resilient enough to get through loss on their own without stages or phases or tasks."

Grief is essential to acceptance of loss and to resuming a full life. Keeping grief submerged is a catalyst for creating emotional or physical problems in the future.

While grieving is a painful process, it is worthwhile to endure to achieve a state of well-being.

*Dianne L. Needham*

*See also* Depression; Immune System/Lymphatic System; Insomnia; Stress.

### References

Bonanno, George A. *The Other Side of Sadness: What the New Science of Bereavement Tells Us about Life after Loss.* New York: Basic Books, 2009.

Bower, Julienne E., et al. "Finding Positive Meaning and Its Association with Natural Killer Cell Cytotoxicity among Participants in a Bereavement-Related Disclosure Intervention." *Annals of Behavioral Medicine* 25, no. 2 (2003): 146–55.

Elisabeth Kubler-Ross Foundation, www.ekrfoundation.org/.

Grief.com—David Kessler. "Public Grief," http://grief.com/public-grief/.

Hirsch, Michael. "Coping with Grief and Loss." *Harvard Special Health Report* (Annual 2007): 4.

Hospice Foundation of America. "An Introduction to Grieving," www.hospicefoundation. org/pages/page.asp?page_id=78811.

Konigsberg, Ruth Davis, "New Ways to Think about Grief." *Time,* January 24, 2011, www. time.com/time/magazine/article/0,9171,2042372,00.html.

Marasco, Ron, and Brian Shuff. *About Grief: Insights, Setbacks, Grace Notes, Taboos.* Lanham, MD: Ivan R. Dee, 2010.

Mayo Clinic. "Complicated Grief," www.mayoclinic.com/health/complicated-grief/DS01023/ DSECTION=symptoms.

Reiss, Michele A. *Lessons in Loss and Living: Hope and Guidance for Confronting Serious Illness and Grief.* New York: Hyperion, 2010.

## GUIDED IMAGERY

Guided imagery is one of many complementary or alternative techniques to improve wellness and reduce disease. It is well known that negative, anxious, worrisome, and other similar thoughts can create unwanted feelings of stress and agitation both physically and mentally. This phenomenon is possible due to the constant interaction between mind and body. Fortunately, positive, pleasant, and peaceful thoughts can achieve the opposite—calmness and relaxation. Whereas negative emotions and thoughts are scientifically linked to states of illness, cultivating positive emotions and thoughts promotes well-being. Guided imagery is one technique to achieve that desirable endpoint.

Surprisingly, despite its relatively straightforward nature and ease of use, as few as 3 percent of Americans practice guided imagery (Barnes, Powell-Griner, McFann, & Nahin, 2004). Guided imagery typically involves creating a scene in your mind's eye to decrease stress and increase your level of relaxation. This technique is typically rehearsed both in the absence and in the presence of stress. In the absence of stress, it contributes to improved mood and relaxation; in the presence of stress or in anticipation of stress, it can be used to lessen the effects of stress and help the individual maintain focus.

It is usually recommended that someone practice the technique when he or she is not stressed in order to train the body and mind to relax while using the technique. This also familiarizes the individual with the technique so it can be used easily during times of stress, since using a familiar technique is easier than trying to learn a new technique when under emotional pressure.

The process of guided imagery achieves positive relaxation effects largely through manipulating physiological processes, including decreased heart rate, blood pressure, and circulating stress hormones. Imagery is usually guided by someone else initially (via a therapist or audio recording), but as the individual becomes more comfortable with the technique, he or she may prefer to move toward self-guided imagery instead. The primary challenge with self-guided imagery is that individuals tend to make the pace too fast during their imagery time. It is often beneficial to use an external guide until the pace and tempo of a relaxing imagery technique becomes familiar.

Although creating a scene may seem to be a purely visual process, guided imagery is actually much more sophisticated. The visual part is clearly important, but guided imagery is optimal when it involves all senses. Because more senses are involved in the imagery, more brain areas are activated during a multisensory guided imagery process, and this will produce the desired effects. Involving all senses in the imagery will also be more powerful in increasing positive emotions and thoughts and decreasing negative emotions and thoughts. The individual should try to place oneself in the scene he or she is imaging, rather than looking at the scene as if viewing it on a television set. Specifically, a scene should be chosen that includes sights, sounds, tastes, physical sensations, and scents. Consider the following example:

Imagine yourself walking along the shoreline on a white-sand beach. With each step you take, you hear the crunch of the sand beneath your feet, and you feel the warm crystals of sand sneak between your toes. The sun is out, and you feel its warmth on your back and shoulders through your lightweight shirt. There is an occasional cool breeze that makes the temperature perfect and wafts the smell of the salty water toward you. You can taste the tang of the salt in the air. With every long, slow stride you take, you breathe a deep breath and realize how relaxed you feel as you walk on the beach. You can hear a few seagulls far away calling to each other, and you watch every wave as it comes to the shore and recedes once again into the ocean. You stop for a moment in your walk along the beach to go to the water. As you get closer, the ground beneath you feels cool and damp, and your footsteps on the sand grow softer. The sound of the waves grows louder, and the scent of the saltwater grows stronger as you get closer to the ocean. Finally, as you exhale a sigh of relief and relaxation, a wave gently covers your feet, washing all the sand from between your toes. The water is warm and crystal clear, and it looks frothy as it washes back out to sea and away from your feet. As you stand, your feet sinking into the sand while you listen to the waves and the birds, you feel more calm and relaxed with each breath you take and with each cleansing wave that washes over your feet.

**History** The use of guided imagery has a long history before its common use in psychotherapy. Scripts like this one are readily available in books and online resources, which can be found by doing a search on the Internet for "guided imagery script." Alternatively, one can use a favorite relaxing vacation spot as a template to create a personalized script.

Prior to the existence of psychotherapy, guided imagery was practiced in indigenous cultures (e.g., Native Americans), religious groups (e.g., Jewish, Christian), and ancient medicine (e.g., Chinese medicine) as a spiritual practice and way of healing (Utay & Miller 2006, p. 40). Therefore, this method has a longstanding history of being used to achieve wellness. In more recent history, guided imagery began to emerge in psychotherapy practices with individuals such as Sigmund Freud, who emphasized imagery found in dreams.

Due to the powerful emotional, physical, and spiritual effects resulting from using imagery in these historical ways, guided imagery is now applied to more than relaxation and stress management. It has been used successfully in rehabilitative medicine, health care, sports training, academic performance, and other domains in addition to psychotherapeutic contexts (Utay & Miller, 2006). Guided imagery is effective in rehabilitative medicine with stroke patients to recover motor functioning and reduce pain. Multiple studies have also shown it to be effective in stimulating the immune system (for cancer) or quieting the immune

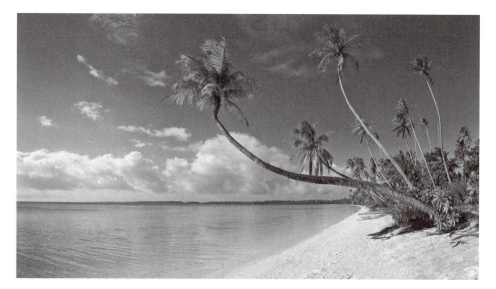

Palm trees grow on a tropical white sand beach. The process of guided imagery can offer many relaxing effects from visualizing calm scenes of peaceful places like this. (Vladoskan/Dreamstime.com)

system (in rheumatoid arthritis), and increasing blood flow to an area (for wound healing) (Trakhtenberg, 2008).

**New Applications**   In sports and athletic performance, guided imagery can be used for a number of purposes. These may include improving a performance, reducing the effects of pain during performance, and promoting healing after an injury has occurred (Utay & Miller, 2006). It has become so popular that the U.S. Olympic team now regularly uses guided imagery to reduce performance anxiety and improve athletes' skills.

Guided imagery can also be used effectively to reduce anxiety surrounding academic tasks, such as taking exams or delivering public speeches and presentations. Within the context of psychotherapy, guided imagery is often included in treatment plans that target grief, anxiety, eating disorders, addictions, and anger, among other disorders.

Guided imagery may be combined with other approaches, such as meditation, prayer, yoga, and hypnosis, to help the individual reach his or her goals. For example, a recent study showed improvements in quality of life (e.g., sleep, family functioning, pain, emotional well-being) with a combined treatment of guided imagery and other alternative therapeutic approaches (Fernros, Furhoff, & Wandell, 2008).

Guided imagery has a role in everyday life as a stand-alone technique for mood improvement, stress reduction, motivation (e.g., by envisioning a positive outcome for the future), and exploration of various ways to approach a problem. The use of guided imagery can have impressive effects on wellness directly through its positive effects on stress and physiological hyper- or hypo-arousal (e.g., during fear or in preparation for athletic performance, respectively). Indirect effects of guided imagery also contribute to overall wellness as well. For example, the use of guided imagery may help an individual relax his or her mind and muscles after a stressful day, which can lead to improved sleep. Improved sleep boosts immune functioning, memory skills, mood, and ability to cope with future stressors, among other desirable outcomes. Given the immediate and long-term benefits of guided imagery, as well as its accessibility and ease of implementation, it is a skill that should be considered for regular use by anyone with an interest in improving health and overall wellness.

*Amanda Wheat and Amy Wachholtz*

*See also* Cancer; Meditation; Psychosomatic Health Care; Traditional Chinese Medicine; Yoga.

## References

Barnes, Patricia M., Eve Powell-Griner, Kim McFann, and Richard L. Nahin. "Complementary and Alternative Medicine Use Among Adults: United States, 2002." *Advanced Data from Vital and Health Statistics* 343 (2004): 1–20.

Fernros, Lotta, Ann Karin Furhoff, and Per E. Wandell. "Improving Quality of Life Using Compound Mind-Body Therapies: Evaluation of a Course Intervention with Body

Movement and Breath Therapy, Guided Imagery, Chakra Experiencing and Mindfulness Meditation." *Quality of Life Research* 17 (2008): 367–76.

Utay, Joe, and Megan Miller. "Guided Imagery as an Effective Therapeutic Technique: A Brief Review of Its History and Efficacy Research." *Journal of Instructional Psychology* 33 (2006): 40–43.

Trakhtenberg, Ephraim C. "The Effects of Guided Imagery on the Immune System: A Critical Review." *International Journal of Neuroscience* 118 (2008): 839–55.

# H

## HEAD START AND HEALTHY START

Head Start and Healthy Start stand among the most successful public health initiatives in U.S. history. These two federal programs can be found under the U.S. Department of Health and Human Services, in the Maternal and Child Health Bureau, Health Resources and Services Administration. These two programs provide grants and support for a range of federal and state partnerships that ultimately benefit the children of low-income families. However, these programs also face continued budget cuts as the fight over federal spending continues in Washington.

The programs are based on the premise that community-driven, grassroots efforts fill a basic, fundamental need: addressing multiple factors concerning maternal, child, and family nurture, nationwide. These community-driven neighborhood partnerships support lower-income families; the partnerships work together with local staff to provide excellent care, education, and development for infants, children, expectant mothers, and extended families nationwide, in a variety of diverse situations and circumstances.

Head Start's initial planning committee set down seven goals in 1965. More than 40 years later, these still serve as the basis for this program's mission and values.

1. Improving the child's physical health and physical abilities.
2. Helping the emotional and social development of the child by encouraging self-confidence, spontaneity, curiosity, and self-discipline.
3. Improving the child's mental processes and skills, with particular attention to conceptual and verbal skills.
4. Establishing patterns and expectations of success for the child that will create a climate of confidence for future learning efforts.
5. Increasing the child's capacity to relate positively to family members and others, while at the same time strengthening the family's ability to relate positively to the child and his problems.

6. Developing in the child and his family a responsible attitude toward society, and encouraging society to work with the poor in solving their problems.
7. Increasing the sense of dignity and self-worth within the child and his family.

As two popular public health initiatives, Head Start and Healthy Start have their beginnings in the Economic Opportunity Act of 1964, in President Lyndon B. Johnson's War on Poverty. Head Start was started in 1965, and considered by many to be an "educational experiment."

In 1964, the United States Congress gave the newly founded Office of Economic Opportunity (OEO) broad powers to campaign against poverty on a diverse number of fronts. Many of these innovative programs did not have staying power, for one reason or another. Included among these short-circuited programs was the Community Action Program, which centered its focus on efforts to organize and employ adults at or under the poverty line.

The OEO director, Sargent Shriver, was also President Johnson's general in the War on Poverty. He puzzled over why the nationwide grassroots efforts of the Community Action Program were having difficulty. He then asked the research division of OEO to take a closer look at the total problem of poverty in the United States, and also to suggest additional recommendations for ways to address poverty, yet again.

The research division prepared a pie chart to give a visual representation of poverty. This chart clearly showed Shriver that almost half of the people at or under the poverty line in the United States were children, and most of these were under the age of 12. Shriver said, "It was clear that it was foolish to talk about a 'total war against poverty' [a phrase President Johnson used], if you were doing nothing about children" (Ziegler & Muenchow, 1992).

Thus, the decision was made to develop a federal program specifically to benefit lower-income children, to provide for their nurture and educational encouragement. As a former teacher, Johnson fully supported this program. He believed that education held the key to lifting individuals and families from the cycle of poverty.

The Head Start Planning Committee soon followed. Its discussions focused on positive motivation and parental involvement, along with structuring long-lasting change in these children's day-to-day environment. And as a precursor to what eventually became a stand-alone program (Healthy Start), the original planning committee placed "improving the child's physical health" first on the list of the Head Start program's objectives.

Parental involvement was stressed at the very beginning of the planning, and has been an integral part of each Head Start program ever since. As the original planning document stated, "Parents should be involved both for their own and their children's benefit. These parents need success experiences along with their children." Thus, positive motivation for the whole family was an important part of the program. Projects designed to help these children from vulnerable or disadvantaged backgrounds also assist their parents and other caregivers, who can have the opportunity to successfully complete projects as much as their children. This contributes to create feelings of positive well-being and good self-esteem for everyone involved.

The Johnson administration immediately decided to start with a nationwide Head Start program, set to serve 100,000 children. This was highly unusual, since there had been no smaller pilot or test program. The First Lady, Lady Bird Johnson, accepted the invitation—challenge—to serve as Head Start's honorary chairperson. In 1965, the mounting attention of the country was held chiefly by the Vietnam War. A hopeful, positive opportunity to benefit the nation's infants and preschoolers was a welcome change for the Johnson administration. Mrs. Johnson's inaugural tea was a tremendous success, and a large number of community groups signed up to sponsor Head Start programs across the country.

In the beginning, this was seen as an eight-week summer program. The initial financial request for the summer program soon tripled, and continued to accelerate until $90 million were budgeted, and 500,000 children were set to be enrolled. Then, three months before the first program opened, the president announced he had "budgeted $150 million for fiscal 1966 to put Head Start on a year-round basis" (Ziegler & Muenchow, 1992). Thus, many of the summer programs very soon became nine-month, half-day programs.

After several years and a considerable amount of growth and success, Head Start was moved to the Office of Child Development in the federal Department of Health, Education, and Welfare. The transition from summer programs to nine-month programs and funding cuts caused some decrease in the total number of children enrolled during the early 1970s. However, funding soon increased in the mid- to late 1970s. By 1979, the annual budget for all Head Start activities was $680 million. Ten years later, services were provided to more than 450,000 children, and the budget was increased to $1.2 billion (Ziegler & Muenchow, 1992).

Head Start was revitalized by the Human Service Reauthorization Act in 1990, and was expanded further by the Head Start Reauthorization Act of 1994. This act required development of quality standards for many aspects of the program, including performance measures. It also led to the development of family-centered programs for infants and toddlers in 1995 and the beginning of the Early Head Start Program. The first Early Head Start grants totaled $47 million. Congress began the new program as a response to many studies that indicated early intervention enhances infant and child development. This new initiative had three basic goals:

1. To promote healthy prenatal outcomes for pregnant women,
2. To enhance the development of very young children, and
3. To promote healthy family functioning.

Any Early Head Start program had to assess community resources and needs before the grant was awarded. Also required was a research and evaluation plan. This would ensure that a good program model could be located, to optimize successful program outcomes, or in simpler terms, to aid infants, children, mothers, and their families in a variety of ways.

These local partnerships not only assisted infants and children in achieving better health, but also aided parents and other caregivers in improving their parenting skills, and helped the families to reach their own goals, including economic independence.

Healthy Start, which was launched in 1991 as an outgrowth of the Head Start program, deals specifically with the health-based component of the War on Poverty. This includes local outreach, care management, depression screening, and education activities for individuals and local families. As with the communities reached by the educationally oriented Head Start, these local communities across the country have several features in common: large minority populations, high rates of unemployment and poverty, and limited availability to medical providers and safe housing.

The Healthy Start Program is very much like Head Start in that it utilizes community-based partnerships to promote maternal, family, and child health and well-being. It is part of the federal Maternal and Child Health Bureau, and is based in the Division of Perinatal Systems and Women's Health. Local Healthy Start programs address a variety of health-related issues:

1. Providing adequate prenatal care,
2. Promoting positive prenatal health behaviors,
3. Meeting basic health needs (nutrition, housing, psychosocial support),
4. Reducing barriers to access, and
5. Enabling client empowerment.

Healthy Start started with 15 test sites, in areas (both rural and urban) where there were communities with infant mortality rates 1.5 to 2.5 times higher than the national average (National Healthy Start Association). These Demonstration Projects showed such promise that infant mortality at these sites was reduced substantially. The federal program has grown to nearly 100 sites, in 38 states, the District of Columbia, and Puerto Rico. Since its inception, this nationwide program has had the benefit of being generally well liked by both the clients and by the local staff.

This widespread network of local consortium services has had a solid success rate. It reaches vulnerable populations, supporting and encouraging them in a variety of health services. However, some local sites do have continuing problems, and struggle to reach immigrant families, new moms from across a variety of cultures, and the increasing number of working moms. Plus, the newer initiatives, which include depression screenings and interconception (or, the period between the birth of one child and conceiving another) programming, have not been quite as well accepted. These pockets of client resistance are roadblocks to specific, positive results, but they are by no means true in the majority of program sites.

One newer initiative of Healthy Start is support for males, especially fathers, within these vulnerable communities. This initiative is fairly new, and as such, not as well known. This innovative effort demonstrates that the Healthy Start government program is willing and eager to expand into more than just prenatal care and screening. In fact, the overall rate of acceptance of all Healthy Start programs is vastly positive, nationwide.

A drawback for the success of both Head Start and Healthy Start comes from some reports of case managers, nationwide. The documentation reports higher than usual levels of mental health issues and substance abuse and addiction among clients and their families. This can be explained, to some extent, by the multiple stressors that directly and indirectly affect individuals and families in poverty. This is magnified by the stresses of caring for infants and small children. With the withdrawal of more and more federal, state, and local funding, both public and private services for individuals with mental health and substance abuse issues are quickly disappearing. The positive mental health of parents and other caregivers remains an important factor in assisting families and serving child development needs: psychological, physical, educational, and in many other ways.

The results of many studies using data from Healthy Start have been positive. For example, low infant birth weight has been on the rise among groups of low-income babies. This tendency has been on the increase in the past two decades, especially among pregnancies of minority women. Several studies show that the beneficial effects of the Healthy Start program decreases infant mortality rates and increases birth weight. This in turn decreases hospitalization costs for the first year of life. Any efforts like this that benefit overall infant and maternal health are seen as a widespread benefit.

Head Start continues to be in the forefront of early childhood development. In 2007, Congress stipulated that every Head Start program across the country revise its Program Performance Standards. This is meant to ensure that these programs that serve lower-income children will continue to have high accountability.

These standards also require a high level of training and professional development. For example, every Head Start class across the country must have at least one teacher with an Early Childhood Education or Child Development college degree. Competent, trained staff is important for effective teaching, instruction, and for reaching the various goals of each individual program. And since certain cultural and other individualized characteristics cause each site to be unique, federal stipulations require every program to develop specific educational and performance standards for its individual site, and to set teacher and staff training goals and benchmarks related to these standards.

Flexibility in program design is much encouraged on the local level. A spectrum of differences in educational and program delivery exist, because of the unique needs and challenges of many program sites across the country. Some Head Start programs in certain areas coordinate and partner with other programs to provide full-day care. However, the services offered to all children remain the same, reflecting the excellent goals of the initial Planning Committee in 1965, which continue to stress the involvement of families and the local community.

Studies done on Head Start over the years have caused debate in the educational, sociological, and governmental communities. Do these programs provide lasting benefits or not? Results have been mixed, but overall positive. Several studies done in the 1980s and 1990s documented a "fade-out" effect for school-aged children who had participated in Head Start programs. However, researchers later questioned whether this effect was due to the preschool experience, or rather due to the poor schooling the children went on to receive in elementary school. Some researchers also note that Head Start preschoolers are often disadvantaged in a number of areas. Some children are more motivated once they get into the program. Parents can also be more effective in seeing their children enrolled in scarce Head Start spaces. Comparisons with various groups of preschoolers are made more challenging, even difficult, as a result.

Looking at a purely dollars-and-cents cost analysis study, recent researchers came to the conclusion that Head Start programs were beneficial, overall. (Both Head Start and Early Head Start programs were included in this study.) These results negate critics who argue that only intensive and expensive efforts in early childhood education can be beneficial. The children studied not only had short-term improvement, but also some long-term improvement as well. These areas of improvement were educational, as well as helpful in terms of health outcomes and even in crime reduction.

Overall, this set of programs, including Head Start, Early Head Start, and Healthy Start, has been a source of public and governmental concern for decades since low-income families continue to be present in the U.S. population. Head Start must be reauthorized by Congress every five years. This program has its detractors, and has had for decades. But Head Start and Healthy Start decades later continue to give low-income children, a disadvantaged and mostly voiceless group among American society, a helping hand and a positive opportunity to learn, explore, succeed, and be nurtured.

See the U.S. Department of Health and Human Services' Health Resources and Services Administration (www.hrsa.gov) for further information on Head Start, Healthy Start, and related federal programs. For specific information on where to find local Head Start or Early Head Start programs, contact the Early Childhood Learning and Knowledge Center at the Department of Health and Human Services. For more information on local Healthy Start programs, contact the National Healthy Start Association, Inc., at info@national healthystart.org.

*Elizabeth Jones*

*See also* Medicaid.

### References

Butler, Alice, and Melinda Gish. Domestic Social Policy Division. "Head Start: Background and Funding." Report for Congress, updated February 5, 2003. Congressional Research Service, the Library of Congress.

Health Resources and Services Administration, U.S. Department of Health and Human Resources. "Maternal and Child Health." www.hrsa.gov.

Kotelchuck, M. "Evaluating the Healthy Start Program: A Life Course Perspective." *Maternal and Child Health Journal* 12 (2010): 649–53.

Ludwig, J., and Phillips, D.A. "Long-Term Effects of Head Start on Low-Income Children." *Annals of New York Academy of Sciences* 1136 (2008): 257–68.

Maternal and Child Health Bureau, Health Resources and Services Administration. "About MCHB." http://mchb.hrsa.gov/about/dhsps.gov.

National Healthy Start Association. "The Healthy Start Program." www.healthystartassoc. org/hswpp6.html.

Pennsylvania Head Start Association. "Head Start History: 1965–Present." www.pahead start.org.

Razzino, B.E., M. New, A. Lewin, and J. Joseph. "Need for and Use of Mental Health Services among Parents of Children in the Head Start Program." *Psychiatric Services* 55, no. 5 (May 2004). http://ps.psychiatryonline.org.

Ziegler, E., and Muenchow, S. *Head Start: The Inside Story of America's Most Successful Educational Experiment.* New York: Basic Books, 1992.

# HEALTH AND MEDICAL TOURISM

It is no secret that health care all the world over is a source of great frustration for sick patients. A sizeable number of patients from every country will find themselves dissatisfied with the cost, availability, or legality of various forms of health care. In a world where international travel is becoming increasingly accessible for the masses, traveling overseas to obtain health care has grown into a modern-day industry worth billions. For many centuries, health tourism was primarily about stress relief and general well-being, but today patients travel seeking increasingly complex care such as Lasik eye surgery or cosmetic surgery.

The concept of health tourism is not a new one. In the 15th century, the wealthy would travel to distant medicinal spas and seasides to improve their health and reduce stress (Cook, 2008). The concept of these medicinal healing spas or sunny destinations as a way to rejuvenate the self has continued today and is recognized as leisure tourism.

Thus, while health tourism in general is not a modern phenomenon, the present-day manifestations such as stem cell therapy or organ transplantation in foreign countries represent a distinct and new form of health tourism or medical tourism. *Medical tourism* is a term originally coined by the medical tourism industry to denote the practice of traveling overseas for the purpose of receiving medical care (not including leisure tourism for general well-being or stress relief). More and more, such medical care is provided alongside a vacation package—such that a patient or medical tourist can have a procedure done and then relax or sightsee in the destination nation before returning home.

Although in theory, foreign medical services offered to international patients could run the full gamut of procedures, in practice a few services tend to be the most popular. Cosmetic surgeries are very popular, since they often are not covered by private or public insurance. Other popular procedures include, but are not limited to, hip replacement, knee replacement, in vitro fertilization, Lasik, dental procedures, and most other elective surgeries (Burkett et al., 2007). Generally

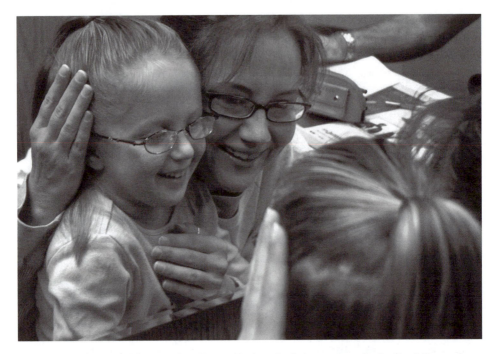

Rylea Barlett, left, and her mother, Dawn Barlett, look in a mirror in Joplin, Missouri, on November 21, 2007. Rylea, who was born blind, traveled with her mother to China for experimental stem cell injections that resulted in her gaining vision. (AP/Wide World Photos)

speaking, procedures with the greatest cost differential between developed and undeveloped countries, or those that are often uninsured or unavailable in developed countries, are the most popular.

**Who Travels Abroad for Care and Why?** In its early years when technology and skill were still relatively bound by geographic and national borders, medical tourism primarily involved travel from developing countries to developed countries for care due to a lack of technology and expertise. The conjoined Burmese twins, Lin and Win, offer an exemplary example of this—the expertise to separate them simply did not exist in Burma. This led them to Canada where the twins were successfully separated in the mid-1980s (Crozier & Baylis, 2010). In the 1990s, the trend shifted toward travel from one affluent country to another, either seeking lower costs or shorter wait times. In the 21st century, increasingly affordable air travel and the ability of developing nations to offer advanced-level care has seen a reversal of the previous trend—the bulk of medical tourists now travel from developed nations to developing nations (Crozier & Baylis, 2010).

The exact reasons why contemporary travelers seek care in developing nations vary from country to country, but can generally be broken down into three major categories: cost, wait times, and legal availability (Horowitz et al., 2007). Travelers from countries where cost is a significant barrier to obtaining health care, such as the United States, see many outbound medical tourists heading overseas for care because that care is unaffordable at home. For example, a complicated open heart surgery can cost as much as $150,000 in the United States or $70,000 in Britain, but only $10,000 in India, even from highly trained surgeons at state-of-the-art facilities. It is common for many other procedures to be at least 75 percent cheaper in India or other popular medical tourism destinations compared to the United States (Connell, 2006). However, even these discounted costs are often unaffordable for the poorest segments of the U.S. population. Thus, American medical tourists driven by cost factors from their own country are often middle class, since the poor are unable to afford it and the wealthy have no need for it.

Another major category of medical tourists are those from countries with universal coverage such as Canada or the United Kingdom. In these countries, wait times for care can often be very long for nonemergency procedures. For example, wait times for a hip replacement can be as long as a year in some areas of Canada. Despite being nonemergency, the delay can often be painful and debilitating for patients with severe consequences for quality of life. Similar to America, low-income individuals are unable to afford overseas care. Therefore, patients tend to be anywhere from middle class to the very upper class, and those with the resources to pay for out-of-pocket care may elect to travel overseas to jump the queue.

The last major reason for patients to seek overseas care is legality. Some procedures, such as stem cell therapy, are not approved in developed nations for a lack of evidence regarding safety and efficacy. Other procedures are not approved for ethical reasons in the home country, most notably purchasing organs for a transplant or ova for fertility treatment (Crozier & Baylis, 2010). Medical tourists for these types of procedures can be from any demographic background capable of paying for the procedures. Of course, this form of medical tourism attracts the most ethical criticism when legal issues come into play.

As with any development, numerous groups stand to gain from the rise in medical tourism. The first and most obvious group is patients. Patients stand to benefit by saving money, bypassing waiting lists, and obtaining access to potentially beneficial procedures unavailable to them at home. However, they are certainly not the only ones who may benefit. If the patients originate from nations that provide universal health coverage (which most Western countries do), an overseas medical procedure paid out of pocket by the patient represents a decreased burden on the health care system at home, shortening wait lists and leaving more resources to treat other patients.

Parties in destination nations also stand to gain from medical tourism. The clinicians and hospitals that treat the medical tourists gain an incredibly valuable source of business since medical tourists are typically wealthier and pay much more than local patients. For instance, traditional tourism package vendors benefit greatly since medical tourism is often accompanied by some traditional leisure and sightseeing. Furthermore, almost 83 percent of medical tourists travel with a companion, leading to even greater tourism expenditures (Medical Tourism Association, 2009). The combination of revenue for hospitals and for tourism-related venues generates significant economic output for the developing destination nation.

This leads to generalized economic growth as well as an increase in tax revenue for the destination nation's government. These governments clearly see medical tourism as beneficial to their economies. For example, India heavily promotes itself as a provider of medical tourism and has even started to issue a new medical visa for foreign patients to ease the process of entering the country for medical care. Clearly, these steps are successful; medical tourism is projected to be worth $2.2 billion, or approximately 1 percent of India's entire GDP by 2012. Another major player in medical tourism, Thailand, owes approximately 0.5 percent of its GDP to medical tourism, which is an eighth of the overall medical expenditures in the country (Crozier & Baylis, 2010). The large amount of revenue generated by medical tourism has the added benefit of drawing expatriate clinicians back to their home countries, many of whom have Western degrees and training, thus attracting even more patients and money in a positive feedback cycle.

**Who Loses from Medical Tourism?**   Interestingly, the groups that can and do benefit from medical tourism are often the same ones that may suffer from it. Although patients gain a lot in terms of money and shortened wait lists, health care providers in destination nations may not be as well trained or as skilled as providers in the patients' home countries, leading to substandard care. To fight this perception, many hospitals that target medical tourists have sought accreditation from well-known Western accrediting bodies, such as Joint Commission International (JCI) (York, 2008).

Another factor exacerbating the risk is the concern patients have should anything go wrong before, during, or after their operation when they are far from home in an unfamiliar locale. In such an event or in cases of malpractice, patients may not have access to the same legal remedies they are accustomed to. In other words, patients may forego the opportunity to seek compensation should their procedures go awry.

There have also been questions raised about the risks of travel and long-haul flights shortly following major operations, which leaves any complications from the surgery to the home country's health care system. It is worth noting that while these are all legitimate concerns, the great majority of medical tourism facilities do, in fact, continue to stay in touch with patients after they return home, sometimes even paying for return airfare should follow-up procedures become necessary. This phenomenon is driven by a combination of ethical and market factors. Ethically, physicians typically feel an obligation to their patients whether they are local or international. From a market point of view, it is in the hospitals' best interest to keep their patients happy, since many of their future patients will come from word-of-mouth referrals and a little negative press can greatly reduce business (Shetty, 2010).

A less common concern, but one of significant note, occurs with patients who seek overseas care for procedures that are not approved in their home country. Sometimes these procedures are simply unproven, other times outright dangerous. Desperation may lead patients in dire circumstances to seek such care to their ultimate detriment. A notable case of this occurred when an Israeli boy traveled to Russia for stem cell therapy, which was not approved in the United

Kingdom because it is deemed unsafe and ineffective. The boy subsequently developed tumors in the brain and spinal cord as a result of the stem cell injections (Crozier & Baylis, 2010). Despite such cautionary tales, patients continue to go abroad seeking unproven treatments, leading to increased opportunity for harm.

The economy of the patient's home country can either win or lose from medical tourism. In countries without universal coverage or where medicine is practiced under a market model rather than a social model, the loss of patients overseas represents lost dollars. Medical tourism is, fundamentally, a form of outsourcing, meaning that health care providers in the patients' home countries lose business. In practice this does not tend to be a major issue since most developed nations with large numbers of medical tourists also face physician and nursing shortages, but it is nevertheless grounds for economically ideological criticism.

Lastly, poor patients in destination, developing nations are often harmed by medical tourism. Despite generating large amounts of revenue, medical tourism has the effect of drawing health care providers and hospitals away from local patients in order to care for the medical tourist patients. In nations such as Thailand, where local health care resources are already severely strained, medical tourism has only served to amplify the problem. Some governments have attempted to reverse this trend by taking advantage of the economic gains from medical tourism to offer care to the impoverished, although so far with little success.

One notable example of such a program occurred just after the turn of the 21st century, when the Indian government sold land to private hospitals (catering to medical tourists) at heavily subsidized prices in exchange for promises that the hospitals would provide some free care to local patients. While certainly well intentioned, a lack of government oversight led to the complete failure of the program. Subsequent research concluded that the majority of these hospitals failed to live up to their promise and most provided far less free care to local patients than initially promised. Many provided none at all (Shetty, 2010). Despite the present deleterious effect that medical tourism imposes on impoverished patients in developing nations, programs such as these nevertheless provide hope for the future. With stricter controls to enforce promises made by hospitals or direct action using medical tourism–generated monies, developing countries' governments may be able to improve access to health care and other social services for their peoples.

**Ethical Criticisms** Numerous ethical issues plague the discourse around medical tourism. Firstly, as previously discussed, medical tourism currently harms local patients in destination nations. This raises questions about whether or not medical tourism is a form of Third World exploitation. Along with other ethical questions about Third World exploitation such as sweat factories, the tug and pull of the debate revolves around the merits of the economic growth spurred by medical tourism versus taking advantage of poor, developing nations and their people. Further complications exist when the medical procedure in question is banned for ethical reasons. For example, purchasing organs for transplantation may not be illegal, or may only be poorly enforced in many developing countries. However, there still exists great potential for exploiting the poor for their organs, by desperate and wealthy individuals in the developing world, a practice that is widely banned in developed countries for ethical reasons. This is considered to be an unethical practice, but it continues nevertheless because these patients are often in such critical situations themselves. Since such things are difficult to enforce across borders without completely restricting international travel, ethical governments have yet to come up with a good way to prevent such abuses.

The potential for exploitation of the desperate goes in both directions. Since patients may themselves be desperate for care, they may turn to ineffective procedures not approved in their own countries. This opens the door for providers in developing countries to entice patients into spending large sums of money on ineffective care while providing false hope.

The last ethical issue exists only in societies with universally equal health coverage such as Canada. Such countries place moral value on every citizen having equal access to care. Therefore, the ability of the relatively more wealthy to buy care overseas and "skip the queue" creates a moral dilemma. Like the issue of exploitation, it is one that currently has little recourse but merits mentioning.

**The Future of Medical Tourism**   Although specific number estimates vary, it is clear that medical tourism is on the rise. Driven by a combination of health care access issues in developed countries and its large economic potential, some estimates project 5 million medical tourists (including companions) with a global value of $60 billion by 2012. Growth in Asia alone is presently at 20 percent per year, with the majority of that growth occurring in India and to a lesser extent, Thailand (Horowitz et al., 2007). As more and more hospitals in the developing world receive international accreditation from bodies like JCI, patients will have ever-increasing options for quality care abroad.

Furthermore, employers and insurance companies have also started exploring international medical care. Increasing numbers of insurers (private, employers, and governments) have begun to offer incentives for enrollees to travel overseas for care. For example, a grocery store chain in Maine now offers fully paid trips to Singapore for knee and hip replacements for the employee/patient as well as a companion thereby sharing the cost savings with the patient (McGinley, 2008). Even government insurers have outsourced care. For example, in 2002 the National Health Service (NHS) in the United Kingdom initiated the Overseas Commissioning Scheme, whereby NHS hospitals could outsource their patients to nearby countries to reduce wait times and costs (Hanna et al., 2009).

For developed countries, the rise in medical tourism is a red flag signaling problems in their own health care systems. They must ask themselves if citizens seek care overseas, does it mean they are unable to access needed care at home? As governments respond and seek to alleviate access issues in their countries, the rise in medical tourism may taper off. This may be a good sign for patients in the developed world as medical costs are forced lower in order to compete and wait lists are shortened.

Finally, providers in destination, developing nations will continue to grow as the market grows. The real question in developing nations is what will happen to the local patient populations. Governments hold the power to capitalize on medical tourism as a way to improve health care services for their own impoverished citizens. If they choose not to, then as medical tourism rises, local patients will see decreasing access to medical care as resources are drawn away to care for medical tourists.

Ultimately, irrespective of harms or ethical issues, it is clear that in our ever-increasingly global society, medical tourism is here to stay. It is a reality of modern health care that all relevant parties—governments, insurers, clinicians, and patients—will need to recognize and adapt to accordingly. As they do, they will need to address the ethical concerns associated with medical tourism to assure their best interests and provide, or access, the best health care possible for their own citizens and the international community.

*David Chen*

*See also* Health Insurance; Spas, Medical.

### References

Burkett, Levi, et al. "Medical Tourism: Concerns, Benefits, and the American Legal Perspective." *Journal of Legal Medicine* 28 (2007): 223–45.

Connell, John. "Medical Tourism: Sea, Sun, Sand and . . . Surgery." *Tourism Management* 27 (2006): 1093–1100.

Cook, Peta. "What Is Health and Medical Tourism?" Annual Conference of the Australian Sociological Association, University of Melbourne, Victoria, December 2–5, 2008.

Crozier, G., and Francoise Baylis. "The Ethical Physician Encounters International Medical Travel." *Journal of Medical Ethics* 36 (2010): 297–301.

Hanna, Sammy, et al. "Sending NHS Patients for Operations Abroad: Is the Holiday Over?" *Annals of the Royal Surgeons of England* 91, no. 2 (2009): 128–30.

Horowitz, Michael, et al. "Medical Tourism: Globalization of the Healthcare Marketplace." *Medscape General Medicine* 9, no. 4 (2007): 33.

McGinley, Laurie. "Health Matters: The Next Wave of Medical Tourists Might Include You." *Wall Street Journal,* 2008. http://online.wsj.com/article/SB120283288380762505.html.

Medical Tourism Association. "Surveys, Quotes." 2009. www.medicaltourismassociation. com/en/surveys-quotes.html.

Shetty, Priya. "Medical Tourism Booms in India, but at What Cost?" *The Lancet* 376 (2010): 671–72.

York, Diane. "Medical Tourism: The Trend toward Outsourcing Medical Procedures to Foreign Countries." *Journal of Continuing Education in the Health Professions* 28, no. 2 (2008): 99–102.

## HEALTH INSURANCE

Health insurance is designed to finance the U.S. health care system. Unlike most other industrialized countries, many of which have publicly financed health care systems, the United States maintains a complex system that includes private health insurance for many people, government-funded health insurance for others, and no health insurance for many, including children.

The complexity of this system when compared to many other countries in the world makes it difficult to describe in simple terms or for people to understand and use effectively. In addition, in 2010, new legislation, the Patient Protection and Affordable Care Act (PPACA), also known by the Obama administration as the Affordable Care Act, was passed. This act seeks to place a number of requirements on health insurance companies in the United States and will over time modify some aspects of how health insurance and access to health care services will work in the United States. While a few provisions begin as soon as 2010, the major provisions of this health care legislation start in 2014. Republicans opposed to the law, who are running for office in Congress and for president in 2012 elections, vow to work to overturn it, considering it unnecessary and a type of socialism.

The impact of this new legislation and its effect on providing health care coverage for uninsured Americans is still uncertain. No matter what happens, however, Americans should understand general health insurance terminology, basic facts, and the history of health insurance. It is also important to note that PPACA changes may affect the major types of health insurance available in the United States. However, what that will mean for Americans both with and without health insurance also remains unclear.

**Basic Insurance Facts and Terms**   Health insurance is a specialized type of insurance generally defined as a financial mechanism to manage or control financial exposure to risk over illness or accidental injury. Thus the concept of risk is central to a definition of insurance. Standard insurance texts usually define *risk* as the possibility of an adverse deviation from a desired outcome that is expected or hoped for. A simpler definition often used is possibility of loss. Combined, the insurance definition of risk means a way to manage exposure to risk due to injury or illness and to protect against the possibility of loss.

Insurance also works to shift the risk from an individual to a group and for all members of a group to share the loss on some type of equitable basis. These ideas apply well to several types of insurance, such as automobile insurance or homeowners insurance. However, in the case of health insurance today, it violates some basic principles of insurance. For example, the loss covered is supposed to be something unusual that can possibly be avoided. Yet health insurance is now expected to cover regular events including a visit to a doctor's office or immunizations. These are not unusual or avoided events. Similarly, most good coverage now includes prescription drug costs, which for many people pays for routine medications taken to manage chronic conditions. Again, these are lifelong conditions rather than an unusual health problem that occurs infrequently.

Since other types of insurance generally cover major costs, the trend in automobile and home insurance is to have higher and higher deductibles. Health insurance by contrast has shown a growth in what is described as "first-dollar" coverage, meaning most costs are covered except for modest deductibles or co-payments on many employer-provided health plans, making health insurance a very different product when compared to other forms of insurance.

The terms *copayment* and *deductible* are confusing for many Americans. A *copayment* is the amount each person must pay every time she receives services, such as a required $10 or $15 payment for a visit to a doctor's office or a $20 or $30 copayment for a prescription medication. In the last few years, copayments have been rising on many insurance plans, often doubling or tripling from $10 to $20 or even $30. Many health plans have also increased copayments for prescription drugs, with a smaller payment for generic drugs and much larger payments for brand-name prescription medications.

A deductible is very different from a copayment. The *deductible* is a predetermined amount that must be paid before insurance funds are available. In some plans, a person must pay the first $500 of health care costs before her health insurance will pay any bills or costs. Generally, employer-based health insurance plans that offer smaller deductibles, or, in many cases, no deductibles are considered more advantageous for the employees, especially if they offer modest copayments. Unfortunately, many businesses have had to turn to higher deductibles and copayments in their employee health insurance plans to offset rising health care costs and their own shrinking profits.

**History of Health Insurance**   The history of health insurance in the United States started as early as 1850 with commercial companies, including Franklin Health Insurance Company of Massachusetts and Travelers Insurance companies. These new policies were designed to cover the loss of income due to serious illness. In the first plans, the actual costs of physician services were not expensive and were not considered part of the insurance coverage.

Similarly, hospitals were viewed as a place of last resort to obtain health care, used mostly by the poor, so insurance plans did not include hospital expenses either. What became a major health insurance model began in Dallas, Texas, in 1929 when Baylor Hospital contracted with a group of teachers to provide coverage for certain hospital expenses. This eventually became Blue Cross hospital insurance coverage.

Health insurance coverage for individuals grew slowly during the Depression of the 1930s, but increased during World War II as some major companies offered it as an additional benefit for workers. This was attractive to workers because wage increases were regulated during the war, but health insurance was not included in any government wage and price controls.

By 1950, more than 50 percent of Americans had health insurance, generally obtained through their jobs. During the next decade, this figure expanded as Blue Cross (hospital) and Blue Shield (physician) plans were created in most states and coverage was offered to the majority of municipal and state workers as well as public school employees. In addition, the growth of labor unions in the 1950s meant most industrial workers also received health insurance as a work benefit.

Passage of the Medicare program in 1965 got a boost from the lack of coverage for the elderly and the fact that people were losing their health insurance coverage when they retired. Medicare is a federal health insurance program that provides government health insurance for Americans who quality for and receive

Social Security. At the same time, the Medicaid program was passed as a joint state-federal effort (as were most welfare programs in the United States at that time) to provide coverage for people who received federal welfare payments.

Health care insurance coverage rates continued to rise through the 1970s. Since that time changes in the economy and the loss of manufacturing jobs, along with the later growth of service sector jobs that fail to include health insurance, has meant that rates of increases in private health insurance have slowed or even declined at various points over the past 30 years.

**Coverage and Costs**   The type of health insurance people have and what it covers changed a great deal in the past 50 years. In the 1960s, most private coverage was either from Blue Cross/Blue Shield plans or for-profit health insurance companies. That has changed as consolidation in the provision of health insurance has increased. Blue Cross/Blue Shield plans in various states are still important providers of health care insurance. However, some of these plans are no longer nonprofit and have been converted into for-profit companies. In addition, major for-profit companies such as Cigna and United Health Care, both providers of traditional types of health insurance and managed care plans, have increased in size. Managed care service providers such as Kaiser have also grown.

For working-aged people health insurance comes mainly through their employer. A serious concern for many people is that, if they lose their jobs, they lose their health insurance coverage. Employers may choose to subsidize the costs of health insurance and a few still provide coverage for the workers and families at low costs, but, in general, the cost of health insurance has been increasing for the last two decades. Employers have dealt with those large increases by transferring more and more of those costs to their employees, especially for family coverage. Although legislation now requires that people can continue their coverage for 18 months after they lose their job, any employer subsidy is lost, making the costs even higher and can result in the loss of insurance for some individuals.

One major change since the passage of Medicare and Medicaid in 1965 has been the role government plays in the provision of health insurance. Almost all Americans over the age of 65 now have Medicare as long as they or their spouse worked long enough to qualify for Social Security payments. However, Medicare is considered by some to be a limited program because it does not cover long-term care services, and only recently has begun paying drugs costs. Prescription drugs must be paid for through a complicated addition to Medicare in which people purchase a drug plan to supplement their basic Medicare coverage. The drug plans are administered by private companies but regulated by the government. Still, with concerns being raised over the PPACA, the federal Medicare program remains the major purchaser of health care services for people over 65.

In most U.S. hospitals Medicare is the major payer of hospital bills. Medicaid has become an important program for low-income Americans, and the addition of the SCHIP (State Child Health Insurance Program) in 1998 to provide health care insurance for children of the working poor (those whose incomes are too high to qualify for Medicaid) has meant that children are now more likely to have health insurance than are other age groups except those 65 years and over. One illustration of the importance of the growth in government programs is that in 1960, before the passage of Medicare and Medicaid, government funds paid for about 24 percent of health care costs, mostly through coverage for those in the military, veterans, and through county hospitals and public health programs for the poor. Forty years later, by 2005, 46 percent of the nation's health care dollar came from Medicare, Medicaid, SCHIP, and other government programs (Kronenfeld, 2006; Blue Cross and Blue Shield Association, 2010). Limitations and issues concerning these same government programs are part of the new PPACA legislation.

**Who Has Health Insurance**  In the last few years, the number of people without health insurance in the United States has been increasing, from 46.3 million in 2008 to 50.7 million in 2009, while the percentage increased from 15.4 percent to 16.7 percent over the same period. The number of people covered by private health insurance decreased from 201.0 million to 194.5 million from 2008 to 2009. Comparable health insurance data have been collected since 1987, showing this is the first year in which the number of people with health insurance decreased. As mentioned earlier, some people are covered by private health insurance, often through their work, and others have government-based health insurance. In contrast, the number covered by government health insurance increased from 87.4 million to 93.2 million. These trends are part of what has led to a call for reform in health care and health insurance, and for ways to stem rising health care costs.

Rates of health insurance coverage are linked to important social and demographic characteristics. Generally, children are more likely to have health insurance than adults, with about 10 percent of children under 18 still lacking health insurance in 2009, a figure similar to 2008. For children living in poverty, more are uninsured (15.1%). As household incomes increase, the percentage of people without health insurance decreases. In 2009, 26.6 percent of people in households with annual incomes less than $25,000 had no insurance in contrast with only 9.1 percent in households with incomes of $75,000 or more.

**Impact of Reform Legislation**  Under the administration of President Obama two important expansions to health insurance have passed. The first was an extension and expansion of SCHIP, approved early in the Obama term. The major focus on health for the first part of the Obama presidency has been on a large, major health reform effort, which resulted in health insurance PPACA reform signed on March 23, 2010. The PPACA legislation, when fully implemented, is expected to guarantee health insurance coverage for an additional 32 million uninsured Americans.

Major coverage expansion begins in 2014, with the controversial requirement that most people purchase health insurance, although a number of important provisions begin sooner. For example, in October 2010, insurers had to remove lifetime dollar limits on policies, while subsidies became available to small businesses to provide coverage to employees. Insurance companies were also barred from denying coverage to children with preexisting conditions. It also became possible for children to remain covered by their parents' insurance policies until age 26. Plans must offer preventive services with no out-of-pocket expenses such as deductibles and copayments for those services.

Other PPACA changes will begin gradually. In 2011, grants will be available to small employers to encourage wellness programs and preventive health care. Some tax changes begin in 2011. For Medicare, a number of changes linked to prevention and drugs will begin in 2012. For Medicaid, the government will begin creation of demonstration programs to point out cost-effective ways of providing care. Those changes may include the use of bundled payments for episodes of care including hospitalizations. For Medicare, Independence at Home demonstration programs will also be created. These programs allow health care professionals the option of providing primary care services for Medicare beneficiaries in their homes, as well as some changes in hospital payment. An independent advisory board will be created to make recommendations for other cost-saving measures. In 2013, more tax changes become law including increased taxes for Medicare high earners.

The largest changes are expected to occur in 2014. That is when individual insurance coverage mandates take effect and when individuals will need to obtain "qualifying" health insurance coverage through their employer, or through Medicare, Medicaid, Veterans Administration coverage, or a privately purchased plan. Individuals who do not have coverage will face tax penalties. In addition to the mandate on individuals, companies with more than 200 employees must offer health plans to their employees, and smaller companies (more than 50) must provide some coverage.

Insurance exchanges will be created as a way for small businesses and individuals to compare costs of different plans and help people meet the mandates. There are also some additional modifications to Medicare scheduled to begin in 2014, including the establishment of payment advisory boards, which experts believe will be critical in holding down rising costs of overall medical care. Medicaid will expand its coverage to all Americans under 65 with incomes up to 133 percent of the federal poverty level, with states receiving funds to help pay for this.

Due to the gradual implementation of this legislation, it will be years before the real impact can be accurately assessed. Supporters and critics agree (Cutler, 2010) the true measure of health care reform's success is whether it drives down medical costs over the long term. Another important measure of success will be whether more people are able to obtain health care insurance. Most experts agree the reforms will create new rules for all groups in health care, especially for health insurance companies. Others suggest litigation as well as regulatory proceedings will ultimately determine the final shape of the new health care rules. In August 2011, the 11th Circuit U.S. Court of Appeals in Atlanta declared the law's "individual mandate" feature, which requires that all Americans carry health insurance, unconstitutional, suggesting to many that there will ultimately be a Supreme Court case to determine the law's constitutionality. The Supreme Court is expected to hear a case by June 2012. There may also eventually be some modifications in the legislation, as a result of the Republicans gaining control over the House of Representatives in the 2010 elections. Several new representatives immediately announced plans to modify or even repeal the PPACA, or at least some of the provisions of the new legislation.

*Jennie Jacobs Kronenfeld*

*See also* Medicaid; Medicare.

### References

Blue Cross and Blue Shield Association. *Healthcare Financing Trends.* October 2010. www.bcbs.com/blueresources/mcrg/chapter1/MCRG_chap1.pdf.

Cutler, David. "Analysis and Commentary: How Health Care Reform Must Bend the Cost Curve." *Health Affairs* 29, no. 6 (2010): 1131–35.

Kronenfeld, Jennie Jacobs. *Expansion of Publicly Funded Health Insurance in the United States: The Children's Health Insurance Program and Its Implications.* Lanham, MD: Lexington Press, 2006.

U.S. Census Bureau. *Income, Poverty and Health Insurance Coverage in the United States, 2009.* www.census.gov/newsroom/releases/archives/income_wealth/cb10-144.html.

## HEALTH SAVINGS ACCOUNT (HSA)

One of the newest developments in recent years is the HSA—a tax-advantaged health savings account that may be opened in concert with a high-deductible health care plan. Some employers may offer these, and even contribute money toward them as part of your health care insurance subsidy.

However, this combination of policy + HSA is also available to independent contractors and sole proprietor entrepreneurs. If you work for yourself, consider procuring a high-deductible health care plan (HDHP) and opening an accompanying HSA. While you may not receive an employer subsidy, this combination can keep your out-of-pocket health care expenses down while providing some pretty meaty tax advantages. Ten million Americans are now covered by HSA-eligible insurance plans according to figures from the insurance industry group America's Health Insurance Plans (AHIP).

President George W. Bush signed Public Law 108-173, the Medicare Prescription Drug, Improvement and Modernization Act of 2003 into law on December 8, 2003, creating the first HSAs. His administration called the law a solution to rising health care costs and growing numbers of Americans without health insurance.

Basically, you pay your health care premiums out of your own pocket. Recently, this expense has also become tax deductible for self-employed individuals. Next, you contribute as much (or as little) as you want to your HSA, up to the maximum amount—which tends to increase every year and may be comparable to the amount of your deductible. (In 2009, the maximum was $5,950 for a family, which was raised in 2010 to $6,150.) Once you hit a specific balance, your account may even offer investment options so that you have the opportunity to grow the money you're saving. And every dime you place in this account is also tax deductible.

You may pull from this account balance to pay for all medical expenses up to your deductible, and then pull from it for your percentage of costs beyond the deductible. You may use it to pay for copays, prescription drugs, and even some over-the-counter medications and the like. The list of qualified expenses grows every year and is available at the IRS website.

You can use money from the HSA to pay for braces, contacts, optometrist visits, and many types of health care expenses that may not even be covered under your health care plan. All tax-free. It's almost like siphoning your hard-earned dollars through an account that allows you to pay for nearly all normal health care expenses—things you pay for out of pocket anyway—only now it's tax-free.

The more you contribute to the account, the lower your income tax bill. For self-employed single parents, combine that savings with the deductibility of your premiums, and you pretty much end up paying no taxes on all your health care–related expenses. Better yet, this is not a use-it-or-lose-it account like many employers offer. If you don't use all that you contribute to your HSA in one year, it rolls over to the next year, and the next.

And if you keep contributing every year, which is a great way to lower your income tax bill, and you don't need all that money, you may use it free and clear once you retire (over age 65). Most accounts also offer investment options, and any interest you earn you may also withdraw tax-free (as long as it's for qualified medical expenses or you're over age 65).

An HSA is a tax haven for income. Paired with a high-deductible health care plan, it's a great way to keep your health care expenses down and save money on taxes at the same time. It's also another tax-advantaged way to save for retirement. An HSA is also portable—it belongs to you, not your employer. If you leave your employer, all the money in the account stays with you. Even if you enroll in an HMO plan next, you may no longer contribute to the HSA but you can still access the money for qualified out-of-pocket medical expenses.

You may use it to pay for COBRA or other health care insurance premiums should you become unemployed. You can use it to pay for long-term care insurance premiums or long-term care expenses should you become disabled. Once you hit age 65, you can use it for anything.

Like a qualified retirement savings account, if you use the money for anything but qualified medical expenses (before age 65), you'll get hit with an extra 10 percent tax penalty. So don't use it for anything but health care expenses; with children on board that's usually not a problem.

Another beauty is that you do not have to contribute to the account, or can contribute whenever you want, such as when you know you have health care expenses coming up—like a family visit to the dentist. Put money in a few weeks earlier; check to make sure the money is in your account. Then pay it out when you're at the dentist or when you get your bill.

Or, once you pay your bills, you can contribute to the account and then reimburse yourself with the expenses you paid. Many HSA providers provide checks and even debit cards that you can use like a VISA card at doctors' offices and pharmacies. Some even work at automatic teller machines so you can get cash. Keep all receipts and put them under "HSA Reimbursements" in your tax folder—staple reimbursement receipts to the bills they went toward paying.

If possible, try to use the debit card whenever you can, even to pay an invoice. The direct payout makes administrative tracking easier, plus you may get an ATM or per check charge if you use another method. All of these details will be included in your HSA information packet when you sign up—be sure you know all charges up front so you can utilize the least expensive method for this account.

Keep all of your medical bills and HSA reimbursement receipts. You don't have to submit these with your tax return but you will need them should you get audited.

Who can have an HSA? Any adult, so long as they meet the following criteria:

Have coverage under an HSA-qualified "high-deductible health plan" (HDHP);
Have no other medical coverage (like an employer-sponsored HMO);
Are not enrolled in Medicare;
Cannot be claimed as a dependent on someone else's tax return.

You can, however, have other forms of health insurance policies, such as specific-injury insurance or accident, disability, dental care, vision care, or long-term care insurance.

**Head of Household Tip: Alternate Health Care Coverage**   Instead of paying out premiums for a dental or vision care policy, consider saving that discretionary income in an HSA and paying out only for expenses as needed. The HSA provides both tax advantages and you only pay for what you actually use, unlike an insurance policy.

Contributions to your HSA can be made by you, your employer, or both, up to a certain limit each year. You may deduct your contributions (even if you do not itemize deductions) when completing your federal income tax return.

The HSA is a very good reason to shop for alternate health care policies if your employer's plan seems too expensive. If your family is reasonably healthy, you can save money on premiums by securing a high-deductible plan, and set aside your savings through monthly installments in an HSA to pay for your out-of-pocket health care expenses.

If you decide to forgo employer-sponsored health care insurance, and you'll probably have to show evidence of alternate insurance if you do, be sure and ask for remuneration since your employer is saving money by not subsidizing your plan. You can use this money to help offset your monthly premiums or deposit it into your HSA. Banks, credit unions, insurance companies, and other financial institutions are allowed by law to be trustees or custodians of these accounts. Other financial institutions that handle IRAs are also automatically qualified to establish HSAs.

Learning to evaluate health care insurance plans is a life skill. It's more important than straightening out your golf swing or learning to cook lasagna, so take the time you would normally devote to a less useful task and learn it.

*Kara Stefan*

*See also* Health Insurance.

### References

Gillentine, Amy. "Health Savings Account Insurance Coverage Reaches 10 Million Nationwide." *Colorado Springs Business Journal* (May 19, 2010), http://csbj.com/tag/health-savings-accounts.

"HSA Enrollment Tops 10 Million." *Medical Economics* 87, no. 11 (June 4, 2010): 12.

Huntley, Helen. "Not Yet Eligible for Medicare? Consider HAS." *St. Petersburg Times,* May 26, 2010, 5S.

Internal Revenue Service. "Health Savings Accounts." www.irs.gov.

Keller, Christine L., Gary Lesser, William F. Sweetnam, and Susan D. Diehl. *Health Savings Account Answer Book*. New York: Aspen, 2008.

Pilzer, Paul Zane. *The New Health Insurance Solution: How to Get Cheaper, Better Coverage without a Traditional Employer Plan*. Hoboken, NJ: Wiley, 2007.

Rooney, J. Patrick, and Dan Perrin. *America's Health Care Crisis Solver: Money-Saving Solutions, Coverage for Everyone*. Hoboken, NJ: Wiley, 2008.

Schulte Scott, Jeanne. "Let's Talk about Health Savings Accounts." *Healthcare Financial Management* 60, no. 9 (September 2006): 46.

## HEART HEALTH

The heart is arguably the most frequently mentioned organ in popular music. Tony Bennett left his in San Francisco, Bruce Springsteen said everyone's heart is hungry, and Billy Ray Cyrus sang about a rare cardiac condition known as an "achy breaky" heart, yet few songs refer to the liver, spleen, or pancreas. In Western culture, the heart is the seat of emotion and motivation. It can be broken, changed, crossed, and hardened. It has been purported to be made of wood, glass, stone, and gold, the latter referring to people of unusual morality, compassion, and generosity. Obviously, the heart is a vital organ. Its purpose, however, can be described much less poetically and its importance to health and wellness cannot be overstated.

The heart is a muscle whose sole purpose is pumping blood to the rest of the body through blood vessels. Sapolsky describes the heart as "a dumb, simple mechanical pump" and the blood vessels that pump blood to and from the heart as "nothing more exciting than hoses" (Sapolsky, 2004), hardly the romantic picture painted by poets or country music singers. Nonetheless, viewing the heart functionally as a pump with hoses suggests the need for properly caring for it to ensure it continues working.

In order to function, our bodies require oxygen; blood is the means by which oxygen is transmitted throughout the body. The cardiovascular system is a closed system that coordinates blood flow. From the lungs, blood is bright red and rich with oxygen and travels through arteries throughout the body's tissues. After delivering its oxygen, the blood absorbs waste products and carbon dioxide, which then return through the heart to the lungs, liver, and kidneys via a different set of vessels called veins. Because of the absence of oxygen, the blood in the veins is a darker red (Jackson, 2000).

The heart's mechanical pumping action maintains a continuous cycle of contraction and relaxation or what we typically experience as a heartbeat, beating at least 100,000 times and pumping 3,000 gallons of blood every 24 hours (Randall & Romaine, 2005). A single cycle of contraction and relaxation takes about eight-tenths of a second and occurs in a healthy person between 70 and 80 times a minute (Romaine & DeWitt, 1998).

In addition to its mechanical pumping action, the heart requires a sophisticated electrical system to trigger the cardiac cycle. The

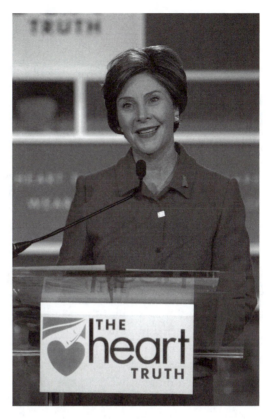

Former First Lady Laura Bush served as the NIH Heart Truth campaign ambassador and worked to support heart health for all Americans. (National Institutes of Health)

electrical patterns that symbolize the cardiac cycle are visible through an electrocardiogram, or EKG, a simple test that is done by attaching electrodes on the surface of the chest and charting the electrical pattern. A person trained to read EKGs will look for patterns indicating either a healthy or problematic heart rhythm. Problems with heart rhythms, or arrhythmias, come in four categories: (1) bradycardia, or a below-normal but steady heart rate; (2) tachycardia, a rapid but steady heart rate; (3) fibrillation, which is a rapid, irregular heart rate where the affected part of the heart is fibrillating, or wiggling, instead of beating; and (4) extra beats (often misinterpreted as skipped beats), that occur before or after regular beats (Randall & Romaine, 2005).

Electrical problems can occur because of irregularities in the ways the heart conducts electrical impulses. One such disorder is Wolf-Parkinson-White syndrome, which involves an extra electrical path that either overrides or competes with normal electrical impulses and often results in dangerous arrhythmias (Randall & Romaine, 2005). However, arrhythmias can also occur when the normal mechanical action of the heart is inhibited by clogs in the coronary arteries or damage to the heart muscle itself.

Electrical or mechanical problems with the heart can lead to a heart attack, which involves the death of heart muscle tissue that occurs when it is deprived of oxygen. *Myocardial infarction* is the technical term for heart attack, and it means heart muscle death (Randall & Romaine, 2005). *Myocardial* refers to heart muscle tissue, while an *infarction* is a medical term that describes the death of any tissue that occurs when it is deprived of oxygen. Heart attack severity can range from mild, where there is little damage to the muscle tissue, to full cardiac arrest, where the heart stops.

The coronary arteries play a key role in keeping the heart supplied with oxygen-rich blood. In its pristine form, coronary arteries, like tiny garden hoses, have smooth inner linings that allow blood to flow freely to the heart. But, like tiny garden hoses that become caked with residue from hard water, cardiac arteries can become occluded, restricting blood flow to the heart. Unfortunately, we do this to ourselves.

When we encounter an acute stressor like an oncoming taxi or an angry boss, our bodies react immediately with the "fight-or-flight" stress response. Among other things, it involves an increase in blood pressure, which is the force with which blood flows through the arteries, so that blood can get to the parts of the body most needed in either fighting or fleeing (Sapolsky, 2004). Once you have fought or flown, your blood pressure returns to normal. The potential for cardiac arteries increases when we are in a chronic state of fight-or-flight. Ongoing financial stress or a difficult work situation results in chronically elevated blood pressure, or hypertension. This puts strain on the blood vessels, forcing them to work harder to regulate blood flow (Sapolsky, 2004).

Hypertension causes a number of problems for heart health. Because hypertension involves an increased force of blood flow, the blood will return to the heart, more specifically the left ventricle, with force enough to cause the muscle tissue around the left ventricle to thicken as it works to regulate the increased force of the blood flow. Eventually, like any muscle that is overdeveloped through strenuous exercise, the heart will hypertrophy or get bigger. The medical term for this condition is *left ventricle hypertrophy,* which can lead to arrhythmias. After controlling for age, "having left ventricular hypertrophy is the single best predictor of cardiac risk" (Sapolsky, 2004).

In addition to having an asymmetrical heart with thickening of the left ventricle, hypertension damages the smooth inner linings of cardiac arteries. As the blood flows through the blood vessels with elevated force, it can cause tears in the tissue. In response to the damage, cells that act as bandages collect around the damaged site. Furthermore, clumps of blood cells that stick together during stress to promote clotting can also collect around the damaged site. These damaged sites also attract cholesterol cells. The resulting covering is a combination of sticky and fatty tissue called plaque that collects over the damaged site. Plaque narrows the opening through which the blood flows. The presence of these plaques is the basis for coronary artery disease (CAD) or atherosclerosis. If the occlusion is narrow enough, there can be a squeezing pressure or pain in the chest commonly called angina. The chest pain warns that the heart muscle is not getting the oxygen it needs; it signals a need to decrease the demand on the heart (Randall & Romaine, 2005). The greater the occlusion, the greater the risk for a heart attack. Hypertension doesn't have symptoms, so blood pressure measurement should be a routine part of a medical examination. For those with hypertension, medication and lifestyle changes like losing weight, exercising, and appropriately managing stress often bring blood pressure into the normal range.

Another indicator of heart health involves the amount of cholesterol circulating in the blood. Cholesterol is a fatty substance created in the body. There are two types of cholesterol: high-density (HDL) and low-density (LDL). HDL cholesterol functions to protect arteries, while LDL cholesterol appears to accelerate the development of arterial plaque (Romaine & DeWitt, 1998). High levels of HDL cholesterol are desirable, while low levels of LDL cholesterol are also desirable.

Cholesterol also comes from the foods we eat. Foods high in saturated fat like red meat, butter, and cheese elevate LDL cholesterol levels. They also "leave fragments of fatty material along the walls of your arteries, like microscopic skid marks. Over time, these build into blockages" (Romaine & DeWitt, 1998). Lowering cholesterol can be accomplished both through medication and reducing the amount of saturated fat in the diet.

When the walls of the coronary arteries are damaged and inflamed, the body sends out a substance called C-reactive protein (CRP), which "migrates to the damaged vessel where it helps amplify the cascade of inflammation that is developing. . . . It helps trap bad cholesterol in the inflamed" area (Sapolsky, 2004). Measurement of CRP levels may be done through a blood test. High levels indicate a high degree of inflammation.

Chronic stress, high blood pressure, and high cholesterol can turn healthy coronary arteries into plaque-filled arteries that restrict blood flow and threaten the electrical integrity of the heart beat. While medications and surgical interventions can address acute crises, there are a lot of lifestyle changes that can prevent or mitigate heart problems. Since chronic stress appears to begin the cascade of environmental factors that damage coronary arteries, learning to manage chronic stress is an important coping skill. Coping skills can be enhanced by developing a stronger social support network, maintaining an appropriate work-life balance, drawing on spiritual or transcendent resources, and recognizing cognitive distortions and tendencies toward perfectionism, among others.

Diet and weight loss are also factors in maintaining good heart health. Since saturated fats are tasty but not heart healthy in large quantities, limiting saturated fat intake is essential. There are good fats that support heart health. Omega-3 fatty acids are believed to be natural blood thinners and are found in certain oily fish like mackerel, herring, and salmon (Jackson, 2000). Foods like peas, beans, lentils, bananas, and oat cereals contain soluble dietary fiber, which prevents cholesterol from being absorbed and lowers cholesterol blood levels (Jackson, 2000). Limiting saturated fat intake is also essential to maintaining a healthy weight.

One measure of body weight is body mass index (BMI). BMI is calculated based on an individual's height and weight, with scores ranging from under 16 to more than 40. Those who score between 18.5 and 25 are in the normal range. In fact, the higher the score, the greater the risk for heart disease. Waist-to-hip ratio is another measure of heart disease risk. Waist-to-hip ratio is "the relationship between the distance around the waist (waist circumference) and the distance around the hips at their broadest point. . . . A waist-to-hip ratio greater than 1.0 in men or greater than 0.8 in women is considered a risk factor for heart disease" (Randall & Romaine, 2005).

Exercise, particularly aerobic exercise, is another way to maintain heart health. In addition to helping with either weight loss or maintaining an ideal weight, it also increases HDL cholesterol, which is believed to protect arteries from plaque build-up, and lowers blood pressure, which also protects arteries. Exercise is also an excellent buffer against stress and heart disease. Additionally, exercise improves mood and may reduce reactivity to psychological stressors (Sapolsky, 2004).

There is certainly much more that can be said about keeping the heart healthy, but the essence of heart health is to keep it pumping regularly and without interruption for as long as possible. Managing stress, maintaining a good diet, losing weight, and engaging in regular aerobic exercise are all ways that can enable us to carry on.

*Kevin J. Eames*

*See also* Aerobic Exercise; Blood Pressure; Body Mass Index (BMI); Cholesterol; Stress.

### References

Jackson, G. *Heart Health at Your Fingertips: The Comprehensive and Medically Accurate Manual on How to Avid or Overcome Coronary Heart Disease and Other Heart Conditions.* London: London Class, 2000.

Randall, O.S., and D.D. Romaine. *The Encyclopedia of the Heart and Heart Disease.* New York: Facts on File Library of Health and Living, 2005.

Romaine, D.S., and D.E. DeWitt. *The Complete Idiot's Guide to a Happy Healthy Heart.* New York: Alpha Books, 1998.

Sapolsky, R. *Why Zebras Don't Get Ulcers.* New York: Henry Holt, 2004.

## HEPATITIS

The word *hepatitis* is a catchall term that refers to any inflammation (*–itis*) of the liver (*hepar*) and does not imply a specific cause or connote contagiousness. Inflammation of the liver is defined as an irritation or swelling of liver cells. Hepatitis is a term that encompasses many different causes. Only hepatitis caused by a *virus* (viral hepatitis) is potentially infectious to others. Consequently, hepatitis from causes other than viruses, such as alcohol (alcoholic hepatitis) or fat (fatty liver hepatitis), cannot be spread through food or by interpersonal or sexual contact.

Hepatitis is generally described using two broad categories. One category refers to how long a person has hepatitis, and the other category refers to what factor caused the hepatitis. Inflammation of the liver that lasts less than six months is known as acute hepatitis. Within six months, people with acute hepatitis are completely healed. The liver typically self-repairs any short-term damage it may have suffered, and no long-term consequences are suffered.

Viral hepatitis A is an example of acute hepatitis. Inflammation of the liver that lasts longer than six months is known as chronic hepatitis. People who progress from acute hepatitis to chronic hepatitis are at risk of developing cirrhosis (severe scarring of the liver that is typically irreversible) and the complications of cirrhosis, such as liver cancer, internal bleeding, and liver failure. Viral hepatitis B and viral hepatitis C can lead to chronic hepatitis.

Hepatitis is also described by its cause. Although hepatitis is most frequently caused by viruses, other stimuli may cause forms of the disease. These include autoimmune liver disease (autoimmune hepatitis), obesity (nonalcoholic fatty liver hepatitis), alcohol (alcoholic hepatitis), and some medications and herbs (toxin-induced hepatitis). This entry only discusses potentially infectious viral hepatitis. A virus is a tiny microorganism that is much smaller than bacteria. Its main activity and goal consists of reproducing more viruses and causing damage. A virus is capable of growth and multiplication only once it has entered a living cell. The main goal of the hepatitis virus is to enter a liver cell, reproduce more hepatitis viruses, destroy the cell, and move on to attack the next liver cell.

**History of Viral Hepatitis**   Viral hepatitis can be traced back to ancient times, when it was believed by scientists that some type of virus existed that attacked the liver, resulting in a yellow discoloration of the skin and eyes, now known as jaundice. From the late 1800s to the early 1900s, scientists believed that there were only two forms of viral hepatitis: infectious hepatitis and serum hepatitis.

In 1963 a major breakthrough in research occurred—the cause of serum hepatitis was identified, and the virus was given the name hepatitis B virus (HBV). It took an additional 10 years for scientists to isolate the cause of infectious hepatitis. This virus was given the name hepatitis A virus (HAV). Around this time, medical researchers realized that other forms of viral hepatitis must exist that were not caused by either HAV or HBV because there were still so many cases of hepatitis that were not the result of one of these two viruses. These cases of unknown viral origin were lumped into the category of non-A non-B (NANB) hepatitis. In 1989 the virus that caused the majority of NANB hepatitis was identified through cloning experiments and was named the hepatitis C virus (HCV).

Although the three most common viruses causing hepatitis are hepatitis A, B, and C, other hepatitis viruses also exist. The hepatitis delta virus (HDV), first isolated in the mid-1970s, was shown to exist only in the presence of HBV. The existence of another hepatitis virus, which is similar to HAV, was suggested throughout the 1980s but was not successfully cloned until 1990, at which point it was named the hepatitis E virus (HEV). Evidence of the existence of a hepatitis F virus (HFV) is, at present, only anecdotal. Hepatitis viruses that do not appear to be significant causes of liver disease are the hepatitis G virus (HGV), discovered in 1995; the transfusion-transmitted virus (TTV), identified in 1997; and the SEN-V, identified in 1999. Other viruses, such as herpes simplex virus and

Epstein-Barr virus, can also attack the liver. However, since the liver is not the principal organ damaged by these viruses, they are considered not to be a significant cause of viral hepatitis. Because approximately 10 percent of hepatitis cases still do not have an identified cause, researchers suspect that one or more as yet unidentified hepatitis viruses may exist.

**Incidence and Prevalence**   In the United States, HAV is the most common cause of acute viral hepatitis. Each year, approximately 134,000 Americans are infected with HAV. In fact, around 33 percent of all Americans have at some point been infected with HAV. Almost 100 percent of people who live in U.S. communities with substandard water and sewage sanitation systems, in addition to people living in economically developing countries such as countries in Africa, Asia, and Latin America, have been infected during childhood.

Approximately 2 billion people worldwide have been infected by hepatitis B, and almost 400 million people worldwide, including 1.25 million people in the United States, are chronic carriers of this virus. Approximately 65 million of those chronically infected will die of the disease. HBV is the single most common cause of cirrhosis and liver cancer worldwide. Hepatitis B is endemic in Southeast Asia, China, and Africa. In these areas of the world, more than 50 percent of the population has been exposed to HBV at some point in their lives. The virus has a relatively low prevalence in North America, Western Europe, and Australia, and accounts for only 5 to 10 percent of all chronic liver diseases in these areas.

HCV is the most common cause of chronic liver disease in the United States. It is estimated that almost 5 million Americans (more than 2% of the U.S. population) and more than 1 percent of the world's population are infected with HCV. Although the incidence of people becoming acutely infected with HCV is decreasing, approximately 8,000 to 12,000 deaths are attributed to hepatitis C each year.

**Hepatitis Transmission**   Hepatitis A virus is transmitted by the enteric or fecal-oral route. Enteric transmission consists of introduction of a virus into the body by way of the digestive tract. It occurs when a virus is present in the feces (fecal) of an infected person, and is then transmitted to another person via ingesting (oral) a small amount of infected stools. HBV, HDV, and HCV are transmitted via the parenteral route, meaning that these viruses are introduced into the body by any way other than via the intestinal tract. HBV is transmitted either through contaminated blood, during sexual contact, or from mother to child during childbirth. HDV only occurs in individuals who already have hepatitis B. HCV is transmitted only by blood-to-blood contact. This includes intravenous drug use, blood or blood product transfusions prior to 1992, and possibly tattoos and body-piercings. Sexual transmission of HCV is very rare, and transmission from mother to child at childbirth occurs in only 3 to 5 percent of cases.

**Symptoms and Signs of Hepatitis**   These may vary greatly. At one extreme, some people are very ill, with jaundice, fever, decreased appetite, abdominal pain, nausea, vomiting, and fatigue. At the other extreme, and more commonly, people with hepatitis may be totally asymptomatic—meaning that they have no symptoms—or may have vague, nonspecific symptoms, such as mild fatigue or flulike symptoms. The severity of symptoms that a person is experiencing often bears no correlation to the amount of damage done to the liver.

The only way to determine the type of hepatitis one has, what caused it, and how much damage has been done to the liver, is through a combination of tests. These include blood tests, such as liver function tests (LFTs) and hepatitis-specific blood tests (such as antibody and antigen tests); imaging studies done by a radiologist, such as a sonogram; and a liver biopsy (removal of a tiny piece of liver tissue using a special needle).

**Treatment and Prevention**  Medications used to treat viruses are known as antivirals. Treatment of acute hepatitis, such as hepatitis A, is mostly supportive. This means that treatment is based upon the symptoms being experienced, and no antiviral medication is typically needed.

Treatment of chronic hepatitis, such as chronic hepatitis B or C, is more complicated and depends on numerous factors. Treatment of hepatitis B may include an injectable medication known as interferon, or one or more oral medications either alone or in combination, known as nucleoside and/or nucleotide analogues.

Typically, hepatitis B cannot be cured, and treatment is lifelong. Treatment of chronic hepatitis C involves the use of pegylated interferon (a once-a-week injectable medication), in combination with an oral medication known as ribavirin, which is taken daily. Treatment lasts for 24 to 48 weeks. Hepatitis C is the only virus that can potentially be cured, with recovery rates greater than 55 percent.

Prevention is, of course, the best treatment for any disease, and fortunately, hepatitis A and B vaccinations are available. The development of the hepatitis B vaccine represents one of the most important advances in medicine. This is the first and only vaccine in history that can simultaneously prevent liver cancer, cirrhosis, and a sexually transmitted disease. This vaccine has been incorporated into the immunization programs of more than 80 countries, and routine hepatitis B vaccination of all newborns in the United States has been in mandatory since 1999. The hepatitis A vaccine has been available since 1995. There is currently no vaccination for hepatitis C.

*Melissa Palmer*

*See also* Vaccinations; Virus.

### References

Boyer, Thomas, Theresa Wright, and Michael Manns. *Zakim and Boyer's Hepatology.* New York: Malcolm Saunders, 2006.

Centers for Disease Control and Prevention. *Viral Hepatitis.* www.cdc.gov/ncidod/diseases/hepatitis/.

Palmer, Melissa. *Dr. Melissa Palmer's Guide to Hepatitis and Liver Disease.* New York: Penguin Putnam Avery Press, 2004.

Schiff, Eugene, et al. *Schiff's Diseases of the Liver.* 10th ed. New York: Lippincott Williams and Wilkins, 2006.

Thomas, Howard C., et al. *Viral Hepatitis.* New York: Wiley-Blackwell, 2005.

World Health Organization. *Hepatitis.* www.who.int/topics/hepatitis/en/.

## HIGH-FRUCTOSE CORN SYRUP

On your next trip to the supermarket, randomly review the lists of ingredients on a number of different processed foods, such as salad dressings, candy bars, sodas, sports drinks, jams, jellies, marinades, condiments, flavored yogurt, cereals, canned foods, breads, pancakes/waffles, and fruit drinks. There is a very good chance you will see the words "high-fructose corn syrup." You may well have heard those words before. But, have you ever considered what high-fructose corn syrup actually is? Most likely, like the vast majority of people, you have absolutely no idea. The goal of this section is to provide more information on high-fructose corn syrup. Since the product has become quite controversial, it is important to offer comments and research findings from various sources. Is high-fructose corn syrup detrimental to one's health and well-being? Should people read ingredient labels carefully and avoid consuming it? Or, is high-fructose corn syrup a useful addition to the marketplace and a product that has been safely used for decades? There are experts and strong opinions on both sides of the issue.

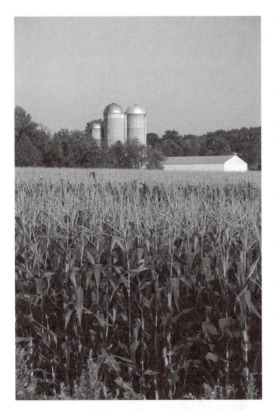

Summer corn grows in a field with the farm in the background. Corn syrup is less expensive to use than sugar and is a main ingredient in high-fructose corn syrup. (Stuart Monk/Dreams time.com)

Before proceeding, it is important to provide a definition. What exactly is high-fructose corn syrup? Truly ubiquitous, high-fructose corn syrup is a sweetener and preservative, which is made from changing the sugar (glucose) in corn syrup to fructose (another type of sugar). So, high-fructose corn syrup is a combination of glucose and fructose.

While high-fructose corn syrup is now found in many foods, until 1957, it did not exist. That year, researchers developed an enzyme (glucose isomerase) that could reconfigure the molecules in corn syrup and turn it into fructose. By the 1970s, the United States was producing large amounts of high-fructose corn syrup, and companies were adding the product to their recipes. It certainly made economic sense to use the sweetener, which is less expensive than sugar. And, it had the added bonus of extending the shelf life of processed foods. Moreover, corn was (and remains) an incredibly abundant crop in the United States.

Today, in the United States, companies make two main types of high-fructose corn syrup. One contains 42 percent high-fructose corn syrup; the other contains 55 percent. The one with 42 percent is about as sweet as sucrose or liquid sugar; the one with 55 percent is sweeter than liquid sugar (Orthodox Union). Table sugar has 100 percent sucrose, which is broken down by intestinal enzymes to 50 percent fructose and 50 percent glucose.

**Critics**   Not everyone sees high-fructose corn syrup as a desirable addition to the array of sweeteners. Many have linked it to a host of medical problems. For example, in a 2009 editorial in the *Townsend Letter,* Alan R. Gaby, MD, reported that he received a cover letter and unsolicited information from the Corn Refiners Association, the national trade association of the U.S. corn refining industry. In essence, the material stated that high-fructose corn syrup was nutritionally the same as sucrose (table sugar). Dr. Gaby began by noting that, "no one on the planet considers sugar to be a health food."

Yet, according to Dr. Gaby, there are other problems with foods that contain fructose. The malabsorption of fructose may result in "gastrointestinal symptoms that mimic irritable bowel syndrome." Furthermore, fructose is a "powerful" reducing sugar. "Reducing sugars promote the glycosylation of tissue proteins, which is a factor both in the complications of diabetes and in the aging process." Dr. Gaby concluded that his reading of the literature on high-fructose corn syrup has led him to believe that the effects "are somewhere between slightly worse than the effects of sucrose and seriously horrible" (Gaby, 2009).

**Excess Weight**   An article in a 2010 issue of the journal *Pharmacology, Biochemistry and Behavior* reported on two studies conducted by researchers from New Jersey and New York. The goal of this research was to learn the effects of high-fructose corn syrup on the body weight, body fat, and circulating triglycerides of rats. (Levels of triglycerides, a type of fat that travels in the blood, should be kept low.)

During the first study, which continued for eight weeks, male rats were divided into two groups. In addition to their standard diets, some rats were given water containing high-fructose corn syrup (half the concentration that would be found in soda) and other rats had water sweetened with regular table sugar (the same concentration found in soda). The researchers consistently found that the rats drinking the water with high-fructose corn syrup gained more weight than the rats drinking the water with sugar (Bocarsly et al., 2010).

The second study investigated the long-term effects of the consumption of high-fructose corn syrup on male and female rats. As in the previous study, researchers monitored body weight, body fat, and circulating triglycerides. This time, the study continued for six or seven months. The findings are certainly noteworthy. When compared to the rats that ate only rat food, the rats that also had access to high-fructose corn syrup had abnormal weight gain, increases in adipose fat, especially in the abdominal area, and elevated levels of circulating triglycerides. All of these factors negatively impact health. The researchers concluded that the "over-consumption of HFCS [high fructose corn syrup] could very well be a major factor in the 'obesity epidemic,' which correlates with the upsurge in the use of HFCS." Thus, the researchers noted, the increasing use of high-fructose corn syrup might be associated with the fact that about two-thirds of the U.S. population is now either overweight or obese (Bocarsly et al., 2010).

In a stunning piece of research presented to the 2010 meeting of the Endocrine Society and described in an article in *Pediatrics Week,* a doctoral student at the University of Bristol in the United Kingdom and her fellow researchers determined that when fructose is present as a child's fat cells mature, more cells mature into belly fat cells. Thus, children who consume high-fructose corn syrup in their sugary beverages, a very common occurrence in childhood, may gain excess weight in their abdominal area. Excess belly fat has been associated with cardiovascular problems and Type 2 diabetes. Moreover, the researchers found that these cells had a reduced ability to respond to insulin ("Fructose Sugar," 2010).

**Elevated Blood Pressure**  In a study conducted at the University of Colorado Denver Health Sciences Center and published in 2010 in the *Journal of the American Society of Nephrology,* researchers examined 4,528 adults 18 years of age or older with no history of high blood pressure (hypertension). Then, they calculated the subjects' intake of fructose (found in table sugar and high-fructose corn syrup). The researchers determined that the people who consumed as little as 74 grams of fructose per day (the equivalent of 2.5 sugary soft drinks) increased their risk of developing high blood pressure. The researchers observed that their findings "suggest that high fructose intake, in the form of added sugar, independently associates with high BP [blood pressure] levels among US adults without a history of hypertension" (Jalal et al., 2010).

In another study, published in 2010 in *Circulation,* Louisiana researchers reviewed the dietary intake of sugar-sweetened beverages, such as sodas with high-fructose corn syrup, and the levels of blood pressure in 810 adults. The researchers found that, over an 18-month period of time, reducing the consumption of as little as one serving per day significantly reduced blood pressure. Similar results were not obtained with diet drinks. The researchers concluded that the reduction in consumption of sugar-sweetened beverages and sugar may be "an important dietary strategy" to lower blood pressure (Chen et al., 2010).

**Early Kidney Disease**  In a cross-sectional analysis published in 2008 in *PLoS ONE,* researchers reviewed the association between the onset of early kidney disease and the consumption of sodas containing high-fructose corn syrup. The cohort (group studied) included 9,358 people who were at least 20 years old and had no history of diabetes. While drinking sodas containing high-fructose corn syrup did not appear to increase the risk of early kidney disease in men, women who reported drinking two or more sodas in the previous 24 hours were 1.86 times as likely to have albuminuria, a marker for early kidney disease. (Albuminuria means that there is an excess amount of a protein called albumin in the urine. Since the kidneys normally filter albumin from the urine, albumin in the urine means that the kidneys are not working as well as they should—a sign of disease.) At the same time, the consumption of one or fewer sodas appeared to cause no harm. The researchers noted that, "the finding of an individual-level association between sugary soda consumption and albuminuria are consistent with the hypothesis that HFCS [high fructose corn syrup] is contributing to the kidney disease epidemic" (Shoham et al., 2008).

**Metabolic Syndrome** In a randomized, controlled trial published in 2010 in the *International Journal of Obesity,* Spanish researchers investigated whether the consumption of high amounts of fructose could cause symptoms of metabolic syndrome, also known as insulin resistance, in healthy adult men, with an average age of 51. (With metabolic syndrome, fat, muscle, and liver cells do not respond well to the hormone insulin. As a result, the pancreas makes excessive amounts of insulin. People with metabolic syndrome also have too much fat around the waist, high levels of blood cholesterol, and borderline or high blood pressure. They have a significant risk for the development of Type 2 diabetes and cardio-vascular disease.)

For two weeks, 74 men, who were mostly overweight, consumed 200 grams of fructose each day. (A typical adult in the United States consumes about 50 to 70 grams of fructose each day.) To avoid gastrointestinal upset, the men were advised to spread this consumption throughout the day. After such a relatively short period of time, the researchers observed increases in levels of triglycerides, blood pressure, and body mass index (BMI) and decreases in high-density lipoprotein (HDL or "good") cholesterol. Twenty-five to 33 percent of the participants developed new-onset metabolic syndrome. These are truly remarkable findings. The researchers commented that, "excessive fructose intake could have a causal role in the current epidemics of hypertension, obesity, and diabetes" (Perez-Pozo et al., 2010).

**Triglyceride Elevations** In a study published in the *Journal of Clinical Endocrinology and Metabolism,* on two separate occasions, researchers from Pennsylvania and California provided 17 obese men and women with identical meals served at the University of Pennsylvania. During one meal, the beverage was sweetened with glucose; during the other meal, the beverage was sweetened with fructose.

The findings were striking. Over a 24-hour period, when the subjects drank the fructose-sweetened beverage, the total amount of triglycerides was almost 200 percent higher. While fructose increased the levels of triglycerides in all of the subjects, the increases were most dramatic in the subjects with metabolic syndrome. So, the subjects who were already dealing with this prediabetic condition had the highest increases in triglycerides. The researchers commented that the consumption of fructose "may exacerbate an already adverse metabolic profile in many obese subjects" (Teff et al., 2009).

**Type 2 Diabetes** At the August 2007 national meeting of the American Chemical Society, which was held in Boston, Chi-Tang Ho, PhD, chair of the Department of Food Science at Rutgers University in New Jersey, and his colleagues presented a report linking Type 2 diabetes to the consumption of carbonated soft drinks that contain high-fructose corn syrup. According to the researchers, soft drinks that are sweetened with high-fructose corn syrup have elevated amounts of reactive carbonyls, reactive compounds that have the potential to activate cell and tissue damage that may result in Type 2 diabetes.

During their investigation, the researchers tested 11 different soft drinks that contained high-fructose corn syrup. The beverages had "astonishingly high" levels of reactive carbonyls. Table sugar does not contain these reactive carbonyls. Dr. Ho said that people with Type 2 diabetes have higher levels of reactive carbonyls in their blood, and these have been associated with diabetes complications. From his study, Dr. Ho determined that one can of soda has about five times the concentration of reactive carbonyls found in the blood of people with Type 2 diabetes. (On an interesting side note, the researchers found that a compound contained in green tea lowered the levels of reactive carbonyls in carbonated soda with high-fructose corn syrup by up to 50 percent.) Dr. Ho noted that people living in the United States consume far too much high-fructose corn syrup, and there is a growing amount of evidence against it (Medical News Today).

**Liver Disease and Type 2 Diabetes**  In a study published in 2008 in the *American Journal of Physiology—Gastrointestinal and Liver Physiology,* researchers from Saint Louis University in Missouri fed male mice a diet that was high in fat, trans fats, and high-fructose corn syrup. In addition, the mice were prevented from exercising. Other mice, that ate alternative combinations of foods, served as controls. In short, the goal of the researchers was to have the mice emulate the fast food and sedentary lifestyle followed by many Americans, and then observe the consequences of these actions.

Though the researchers were fairly certain that they would see health concerns by the end of the 16-week study, after only a few weeks, the experimental group of mice began to show evidence of serious health problems. The mice were developing liver disease and the early stages of Type 2 diabetes. At the end of 16 weeks, the experimental group weighed 42 percent more than the control group of mice that were fed standard mice food and water without high-fructose corn syrup. According to the researchers, there are data to support the fact that fructose suppresses the feeling of fullness. This stands in contrast to fiber-filled foods, which make people feel full fairly quickly (Tetri et al., 2008).

In a study published in 2010 in *Hepatology,* researchers from Duke University, Johns Hopkins University, and the University of Colorado reviewed the association between consumption of high-fructose corn syrup and scarring of the liver (fibrosis) in patients with nonalcoholic fatty liver disease. The cohort included 427 adults. Only 19 people with liver fibrosis reported that they did not consume beverages with high-fructose corn syrup. On the other hand, 52 percent consumed between one and six servings of beverages with high-fructose corn syrup each week. Twenty-nine percent reported consuming these beverages every day. Since increased fibrosis of the liver appeared to be related to the consumption of high-fructose corn syrup, the researchers noted that they have identified a "readily modifiable environmental risk factor that may ameliorate disease progression in patients with NAFLD [nonalcoholic fatty liver disease]" (Abdelmalek et al., 2010). Thus, people with nonalcoholic liver disease may be advised to reduce or eliminate their consumption of beverages with high-fructose corn syrup.

**Pancreatic Cancer**  In a study published in 2010 in *Cancer Research,* researchers from the David Geffen School of Medicine at the University of California, Los Angeles, cultivated human pancreatic tumors in Petri dishes. They added glucose to one set of cells and fructose to another. The researchers found that the pancreatic cells were able to differentiate between the two types of sugar, and they metabolized the sugars differently. While they already knew that cancer cells were supported by glucose, they noted that the cancer cells used fructose to proliferate. The researchers wrote that their findings have "major significance for cancer patients given dietary refined fructose consumption and indicate that efforts to reduce refined fructose intake or inhibit fructose-mediated actions may disrupt cancer growth" (Liu et al., 2010).

**The Question of Mercury**   In January 2009, two different bombshell reports were released. The Institute of Agriculture and Trade Policy issued "Not So Sweet: Missing Mercury and High Fructose Corn Syrup," which described how researchers had found the toxin mercury in almost one-third of the brands of foods that listed high-fructose corn syrup as the first or second ingredient. These brands included Yoplait, Hershey's, Hunt's, Quaker, and Manwich. While most of the beverages tested did not have mercury, mercury was found in snack bars, yogurt, chocolate syrup, barbecue sauce, strawberry jelly, chocolate milk, and catsup. Many of these foods are marketed to children (Institute for Agriculture and Trade Policy).

Second, an article in *Environmental Health* revealed that mercury was found in 9 out of 20 tested samples of commercial high-fructose corn syrup, which came from three different manufacturers. How can that be? During the process of manufacturing high-fructose corn syrup, mercury-grade caustic soda may be used to separate cornstarch from the kernels. Also known as sodium hydroxide or lye, caustic soda is produced in industrial chlorine (chlor-alkali) plants (Dufault et al., 2009). Since Americans tend to consume large amounts of high-fructose corn syrup, there remains concern that they may be harmed by mercury. Of particular worry is the possible harm to children.

According to the institute report, manufacturers of high-fructose corn syrup "don't need to buy mercury-grade caustic soda." It is not necessary to use mercury to produce high-fructose corn syrup. "While most chlorine plants around the world have switched to newer, cleaner technologies, some still reply on the use of mercury" (Institute for Agriculture and Trade Policy).

**HFCS Supporters**   Of course, the Corn Refiners Association, the previously mentioned national trade organization that represents the industry, strongly supports high-fructose corn syrup. The website of the organization lists a number of benefits derived from high-fructose corn syrup. For example, "in addition to providing sweetness at a level equivalent to sugar, high fructose corn syrup enhances fruit and spice flavors in foods such as yogurt and spaghetti sauces, gives chewy breakfast bars their soft texture and also protects freshness. High fructose corn syrup keeps products fresh by maintaining consistent moisture" (Corn Refiners Association).

The Corn Refiners Association notes that high-fructose corn syrup is a natural product made from corn. "High fructose corn syrup contains no artificial or synthetic ingredient or color additives." It does not cause people to become obese. "U.S. Department of Agriculture data show that per capita consumption of high fructose corn syrup is actually on the decline, yet obesity and diabetes rates continue to rise. In fact, obesity rates are rising around the world, including Mexico,

Australia, and Europe, even though the use of high fructose corn syrup outside the United States is limited" (Corn Refiners Association).

The website mentions two studies presented to the 2010 annual meeting of the Endocrine Society by James Rippe, MD, a prominent cardiologist. In the double-blind studies, 63 overweight and obese people were placed on the "weight-stable" American Dietetic Association exchange diet for 10 weeks. As part of their daily food intake, the subjects consumed either 10 or 20 percent table sugar or high-fructose corn syrup in their milk. At the beginning and end of the trials, the researchers measured body mass, body composition, waist circumference, and they took fasting blood samples. The researchers found "no difference between table sugar and high fructose corn syrup on weight gain or any changes in risk factors for metabolic syndrome or insulin resistance" (Corn Refiners Association). It should be noted that these studies were funded by an unrestricted education research grant from the Corn Refiners Association.

Another supporter of the use of high-fructose corn syrup is John S. White, PhD, founder and president of White Technical Research in Argenta, Illinois. Dr. White has written a number of articles on the topic, including one that was published in a 2008 issue of the *American Journal of Clinical Nutrition*. In this article, Dr. White said that high-fructose corn syrup "is not meaningfully different in composition or metabolism from other fructose- glucose sweeteners like sucrose, honey, and fruit juice." And, high-fructose corn syrup, according to Dr. White, is not "uniquely" responsible for the high rates of obesity. Dr. White acknowledged that research using extremely high amounts of fructose, "especially when fed as the sole carbohydrate source," has resulted in "metabolic upset," but he noted that, "there is no evidence that the common fructose-glucose sweeteners do the same." As a result, the "studies using extreme carbohydrate diets may be useful for probing biochemical pathways, but they have no relevance to the human diet or to current consumption." Dr. White maintained that the connection between high-fructose corn syrup and obesity "is neither supported in the United States nor worldwide" (White, 2008).

A year later, in 2009, Dr. White wrote a similar article for the *Journal of Nutrition*. In this piece, he emphasized his belief that the researchers who have presented "data gathered under extreme experimental methods" mislead those who are "uninformed." Such data fail to account for the far more modest amount of high-fructose corn syrup in actual human diets. Eventually, an atmosphere of distrustful is created, causing people to shun "what, by all rights, should be considered a sage and innocuous sweetener" (White, 2009).

**Other Experts Show Support for HFCS**   In an article published in 2009 in the *Journal of the American College of Nutrition,* members of the American Medical Association's Council on Science and Public Health offered a comprehensive review of high-fructose corn syrup. They acknowledged that some researchers have found that "fructose has been directly associated with adverse health outcomes." However, the members of the council wrote that "most caloric sweeteners contain fructose, and there is little evidence, at present, that HFCS [high fructose corn syrup] contributes more to obesity or other conditions than sucrose does." So, all types of sugar may well play a role in obesity. In some ways, high-fructose corn syrup is better than sugar. "Compared to sucrose, HFCS provides foods with better flavor enhancement, stability, freshness, texture, color, pourability, and consistency." The council members concluded that there is currently "insufficient evidence to ban or otherwise restrict use of HFCS or other fructose-containing sweeteners in the food supply or to require the use of warning labels on products containing HFCS." Still, "dietary advice to limit consumption of all caloric sweeteners, including HFCS, is warranted" (Moeller et al., 2009).

Two papers, both published in 2010, from researchers at the University of Lausanne in Lausanne, Switzerland, also offered support for the safe use of high-fructose corn syrup. The first, published in *Physiological Reviews,* agreed that the testing of high-fructose corn syrup in animals has resulted in a number of medical problems such as obesity, Type 2 diabetes, and high blood pressure. However, the results of tests in humans are "less compelling." While it is true "that very high fructose intake can have deleterious metabolic effects in humans as in rodents, the role of fructose in the development of the current epidemic of metabolic disorders remains controversial." What is clear, the researchers noted, is that the high intake of all types of sweetened beverages is "associated with a high energy intake, increased body weight, and the occurrence of metabolic and cardiovascular disorders." At the same time, "there is . . . no unequivocal evidence that fructose intake at moderate doses is directly related with adverse metabolic effects." Furthermore, "there is . . . no direct evidence for more serious metabolic consequences of high fructose corn syrup versus sucrose consumption" (Tappy & Lê, 2010). The second report, which was published in *Nutrition,* repeated the contention that there is "only limited evidence that fructose per se, when consumed in moderate amounts, has deleterious effects." According to the researchers, it is far more likely that the development of metabolic syndrome is a result of excess caloric intake. "Consumption of sweetened beverages is however clearly associated with excess calorie intake, and an increased risk of diabetes and cardiovascular diseases through an increase in body weight. This has led to the recommendation to limit the daily intake of sugar calories" (Tappy et al., 2010).

In a study that was published in 2008 in *Bone,* West Virginia University researchers investigated the effects of different sugar-sweetened beverages on bone mass and strength. Adolescent female Sprague-Dawley rats were randomly assigned to consume deionized distilled water (control) or deionized distilled water that contained glucose, sucrose, fructose, or high-fructose corn syrup. At the end of eight weeks, a number of different bone measurements were taken. The researchers found that the "differences in bone and mineral measurements appeared most pronounced between rats drinking glucose versus fructose-sweetened beverages." And, "the results suggested that glucose rather than fructose exerted more deleterious effects on mineral balance and bone" (Tsanzi, Light, & Tou, 2008).

Earlier a study was presented in which high-fructose corn syrup was found to elevate levels of triglycerides in the blood. Another article, published in 2009 in the *Journal of Nutrition,* offered different findings. The researchers, who included the previously mentioned Dr. Rippe, agreed that excess fructose consumption may be "detrimental" to metabolic health. But, they added that high-fructose corn syrup "does not seem to be any more insidious than other caloric sweeteners." All sweeteners contribute to weight gain, and "rates of overweight and obesity have been on a steady rise for decades" (Angelopoulos et al., 2009).

The negative toll that all types of sugar consumption takes on human lipid levels was stressed in a cross-sectional study that was published in 2010 in *JAMA: The Journal of the American Medical Association*. Researchers from a variety of locations assessed the diets and lipid profiles of more than 6,000 U.S. adults. The adults, who were living within their communities and eating their normal diets, were divided into groups according to their consumption of sugars—less than 5 percent of calories, 5 percent to less than 10 percent, 10 percent to less than 17.5 percent, 17.5 percent to less than 25 percent, and 25 percent or more of total calories.

The researchers determined that, on average, the daily consumption of sugar represented 15.8 percent of the total caloric intake. That figure is appreciably higher than the 10.6 percent calculated in 1977–1978. The researchers also found a significant association between increased intake of sugar-sweetened foods and reduced HDL cholesterol levels and elevated triglycerides. There was clear evidence that higher sugar consumption compromised cardiovascular health (Welsh et al., 2010).

**What Should People Do?** It is very evident that the majority of people need to reduce their consumption of all types of sugar. As for high-fructose corn syrup, more studies are needed. However, without a doubt, everyone should reduce their consumption of soda, fast food, and all types of processed or refined foods. The rates of overweight and obesity are only fueling the costs of health care in the United States. And, they are causing people to become chronically ill at younger ages. A diet containing higher amounts of fruits and vegetables automatically contains lower levels of sugar. That is a diet everyone should follow.

The Corn Refiners Association, an association representing high-fructose corn syrup manufacturers, has petitioned the FDA for a product name change. It wants to call the ingredient "corn sugar," which it suggests will better communicate the product and clear up any consumer confusion. The FDA can take six months to respond, and if the name change is accepted the process to implement the change may take up to another 18 months. If accepted, consumers could see the new name in 2012.

*Myrna Chandler Goldstein*

*See also* Cancer; Diabetes; Hypertension; Obesity.

### References

Abdelmalek, Manal F., Ayako Suzuki, Cynthia Guy, A. Unlp-Arida, R. Colvin, R.J. Johnson, and A.M. Diehl. "Increased Fructose Consumption Is Associated with Fibrosis Severity in Patients with Nonalcoholic Liver Disease." *Hepatology* 51, no. 6 (June 2010): 1961–71.

Angelopoulos, Theodore J., Joshua Lowndas, Linda Zukley, et al. "The Effect of High-Fructose Corn Syrup Consumption on Triglycerides and Uric Acid." *Journal of Nutrition* 139, no. 6 (June 2009): 1242S–45S.

Bocarsly, Miriam E., Elyse S. Powell, Nicole M. Avena, and Bartley G. Hoebel. "High-Fructose Corn Syrup Causes Characteristics of Obesity in Rats: Increased Body Weight, Body Fat and Triglyceride Levels." *Pharmacology, Biochemistry and Behavior* 97, no. 1 (2010): 101–106, doi: 10.1016/j.pbb.2010.02.012.

Chen, L., B. Caballero, D.C. Mitchell, et al. "Reducing Consumption of Sugar-Sweetened Beverages Is Associated with Reduced Blood Pressure: A Prospective Study among United States Adults." *Circulation* 121, no. 22 (June 8, 2010): 2398–2406.

Corn Refiners Association. www.SweetSurprise.com.

Dufault, Renee, Blaise LeBlanc, Roseanne Schnoll, et al. "Mercury from Chlor-Alkali Plants: Measured Concentrations in Food Product Sugar." *Environmental Health* 8, no. 2 (January 26, 2009): 2+.

"Fructose Sugar Makes Maturing Human Fat Cells Fatter, Less Insulin-Sensitive." *Pediatrics Week,* July 10, 2010, 162.

Gaby, Alan R. "Editorial: High-Fructose Corn Syrup Propaganda." *Townsend Letter* 309 (April 2009): 83.

Institute for Agriculture and Trade Policy. "Not So Sweet: Missing Mercury and High Fructose Corn Syrup." 2009. www.iatp.org.

Jalal, Diana I., Gerard Smits, Richard J. Johnson, and Michel Chonchol. "Increased Fructose Associates with Elevated Blood Pressure." *Journal of the American Society of Nephrology* 21 (2010).

Liu, H., D. Huang, D.L. McArthur, et al. "Fructose Induces Transketolase Flux to Promote Pancreatic Cancer Growth." *Cancer Research* 70, no. 15 (August 1, 2010): 6368–76.

Medical News Today. August 2007. www.medicalnewstoday.com.

Moeller, Suzen M., Sandra Adamson Fryhofer, Albert J. Osbahr III, and Carolyn B. Robinowitz. "The Effects of High Fructose Syrup." *Journal of the American College of Nutrition* 28, no. 6 (2009): 619–26.

Perez-Pozo, S.E., J. Schold, T. Nakagawa, et al. "Excessive Fructose Intake Induces the Features of Metabolic Syndrome in Healthy Adult Men: Role of Uric Acid in the Hypertensive Response." *International Journal of Obesity* 34, no. 3 (March 2010): 454–61.

Shoham, David A., Ramon Durazo-Arvizu, Holly Kramer, et al. "Sugary Soda Consumption and Albuminuria: Results from the National Health and Nutrition Examination Survey, 1999–2004." *PLoS ONE* 3, no. 10 (October 17, 2008): e3431.

Tappy, L., and K.A. Lê. "Metabolic Effects of Fructose and the Worldwide Increase in Obesity." *Physiological Reviews* 90, no. 1 (January 2010): 23–46.

Tappy, L., K.A. Lê, C. Tran, and N. Paquot. "Fructose and Metabolic Diseases: New Findings, New Questions." *Nutrition* 13 (2010).

Teff, Karen L., Joanne Grudziak, Raymond R. Townsend, et al. "Endocrine and Metabolic Effects of Consuming Fructose- and Glucose-Sweetened Beverages with Meals in Obese Men and Women: Influence of Insulin Resistance on Plasma Triglyceride Responses." *Journal of Clinical Endocrinology and Metabolism* 94, no. 5 (2009): 1562–69.

Tetri, L.H., M. Basaranoglu, E.M. Brunt, et al. "Severe NAFLD with Hepatic Necroinflammatory Changes in Mice Fed Trans Fats and a High-Fructose Corn Syrup Equivalent." *American Journal of Physiology—Gastrointestinal and Liver Physiology* 295, no. 5 (November 2008): G987–95.

Tsanzi, Embedzayi, Heather R. Light, and Janet C. Tou. "The Effect of Feeding Different Sugar-Sweetened Beverages to Growing Female Sprague-Dawley Rats on Bone Mass and Strength." *Bone* 42, no. 5 (May 2008): 960–68.

Welsh, Jean A., Andrea Sharma, Jerome L. Abramson, et al. "Caloric Sweetener Consumption and Dyslipidemia among US Adults." *Journal of the American Medical Association* 303, no. 15 (April 21, 2010): 1490–97.

White, John S. "Misconceptions about High-Fructose Corn Syrup: Is It Uniquely Responsible for Obesity, Reactive Dicarbonyl Compounds, and Advanced Glycation Endproducts?" *Journal of Nutrition* 139, no. 6 (June 2009): 1219S–27S.

White, John S. "Straight Talk about High Fructose Corn Syrup: What It Is and What It Ain't." *American Journal of Clinical Nutrition* 88, no. 6 (December 2008): 1716S–21S.

## HMO. *See* MANAGED CARE

## HOMEOPATHY

Homeopathy is an alternative medicine that employs the law of similars ("like cures") in its remedies. Instead of confronting an illness using symptom-suppressing drugs, homeopathy treats ailments by introducing the same allergen that is causing the problem. The theory behind this practice states that a small dose of a particular substance will cure the same symptoms that it produces in large doses. If there is a substance that produces symptoms of disease in a healthy person, the same substance in minute amounts can cure those symptoms in a sick person. It is claimed that these remedies, composed of highly diluted plant, animal, and mineral substances, stimulate the body's defenses so that it may heal and protect itself.

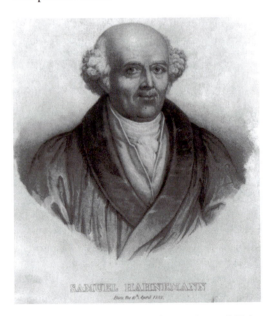

Homeopathy was developed by Dr. Samuel Hahnemann in the late 1700s. (Library of Congress)

This method is used to treat many conditions, and it has been in continuous use in Europe for more than 200 years. It was in the vein of the Hippocratic "law of similars" teachings that German physician Samuel Hahnemann (1755–1843) first developed the technique. He conducted his initial experiment on himself and was able to show that Peruvian bark, which contains quinine, could not only be used to treat malaria, but also caused malarialike symptoms in a healthy person.

Homeopathy is considered a holistic form of medicine that helps the body heal itself. It can be used as a treatment for chronic and acute ailments, and to prevent illness. Instead of suppressing symptoms of disease like conventional allopathic medicine, it introduces minute quantities of allergens. Adherents believe this method encourages the body's immune response to heal itself. There are between 2,000 and 2,500 homeopathic remedies. Each preparation contains minute amounts of an individual substance that is diluted with milk, sugar, or alcohol and then shaken. This process is called potentization and is repeated up to 200 times or more. The further the substance is diluted, the more potent it is thought to be. A remedy may also be administered in pill form, by being placed directly under the tongue, where it can dissolve and easily enter the bloodstream.

When prescribing a remedy, the homeopath considers the patient's personal life, habits, emotions, diet, exercise, sleep patterns, complexion, appetite, moods, libido, posture, environment, and the weather, along with the symptoms she exhibits. While the symptoms may be the same in many people, the treatment for each person will vary. Homeopathic medicine is considered safe for everyone, including babies, but is only to be taken as it is needed. It is used to treat almost every physical condition.

It is administered in emergencies to help with shock or to encourage the healing of injuries, and is also commonly called upon to treat emotional conditions like panic, anxiety, and fear. A typical treatment requires a consultation and a return visit once or twice a month to assess and adjust the prescription. Chronic conditions require extended treatment, while acute disorders may respond after just one visit.

The American Institute of Homeopathy, the United States' oldest medical society, played a significant role in the country at the turn of 20th century, when 15 percent of practicing physicians were homeopaths. At that time, the nation housed 22 homeopathic medical schools, including ones at Boston University and New York Medical College, 100 practicing hospitals, and more than 1,000 homeopathic pharmacies. However, the paramount advancement of conventional pharmaceuticals eventually eclipsed homeopathic medicine. The formation of the American Medical Association, and later the Food and Drug Administration (FDA), allowed allopathic medicine to advance and preside over homeopathy using political and legislative power.

In recent years, homeopathic medicine has experienced a resurgence of popularity. It is widely used and widely available in Western countries. Studies in the well-respected *Journal of Pediatrics* and *Lancet* have proven that it is effective, and a review of multiple studies compiled by the *British Medical Journal* also concluded that the use of homeopathy had positive results. However, it has yet to be accepted as a standard, mainstream form of treatment because there has been no scientific way of explaining how or why it works.

The mystery of homeopathy's function has to do with levels of dilution. The more diluted the tincture, the more powerful the results, yet in these concoctions, the infinitesimally small amounts of a substance can be diluted to the point where no original molecules remain. This leaves questions as to the true chemistry of the substance and how it produces the claimed healing results.

Those familiar with holistic and Eastern medicine profess that the healing effects of homeopathic medicine are caused by a remedy's subtle energy, which influences a person's vital force. Some homeopath proponents have said that the substance leaves a "holographic imprint" of energy in the dilution, which, in turn, acts upon a person's energetic qualities. They claim that this corrects a person's energy field, allowing the body to function with a higher degree of efficiency and to eliminate the manifestation of symptoms. These hypothetical qualities of electromagnetism have not been proven or understood. Similar concepts, such as the chi in traditional Chinese medicine or the *prana* in Ayurveda, are widely accepted as the key to healing in the East. Western science has no parallel concept and does not accept it as a legitimate form of treatment.

*Brian Regal*

*See also* Ayurveda; Immune System/Lymphatic System; Reiki; Traditional Chinese Medicine.

### References

Horrocks, Thomas A. *Popular Print and Popular Medicine: Almanacs and Health Advice in Early America*. Amherst: University of Massachusetts Press, 2008.
MacEoin, Beth. *Homeopathy: The Practical Guide for the 21st Century*. London: Kyle Cathie, 2007.
Starr, Paul. *The Social Transformation of American Medicine*. New York: Basic Books, 1984.

## HUMAN CHORIONIC GONADOTROPIN (HCG)

There are many misconceptions about human chorionic gonadotropin (HCG), especially concerning its use as a diet aid and its use by athletes to counteract anabolic steroid problems. The fact is that HCG is a hormone produced by women during pregnancy. The production of the hormone increases up to the 10th week of pregnancy and then decreases. This early increase makes it useful as the key ingredient in home pregnancy kits where a small stick measures HCG levels in a woman's urine to determine if she is pregnant.

However, thanks to Internet blogs the use of HCG as a diet aid has once again gotten new attention. Today, the form of the hormone has been adapted, making it easier for dieters to use. It now comes in a lozenge that can be placed under the tongue and ingested rather than injected. It was in the 1970s that HGC first awakened public interest as an important partner in a weight-loss plan that combined daily injections of the hormone with a 500-calorie-per-day diet.

The official love affair with HCG was short. By 1974 the Food and Drug Administration (FDA) issued a statement that expressed growing concern about the continued use of HCG in weight-loss clinics around the country, saying there was no evidence that the drug was effective in treating obesity. Doctors said that anyone following a diet that low in calories would lose weight no matter what foods were eaten or injections taken. Problems that developed from the injections included blood clots, headaches, and depression.

At that time the FDA also announced that the drug HCG must bear a label saying it is worthless for weight loss. The report stressed that any active drug can have unexpected adverse reactions. The FDA later issued an alert on the dangers of contaminated HCG reportedly being used by athletes and bodybuilders to counter the effects of steroids.

Officials believe the hormone injections are used by athletes to kick-start the production of testosterone following the completion of a steroid cycle. The steroids, particularly synthetic testosterone, confuse the body and stop normal testosterone production when they are injected. HCG is now banned by all professional sports organizations, but its use continues to be a problem. In 2009, baseball player Manny Ramirez received a 50-game suspension when league officials linked him to HCG use. In the spring of 2010, officials with the National Football League (NFL) suspended linebacker Brian Cushing from the first four games of the season when he tested positive for HCG. Along with its use in pregnancy testing, doctors legitimately prescribe HCG to treat cases of undescended testicles in men or infertility in women.

*Sharon Zoumbaris*

*See also* Steroids.

### References

Ballin, J.C., and P.L. White. "Fallacy and Hazard: Human Chorionic Gonadotropin Diet and Weight Reduction." *Journal of the American Medical Association* 230, no. 5 (November 4, 1974): 693.

"By the Way, Doctor: What Do You Know about the HCG Diet?" *Harvard Women's Health Watch* (May 1, 2010).

"Human Chorionic Gonadotropin." *Gale Encyclopedia of Science.* Farmington Hills, MI: Thompson Gale, 2001.

"Manny Tests Positive, Is Suspended 50 Games." NBC Sports. http://nbscsports.msnbc.com/id/30622607.

Murphy, Austin. "Dopey Ballot." *Sports Illustrated* 112, no. 22, May 24, 2010, 18.

## HUMAN IMMUNODEFICIENCY VIRUS (HIV)

The end result of infection with the human immunodeficiency virus (HIV) is the infectious disease acquired immune deficiency syndrome (AIDS). In June 1981, AIDS was first recognized in the medical literature, but at that time, the causative agent of AIDS was unknown, so the disease was given several names describing either symptoms exhibited by patients or social characteristics of those patients. "Wasting disease," "slim disease," "opportunistic infections," and "Kaposi's sarcoma (KS)" were used singly or together to describe the symptoms.

The disease, first recognized in the homosexual communities of large U.S. cities, was also called "Gay-Related Immune Deficiency (GRID)" and "Gay cancer" to describe a salient identity of patients. By 1984 medical researchers had identified a retrovirus as the causative agent in the disease. In 1986 this virus was named Human Immunodeficiency Virus (HIV), and in 1987 the disease AIDS was defined by the U.S. Centers for Disease Control and Prevention (CDC) and the World Health Organization (WHO) as the end stage of infection with this virus—hence the name HIV/AIDS.

HIV is transmitted by intimate contact between bodily fluids. Over 2 to 10 years, the virus kills key controlling cells of the body's immune system until an infected person has no immunological defenses against many different opportunistic infections and cancers. Because infected and contagious people appear healthy for many years, HIV has spread rapidly in geographic locations where individuals engage in sexual relations with many partners, infected women become pregnant and transmit the virus unknowingly to their babies, and injecting drug abusers share needles. In areas of the world with large populations and few medical resources, the rapid spread of HIV and subsequent epidemic of AIDS has destabilized societies by killing the young adults most likely to become infected and thus leaving children without parents and communities without leadership.

**Effects of the Virus** HIV is a retrovirus, composed of ribonucleic acid (RNA). The term *retro* originates from the property of these viruses to transcribe themselves, via an enzyme called reverse transcriptase, into a DNA form that is then integrated into the invaded cell's genome. The creation of new viruses then becomes a part of the cell's own genetic instructions. In the early decades of the 20th century, the AIDS virus mutated in West Africa from a form that infected only chimpanzees to one that could infect humans.

Retroviruses had been known to cause disease in animals since 1911, when Peyton Rous (1879–1970), a scientist at the Rockefeller Institute for Medical Research in New York City, discovered that a particular type of cancer in chickens could be transmitted by grinding up a tumor and injecting it into another chicken. By the 1970s, the molecular structure of retroviruses was known, but none had ever been identified as causing disease in humans. In 1980 Robert C. Gallo (b. 1937) and his colleagues at the National Cancer Institute, National Institutes of Health, in Bethesda, Maryland, demonstrated the existence of retroviruses that caused cancer in humans by triggering unchecked replication of T cells.

In contrast, HIV, the retrovirus that causes AIDS, kills the helper T cells that regulate the immune system, thus destroying the body's natural defenses against opportunistic infections and cancers. When the initial infection takes place, HIV causes fever, headache, malaise, and enlarged lymph nodes—symptoms similar to those of many other virus infections. These symptoms disappear within a week or two, but the infected individual is highly contagious at this point, with HIV present in large quantities in genital fluids.

For the next 10 years in adults (and approximately 2 years in infants infected at birth), there may be no disease symptoms at all. During this period, however, HIV is destroying the T cells that are the body's key infection fighters, and this decline is measurable. Once the immune system has reached a certain level of disruption, the infected person begins to experience symptoms. Lymph nodes may enlarge again, energy may decline, and weight may be lost. Fevers and sweats may become frequent. Yeast infections may become frequent or persistent, and pelvic inflammatory disease in women may not respond to treatment. Short-term memory loss may be observed. Infected children may grow slowly or have many bouts of sickness.

The CDC defines the advent of full-blown AIDS as the moment when an individual infected with HIV experiences a T cell count below 200 per cubic millimeter of blood (healthy adults have T cell counts of 1,000 or more). This is the point at which the immune system is so ravaged that it cannot fight off bacteria, viruses, fungi, parasites, and other microbes normally kept in check by the immune system.

Symptoms of people with AIDS may include coughing and shortness of breath, seizures, painful swallowing, confusion and forgetfulness, severe and persistent diarrhea, fevers, loss of vision, nausea and vomiting, extreme fatigue, severe headaches, and even coma. Children with AIDS may experience these same symptoms plus very severe forms of common childhood bacterial diseases such as conjunctivitis, ear infections, and tonsillitis. People who develop AIDS also may develop cancers caused by viruses, such as Kaposi's sarcoma and cervical cancer, or cancers of the immune system known as lymphomas. Eventually, the person with AIDS is overwhelmed by the opportunistic infections and cancers and dies. Antiviral drugs are able to suppress the damage to the immune system but not to eradicate the virus. People living with AIDS must take antiviral drugs, which have many side effects, for the rest of their lives.

**Transmission** HIV is not easily transmitted. It is *not* transmitted by hugging, kissing, coughing, using public toilets or swimming in public pools, or sharing eating utensils or towels in the bathroom. Transmission of HIV requires close contact between an infected person's bodily fluids and the blood or other bodily fluids of a noninfected person. The principal way in which AIDS is transmitted is through sexual intercourse—genital, anal, or oral. It is also transmitted easily when injecting drug users share needles, or when needles used in tattooing or body piercing are reused without being sterilized. HIV may be transmitted from mother to child before, during, or after birth, and it may be transmitted in breast milk. Before 1985, when a test for HIV was released, the AIDS virus was also transmitted through contaminated blood and blood products used in surgery or to treat hemophilia.

Education about the routes of transmission, programs to encourage abstinence from sex or faithfulness to one partner, the distribution of condoms and clean needles, and free testing so that people may learn their HIV status have been the major methods by which the transmission of AIDS has been slowed, when such methods have been utilized. Religious taboos against the use of condoms during sex and political views that oppose the distribution of clean needles to drug abusers have inhibited prevention efforts. Cultural resistance to permitting women to refuse unsafe sex and the existence of informal multipartner sexual networks in which individuals do not think of themselves as promiscuous because they have sex with only a few people whom they know well have also hindered the interruption of transmission of HIV.

HIV infection and AIDS are concentrated in places where the methods of transmission are most prolific and where prevention methods are not employed.

It was first identified in the United States, for example, in the gay communities of large cities, where frequent and unprotected sexual encounters took place, enabling rapid spread of the virus. Injecting drug users, communities of whom are often concentrated in large cities, spread the virus to one another through shared needles and to their sexual partners during sex.

In much of Sub-Saharan Africa, in contrast, AIDS is more often transmitted heterosexually. HIV transmission is concentrated along highways traveled by men working far from home and seeking sex with female sex workers. Once infected, the men may unknowingly infect their wives. When the wives become pregnant, their unborn children may become infected as well. Cultural practices that discourage the discussion of sex may lead men to deny infection. Because women in many African cultures have no recognized right to demand that their husbands wear condoms during sex, they have almost no options to protect themselves from infection. A popular superstition that a man will be cured of his HIV infection by having sex with a virgin may lead men to have forcible intercourse with young girls, thus spreading the infection further. In Southeast Asia and in India, the sex trade in large cities has been a principal locus of HIV transmission.

**History of Research**   As soon as epidemiologists understood that AIDS attacked the helper T cells that controlled the immune system, they urged virologists to search for a hitherto unknown virus that fit this description. The only viruses known to attack human T cells were the retroviruses identified by the Gallo laboratory at the National Cancer Institute (NCI) in Bethesda, Maryland.

These viruses were known as human T-cell lymphotrophic virus, Types I and II (HTLV-I and HTLV-II), which caused cancer in humans. Three groups of investigators began searching for retroviruses as possible causative agents of AIDS. In addition to Gallo's group, there were virologist Luc Montagnier's (b. 1932) group at the Pasteur Institute in Paris and medical researcher Jay Levy's (b. 1938) group at the University of California San Francisco (UCSF).

In 1984 Gallo's group published four papers in the journal *Science* that demonstrated a retrovirus as the cause of AIDS. They initially believed that it was in the same family as the other two HTLV viruses; hence, they named it HTLV-III. Montagnier's group at the Pasteur Institute and Jay Levy's at UCSF also identified the causative retrovirus of AIDS at about the same time. They named their viruses, respectively, lymphadenopathy associated virus (LAV) and AIDS related virus (ARV). Within a year, these viruses were shown to be identical. Because the AIDS virus caused destruction of infected T cells instead of the uncontrolled reproduction that occurred in cancer, it was deemed separate from the HTLV family. In 1986 an international group of scientists proposed that the name of the retrovirus that caused AIDS be changed to *Human Immunodeficiency Virus* (HIV).

The first medical intervention developed for the control of AIDS was a diagnostic test adapted from the laboratory assay that confirmed the presence of antibodies to HIV in cell cultures. This enzyme-linked immunosorbancy assay (ELISA) can have false positives, however, so a second test, known as the Western blot, which assays for specific viral proteins, was used to confirm a positive ELISA test. In 1987 the U.S. Food and Drug Administration (FDA) required that both tests be used before someone would be told that he or she was infected with AIDS. Twenty-five years into the epidemic, these diagnostic tests arguably remain medicine's most useful interventions for addressing the AIDS epidemic because they provide a measurable, replicable means to identify infected individuals.

During the two years of intensive laboratory research during which HIV was identified and characterized genetically, information also emerged about the virus that helped suggest which preventive interventions by political and public health leaders might be possible. Within just a few months after HIV was identified, molecular biologists understood that it mutated far too rapidly—up to 1,000 times as fast as influenza virus—for a traditional vaccine to be made against it. Instead of being able to vaccinate against AIDS, political and public health leaders needed to use educational methods aimed at curbing high-risk behavior to slow transmission, a much harder task.

Molecular and genetic studies also identified the key points in the virus's life cycle, which, if interrupted, would halt the spread of the virus. The first was the CD-4+ receptor on the cell wall of the host cell to which the virus attached. Second was the point at which the enzyme reverse transcriptase caused the single-strand RNA virus to make a complementary copy that transformed it into double-stranded DNA.

Third, the enzyme integrase caused the viral DNA to be spliced into the genome of the host cell. Finally came the point at which the enzyme protease cut newly constructed polypeptides into viral proteins in the final assembly of new virus particles. By 1986 intellectual strategies were in place to intervene in each of these four steps, but scientists were not technologically capable of implementing most of them, and a great deal of molecular information about HIV, such as the existence of necessary co-receptors in step 1, was not yet known.

In 1984 some drugs were known to inhibit reverse transcriptase, so this is where the work on an AIDS therapy began. Scientists utilized an anticancer drug-screening program at the NCI to identify potential drugs for use against AIDS. One of these that showed promise *in vitro* was azidothymidine, commonly called AZT. After truncated clinical trials in which AIDS patients showed a clear response to AZT, it was approved for use by the FDA in record time and sold under the brand name Retrovir or the generic name zidovudine. Within a few more years, two additional reverse transcriptase inhibitors, known in chemical shorthand as ddI and ddC, were approved by the FDA for treating AIDS. The reverse transcriptase inhibitors improved the condition of AIDS patients but had a number of toxic side effects and were subject to the development of resistance by HIV.

Other than these antiretroviral drugs, treatments for AIDS focused on existing drugs for treating the opportunistic infections and cancer that people with AIDS developed. In 1995 the first of a new class of antiretroviral drugs was introduced. Known as protease inhibitors, these drugs interfered with the final enzymatic step in the viral assembly process. For a brief period, there was optimism that the protease inhibitors would "cure" AIDS because viral loads—the number of virus particles in a quantity of blood—disappeared. It soon became apparent, however, that HIV was only suppressed and that it rapidly rebounded if the drugs were withdrawn. These drugs, too, caused unpleasant side effects. The combination of reverse transcriptase inhibitors and protease inhibitors known as Highly Active Antiretroviral Therapy, or HAART, is nevertheless the most effective "cocktail" of drugs for long-term therapy against AIDS. Pharmaceutical research still works toward a rationally designed, molecularly based drug with minimal toxicity as a therapy for AIDS, but at present, that goal has not been attained.

In November 2006, WHO reported that 2.9 million people had died of AIDS-related illnesses and estimated that 39.5 million people were living with HIV/AIDS. The WHO also reported that there were 4.3 million new infections in 2006, 65 percent of which occurred in Sub-Saharan Africa. There were also important increases in Eastern Europe and Central Asia.

Research continues on a preventive vaccine and on new antiviral drugs. The most effective means for controlling the epidemic, however, still remains diagnosis of individuals infected with HIV, education about how the virus is spread, and public health efforts to change behavior to minimize the risk of infection.

*Victoria A. Harden*

*See also* Acquired Immune Deficiency Syndrome (AIDS); Bacteria; Cancer; Immune System/Lymphatic System.

## References

Barnett, Tony, and Alan Whiteside. *AIDS in the Twenty-First Century: Disease and Globalization*. 2nd rev. ed. New York: Palgrave Macmillan, 2006.

Campbell, Catherine. *Letting Them Die: Why HIV/AIDS Prevention Programs Fail*. Bloomington: Indiana University Press, 2003.

Centers for Disease Control and Prevention. *HIV/AIDS*. www.cdc.gov/hiv/.

Engel, Jonathan. *The Epidemic: A Global History of AIDS*. New York: Smithsonian/ Harper-Collins, 2006.

Fan, Hung. *AIDS: Science and Society*. 5th ed. Boston: Jones and Bartlett, 2007.

Frontline (PBS). *25 Years of AIDS: The Age of AIDS*. www.pbs.org/wgbh/pages/frontline/aids/cron/.

Grmek, Mirko. *History of AIDS: Emergence and Origin of a Modern Pandemic*. Translated by Russell C. Maulitz and Jacalyn Duffin. Princeton, NJ: Princeton University Press, 1990.

Hunter, Susan. *AIDS in America*. New York: Palgrave Macmillan, 2006.

Hunter, Susan. *AIDS in Asia: A Continent in Peril*. New York: Palgrave Macmillan, 2005.

Hunter, Susan. *Black Death: AIDS in Africa*. New York: Palgrave Macmillan, 2003.

Levy, Jay A. *HIV and the Pathogenesis of AIDS*. 3rd ed. New York: ASM Press, 2007.

Mayo Clinic. *HIV/AIDS*. www.mayoclinic.com/health/hiv-aids/DS00005.

National Institute of Allergy and Infectious Diseases. *AIDS*. www.niaid.nih.gov/publications/aids.htm.

*New York Times. The AIDS Epidemic: AIDS at 20*. www.nytimes.com/library/national/science/aids/timeline.

San Francisco AIDS Foundation. *Milestones in the Battle against AIDS: 25 Years of an Epidemic*. www.sfaf.org/aidstimeline/.

World Health Organization. *HIV Infections*. www.who.int/topics/hiv_infections/en/.

## HUMAN PAPILLOMAVIRUS (HPV)

HPV is the human papillomavirus. It is neither the same as HIV (human immunodeficiency virus) nor HSV (herpes simplex virus), nor is it a new virus. There are more than 100 types of HPV. They have been around for generations. HPV can cause anything from warts on hands, feet, and the genital area to cancer of the head, neck, anal, penile, and cervical regions. Most HPV infections have no signs or symptoms. Therefore, many people are unaware that they are infected and can transmit the virus to a sex partner.

**Who Gets HPV?**  First and foremost, it is important to understand that anyone can get HPV infections, although some HPV infections require genital contact. There are mainly two broad categories of HPV infections. The first category causes warts—cauliflowerlike lesions—to grow on the hands and feet and is spread by skin-to-skin contact. The transmission does not require sexual contact of any kind, and this type does not cause cancer. The second category of infection is caused by sexual contact (not necessarily intercourse) with a partner who is already infected with one or more types of the HPV, some of which can cause cancer. As with any sexually transmitted disease, the chances of getting infected with HPV increase with the number of sexual partners a person has. An infected carrier can live many years without any visible symptoms or illness but can potentially always be an active transmitter to a sexual partner.

*How Common Is HPV?*  According to the CDC, HPV is the most common sexually transmitted disease. Approximately 20 million people are currently infected with the virus in the United States (Myers, McCrory, Nanda, Bastian, & Matchar, 2000). About 6.2 million Americans get a new genital HPV infection each year (Weinstock, Berman, & Cates, 2004). It is estimated that at least 50 percent of sexually active men and women will acquire genital HPV infection at some point in their lives. Some studies even suggest that by age 50, more than 80 percent of women will have acquired genital HPV infections (Myers et al. 2000). Most infections are transient and clear up on their own.

**What Are the Consequences of Having HPV?**  One of three results can occur from HPV infection: First, it is possible to become a carrier of HPV and never show symptoms for the rest of your life. It can take weeks, months, or even years after you are exposed to HPV to show symptoms of genital warts or have an abnormal Pap smear. For this reason, it is impossible for most people to know when and from whom they contracted the virus. In most instances, HPV is a harmless infection that does not result in visible symptoms or health complications. HPV infections are most common in women and men in their 20s, and most infections clear spontaneously. However, even when infected people are not showing symptoms, they could still be capable of passing the virus on to their sexual partners. This is done without any knowledge of whether the virus could take a more aggressive form or what the consequences could be either to them or to their partners.

The second possible outcome involves developing warts on your hands, feet, and anogenital area (around the anus and in the genital area) that could be irritating, visually unpleasant, and embarrassing. These warts almost never develop into precancerous or cancerous lesions.

The third and the most serious outcome of an HPV infection is that it can lead to precancerous and cancerous lesions of the cervix, vulva, vagina, urethra, anus, penis, mouth, and throat. Of these diseases, cervical cancer is the most significant. Currently, FDA statistics show that there are about 500,000 cases of cervical cancer annually around the world, with 250,000 deaths due to this disease.

In addition, one cannot underestimate the emotional toll it can take on a person who contracts HPV. Emotions of guilt, shame, and anger, compounded with the fact that there is no permanent cure, can create significant psychological upheaval.

***Is There a Cure for HPV If I Am Already Infected?*** No. Unfortunately, like all other viral infections, such as the common cold virus or the herpes virus, there is no cure for HPV. The good news is that most HPV infections resolve by themselves.

***Is HPV the Cause of All Cervical Cancers?*** Ninety-nine percent of cervical cancer in women can be directly attributed to HPV (Walboomers, Jacobs, & Manos, 1999). The cause for the other 1 percent is unknown. However, it should be noted that, out of the existing 20 million cases of HPV infections, *very few* actually progress to cervical cancer (NIH, 1996).

***Is There an Approved Vaccine Available Now?*** Yes, *Gardasil* (manufactured by Merck) was approved in June 2006 by the FDA. *Cervarix* (manufactured by GlaxoSmithKline [GSK]) was approved by the FDA in 2009. The current vaccines do not protect against all strains of the virus, but are designed to prevent 70 percent of all cervical cancers. *Gardasil* also protects against 90 percent of genital warts. It is important to note that neither vaccine prevents other sexually transmitted diseases such as herpes, AIDS, or gonorrhea.

***Who Should Get the Vaccine?*** The Advisory Committee on Immunization Practices (ACIP) arm of the CDC approved the vaccine, *Gardasil,* for all girls aged 11–12. The vaccine can be given as early as nine years of age, as well as to females between 13 and 26 years, even if one has already been sexually active. The other vaccine, *Cervarix,* has not yet been approved in the United States.

***Are There Any "Absolute" Ways to Prevent HPV?*** The answer to this is an emphatic *yes,* but it may not be practical or realistic. The only absolute way to prevent HPV is total abstinence by both partners prior to their meeting and commitment to sex with only each other from that point forward. This means both you and your current sexual partner must not have any other sexual partners for your entire lives. This method of prevention clearly has serious limitations for most people.

***Are There Any Tests to Detect HPV before It Leads to Cervical Cancer?*** Yes. For sexually active women, routine Pap smears can detect abnormalities several years before they turn into cancer. Cervical cancer is normally a very slow-growing cancer, and it can take decades from the time you have an abnormal Pap smear to the time you actually get cancer.

Perhaps the above information has already convinced you that the only way to proceed from here regarding the vaccine is a decision between you and your doctor or your child's doctor. However, factual information is not the only factor in making health decisions. In the case of HPV, there are conflicting business interests (drug companies), professional interests (doctors), religious interests (pastors and priests), political interests (politicians and community leaders), and last but not least, parents and teenagers. The topic of sex among teenagers has always been a political hotbed in the United States, creating the perfect recipe for controversy. These different groups have taken numerous steps to forward their agendas, and each group has been met with increasing opposition—with the various parties citing freedom of choice, freedom of speech, and even life, liberty, and the pursuit of happiness as justifications for their arguments.

The questions remain: Why do so many controversies surround the HPV vaccination? If each group claims it is acting in the best interest of women and teenagers, shouldn't we be in total agreement? The answer is *yes*—but even though each group wants to achieve the "big picture" of protecting women and teens, each sees the "correct" path to achieving this goal quite differently.

The benefits of the vaccine are self-evident—according to most scientists, it will irrefutably reduce the occurrence of the second leading cause of cancer in women around the world. Normally, you would think that this kind of medical breakthrough would earn much fanfare and be accepted unequivocally. Not true. On the contrary, the advent of this vaccine for cancer prevention has fallen prey to cultural wars. The vaccine's release has been accompanied by a stormy scientific, moral, and political controversy, entrenched in passionate rhetoric and hidden agendas.

The ACIP voted unanimously to recommend the HPV vaccine to all 11- and 12-year-old girls in June 2006. Soon after, lawmakers in many states wanted to make the vaccine mandatory, in order to ensure early prevention of cervical cancer in girls who were not then sexually active. A new study, approved by the FDA and published in the May 2010 issue of the *Journal of Preventative Medicine,* showed that one-third of American girls ages 13 to 17 have received the HPV vaccine. In 2009 the Food and Drug

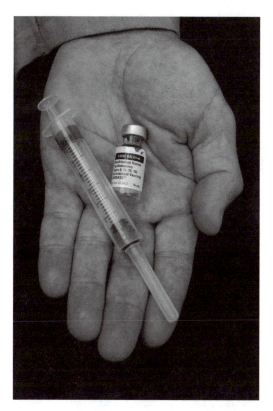

Dr. Donald Brown holds the human papillomavirus vaccine Gardasil in his hand at his Chicago office on August 28, 2006. (AP/Wide World Photos)

Administration (FDA) approved the Gardasil vaccine for boys and men aged 9 to 26 to prevent genital warts associated with HPV. However, the ACIP declined to recommend routine use of Gardasil for men or boys, leaving the decision to physicians whether to vaccinate them or not.

Scientists thought that vaccinating all preteen girls was premature, while conservative parents voiced that mandatory vaccination was immoral and compromised their family values. These varied opinions have led to vocalizations from a number of colorful personalities who have brought the controversy to life and highlighted its numerous pitfalls: the age at which it is recommended, the ethical dilemmas, corporate greed, and public outrage, all of which continue to shape this debate.

*Shobha S. Krishnan*

*See also* Sexually Transmitted Diseases (STDs); Virus.

## References

Loehr, Jamie. *The Vaccine Answer Book: 200 Essential Answers to Help You Make the Right Decisions for Your Child*. Naperville, IL: Sourcebooks, 2009.

Myers, E.R., D.C. McCrory, K. Nanda, L. Bastian, and D.B. Matchar. "Mathematical Model for the Natural History of Human Papillomavirus Infection and Cervical Carcinogenesis." *American Journal of Epidemiology* 151 (2000): 1158–71.

Nardo, Don. *Human Papillomavirus (HPV)*. Detroit: Lucent Books, 2007.

National Institutes of Health. "Cervical Cancer." *NIH Consensus Statement* 14 (1996):1–38.

"One-Third of U.S. Girls Get HPV Vaccine." *Consumer Health News* (June 4, 2010).

Park, Alice. "Why HPV Is Still Not a Straight Shot." *Time* 174, no. 8, August 31, 2009, 49.

Splete, Heidi. "FDA Approves Gardasil Use in Males Aged 9–26." *Family Practice News* 39, no. 19 (November 1, 2009): 22.

Sutton, Amy L. *Sexually Transmitted Diseases Sourcebook: Basic Consumer Health Information about Chlamydial Infections, Gonorrhea, Hepatitis, Herpes, HIV/AIDS, Human Papillomavirus, Pubic Lice, Scabies, Syphilis, Trichomoniasis, Vaginal Infections and Other Sexually Transmitted Diseases*. Detroit: Omnigraphics, 2006.

Walboomers, J.M., M.V. Jacobs, and M.M. Manos. "Human Papillomavirus Is a Necessary Cause of Invasive Cervical Cancer Worldwide." *Journal of Pathology* 189 (1999):12–19.

Weinstock, H., S. Berman, and W. Cates Jr. "Sexually Transmitted Diseases among American Youth: Incidence and Prevalence Estimates, 2000." *Perspectives on Sexual and Reproductive Health* 36 (2004): 6–10.

## HYPERTENSION

Called the silent killer because it carries no obvious symptoms, hypertension is the same as having high blood pressure. Hypertension is an equal opportunity disease that cost the United States more than $76 billion in health care services, medications, and missed days of work according to the CDC ("High Blood Pressure Facts," 2011). It can lead to other serious health problems such as heart attack or stroke and it can happen to anyone; adults, children, people on certain medications, or people who make poor lifestyle choices are all susceptible to hypertension (National Library of Medicine and National Institutes of Health, 2011).

The magic numbers 120 and 80 mean a person has healthy blood pressure. When a person's pressure measures between 120/80 and 139/89, this is prehypertension; 140/90 and higher is hypertension or high blood pressure. The top number represents the force at which blood pushes against the arteries when the heart pumps blood. A person's pressure is at its highest when the heart is engaged in pumping. This is called the systolic pressure. When the heart is at rest—in between beats—blood pressure is lower. The second number represents the diastolic blood pressure (National Library of Medicine and National Institutes of Health, 2011).

The number of adults in the United States with hypertension

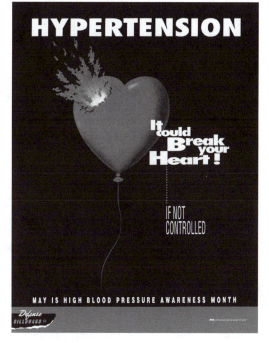

This U.S. Department of Defense poster issued during 1988–2000 warns against the risks of high blood pressure. (Department of Defense)

has steadily increased, with the latest figures from the Centers for Disease Control and Prevention (CDC) showing one out of three U.S. adults has high blood pressure ("High Blood Pressure Facts," 2011). Now studies have found a growing number of young adults are afflicted as well. Two studies, funded through the National Institutes of Health, looked at hypertension rates for men and women ages 24 to 32. One study found that 19 percent of young adults had blood pressure readings in the hypertension range and an earlier, smaller study suggested just 4 percent had hypertension (Rabin, 2011).

The National Longitudinal Study of Adolescent Health or Add Health followed 14,000 individuals beginning in 1995 and reported their results in the spring of 2011. The earlier study by the National Health and Nutrition Examination Survey (NHANES) had found fewer young adults with blood pressure readings of 140/90 or higher. One explanation for the discrepancy is that many young adults do not know they have hypertension. The study authors noted that the number of participants who had been told by a health care provider they had high blood pressure was much closer: 11 percent for Add Health and 9 percent for NHANES (Adams, 2011).

Children who have congenital illnesses or who struggle with overweight issues may have or develop hypertension. While some causes such as congenital heart problems or adrenal disorders cannot be avoided, weight matters can be addressed (National Library of Medicine and National Institutes of Health, 2011).

To get a blood pressure reading, a stethoscope is placed on the crease of the inside of the arm while a special cuff is quickly inflated on the upper part of the arm. The cuff squeezes the arm, and when released slowly, allows the clinician to listen to the patient's heartbeat. There are also digital devices that do the same thing and make it easy for everyone to monitor their blood pressure outside of a doctor's office. This can help consumers know if they need to ask their doctors about medication for hypertension or if the medication on which they have been placed is indeed working.

During the blood pressure reading posture is everything. Research has shown that the most accurate readings are gathered when a person is seated with his back against a chair, both feet are planted firmly on the floor, and the arm used to measure blood pressure is resting on a surface placed at heart level. Relaxing is also recommended (Turner, 2008).

While hypertension can be treated with medication, the best way to avoid and control the condition is to make healthy lifestyle choices. One of the best ways to lower blood pressure is by losing weight and regular exercise. Individuals should always consult their primary care physician before they begin any program of weight loss or regular exercise. At the 26th annual American Society of Hypertension's Annual Scientific Meeting and Exposition, researchers presented a myriad of research in areas such as the benefits of lifestyle practices and barriers to proper hypertension management (American Society of Hypertension, 2011).

Coffee, for example, has been shown to dramatically increase blood pressure in drinkers for a brief period of time. Particularly in men, alcohol consumption has been shown to elevate blood pressure. Even certain professions can increase the risk of hypertension. In U.S. firefighters, the stress from putting out fires seems to elevate the risk of cardiovascular disease, and can cause an exaggerated increase in blood pressure, for those who are not as physically fit (Nephrology News and Issues, 2011).

Another identified cause of hypertension is salt. Particularly in African Americans, salt consumption has been shown to raise blood pressure. Researchers have isolated genes that can predict the risk of developing salt-related high blood pressure. The findings can one day lead to a genetic test to diagnosis the condition (Hironobu, 2006).

Smoking is another contributor to hypertension as nicotine actually raises blood pressure. Stress is also thought to increase blood pressure. Finding ways to positively manage stress and to relax may also succeed in lowering blood pressure numbers.

It is important to know and understand one's blood pressure and take action to control it if necessary. Awareness and control of hypertension can lead people to make healthier lifestyle choices, comply with instructions from physicians, and ultimately save lives.

*Abena Foreman-Trice*

*See also* Blood Pressure; Exercise; Smoking; Stress.

## References

Adams, Rebecca. "One-Fifth of Young Adults May Have High Blood Pressure—or Not." *CQ Healthbeat* (May 26, 2011).

American Society of Hypertension. 2011 Annual Meeting, New York, NY, May 2011. www.ash-us.org/Scientific-Meetings/2011-Annual-Meeting.aspx.

"High Blood Pressure Facts." Centers for Disease Control and Prevention (CDC). March 21, 2011. www.cdc.gov/bloopressure/facts.htm.

Hironobu, Sanada, Junichi Yatabe, Sanae Midorikawa, Shigeatsu Hashimoto, Tsuyoshi Watanabe, Jason H. Moore, Marylyn D. Ritchie, Scott M. Williams, John C. Pezzullo, Midori Sasaki, Gilbert M. Eisner, Pedro A. Jose, and Robin A. Felder. "Single-Nucleotide Polymorphisms for Diagnosis of Salt-Sensitive Hypertension." *Clinical Chemistry* 52, no. 3 (2006): 352–60.

National Library of Medicine and National Institutes of Health. *Medline Plus: High Blood Pressure.* May 29, 2011. www.nlm.nih.gov/medlineplus/highbloodpressure.html.

Nephrology News and Issues. *Studies Highlight Impact of Lifestyle Variations on Hypertension.* May 24, 2011. www.nephronline.com/clinical/article/studies-highlight-impact-of-lifestyle-variations-on-hypertension.

Rabin, Roni Caryn. "Risks: Hypertension Lurking in Young Adults." *New York Times,* May 31, 2011, D6.

Turner, Melly, interview by Abena Foreman-Trice RN, University of Virginia Health System. Charlottesville, VA, August 2008.

## HYPNOSIS

Hypnosis has been defined as "a situation or set of procedures in which a person designated as the hypnotist suggests that another person designated as the patient, client, or subject experience various changes in sensations, perception, cognition, or control over motor behavior" (Kirsch, Lynn, & Rhue, 1993). Popular uses of hypnosis include behavior modification especially in the treatment of phobias, stress reduction, and relief from chronic pain.

Hypnoticlike states (Krippner & Friedman, 2009), which may or may not be completely equivalent to hypnosis as the term is used in the contemporary West, have long been part of religious and healing ceremonies within most ancient and indigenous societies. These frequently employ rhythmic chanting, monotonous drumming, eye fixations, and other techniques to alter consciousness and gain behavioral changes. For example, Egyptian hieroglyphics found on ancient Egyptian temples indicate that hypnoticlike experiences were a common practice among its priests, and healing sanctuaries (called sleep or dream temples) were located throughout ancient Egypt and other ancient cultures, such as Greece. These ancient and indigenous practices continue under what we now call hypnosis in the contemporary West.

**Suggestion or Hysteria?** James Braid (1843–1960) coined the term *hypnosis,* referring to the Greek god of sleep, Hypnos. Braid eventually concluded that the hypnosis was due to suggestion, but Jean Martin Charcot argued that the effects of hypnosis were related to psychopathology, due to his supposition that "hysteria" was largely responsible for the hypnotic experience. The notion that hypnosis reflects psychological abnormality became known as the Charcot School, which influenced both Pierre Janet and Sigmund Freud, the father of psychoanalysis.

In contrast, Hippolyte Bernheim proposed that normal suggestibility could explain the effects of hypnosis. A.A. Liébault supported Bernheim's view that hypnosis was due to normal suggestion and the Liébault-Bernheim theory of hypnosis became known as the Nancy School in which hypnosis was held to be a normal psychological phenomenon related to suggestion and not necessarily related to psychopathology. The Nancy School's stance eventually triumphed, and the controversy between the Charcot and Nancy Schools' perspectives propelled hypnosis from its former fringe associations with mysticism and charlatanism into the scientific domain. Near the end of the 19th century, hypnosis was accepted within the scientific community, as illustrated by William James's (1890) chapter on hypnosis in his renowned book.

**Principles of Psychology**  Freud initially used hypnosis successfully in his healing practices, but later rejected it for his psychoanalytic methods. Due to his rejection, a relatively quiet period for hypnosis ensued until experimental psychologist, Clark Hull (1933), summarized experimental work with hypnosis in his book, *Hypnosis and Suggestibility.* Later, Hull also abandoned the use of hypnosis, which once more fell into another lull period until World War II accelerated interest in hypnosis, when it was used successfully to treat emotional reactions to the war, as well as for dental applications. This led to the growing popularity of hypnosis within psychological and medical settings.

**Professional Associations**  The Society for Clinical and Experimental Hypnosis was established in 1949 and the American Society of Clinical Hypnosis was established in 1957, which are the two major professional hypnosis organizations in the United States. Both societies strongly support the idea that only trained certified professionals should use hypnosis, due to potential adverse side effects for some people, which are associated with their varying capacity for hypnotizability, various personality factors, and especially levels of mental and emotional stability. In 1960, the American Psychological Association officially recognized the American Board of Examiners in Psychological Hypnosis as a certifying board for hypnosis practitioners, and many other mainstream organizations followed suit. However, a cautionary stance on hypnosis remains within most mainstream psychological and medical settings, perhaps because the phenomenon of hypnosis remains mysterious, despite the demonstrated usefulness of hypnosis in various clinical, medical, educational, and other settings from more than 150 years of investigations.

Although a consensus has not been reached on the nature of hypnosis, most theorists have agreed upon broad characteristics of the hypnotic domain. Of course not all persons hypnotized exhibit these characteristics during hypnotic states.

In addition, there are various models of hypnosis, which can primarily be viewed as physiological, psychological, or a mixture of both. These attempt to explain what hypnosis is and how it works by proposing different mechanisms (e.g., atavistic regression, dissociation, hemispheric specificity, modified sleep, role playing, pathological theories, psychoanalytic, suggestion, conditioned behavior response, neurological, systems perspective, social compliance, ego functioning, trait assumptions). One very popular model is Milton Erickson's (1958) naturalistic approach to hypnotherapy, which specifies that all persons possess hypnotic ability and that each person individualistically responds to different hypnotic techniques.

**Modern Hypnosis**   Modern hypnosis focuses predominantly on dissociated control (Bowers, 1992) and neodissociation (Hilgard, 1992) theories. Early in the history of modern hypnosis, Janet (1889) focused his interests on "psychological automatism," a concept proposing that a part of the personality could split off from conscious awareness and autonomously follow a subconscious development. This idea eventually evolved into the concept of dissociation and became the cornerstone in the study of many psychopathological disorders (e.g., amnesia, fugue, somnambulism, multiple personality disorder later renamed dissociative identity disorder).

Although earlier dissociation theory focused on pathological mental processes, Hilgard (1992) formulated a "neodissociation" theory proposing that hypnosis was a condition whereby the normal functioning of the executive ego was temporarily modified by hypnotized persons, who allow their cognition to be externally controlled by the hypnotist. Some empirical studies with automatic writing demonstrate this effect. Hilgard also demonstrated this effect with the "hidden observer" in which the hypnotized person can perform and experience dual roles, simultaneously being both the observer and the observed. The hidden observer, sometimes known as "witness" consciousness, is a metaphor for the information source of a high level of cognitive functioning not consciously experienced by the hypnotized individual. Not all highly hypnotizable individuals experience the hidden observer, but those who experience profound dissociated states often experience the hidden observer.

**Medical Applications**   There are many medical applications of hypnosis. One of the most common is pain management, such as during childbirth or serious burns. Hypnosis is often used in habit control (e.g., smoking cessation, weight loss), and in psychological explorations of memories to help patients connect with their feelings. It should be cautioned, however, that memories retrieved during hypnosis may be confabulated and are not necessarily trustworthy.

Hypnosis is also being applied to reduce symptoms in children and adolescents with Tourette syndrome. In a study published in the July/August 2010 issue of the *Journal of Development and Behavioral Pediatrics,* researchers reported a significant percentage of participants showed improvement in tic control through the use of self-hypnosis (Lazarus & Klein, 2010).

In addition, hypnosis is strikingly similar to what is called meditation, also a group of widely varying techniques used to alter consciousness, and increasingly used within psychological and medical settings. In this regard hypnosis, especially self-hypnosis, offers a potent avenue for transpersonal and spiritual exploration (Leskowitz, 1999). One advantage of hypnosis is that its techniques are secular, whereas most meditation practices are embedded within religious traditions that contain metaphysical assumptions (unnecessary for practical applications), which may discourage those of different religious views from benefiting through their use.

Hypnosis is a fascinating area in which people can exhibit truly amazing abilities, such as regulating various body processes generally thought not to be under control. Although the mechanisms of hypnosis remain unknown, hypnotic responsiveness may be viewed as a continuum. On one hand, it may be based on a rudimentary defensive reaction (e.g., freeze response of a threatened opossum) that was a necessity for survival as our human ancestry evolved, and in that sense may be related to various psychopathologies.

Alternatively, it may be based on evolutionarily strengths that are fundamentally growth-oriented and encoded for situations requiring a more proactive approach to survival (e.g., underlying cooperative efforts, such as food gathering or conflict avoidance, that rely on rapid suggestibility for group coherence in following a leader). Either way, hypnotizability may provide a way to ensure that the human species continues to evolve and survive, even when an immediate threat is not pressing for decisive action. As we learn more about enhancing health and wellness through impressive modern technologies, it is important to keep in mind that hypnosis and other ancient and traditional healing methods are inherently useful and may exceed the effectiveness of high technology approaches.

*Joan H. Hageman and Harris Friedman*

*See also* Meditation; Reiki.

### References

Bowers, K.S. "Imagination and Dissociation in Hypnotic Responding." *International Journal of Clinical and Experimental Hypnosis* 40, no. 4 (1992): 253–75.

Braid, J. *Braid on Hypnotism: The Beginnings of Modern Hypnosis.* Rev. ed. New York: Julian, 1960. [Original work published 1843].

Erickson, M.H. "Naturalistic Techniques of Hypnosis." *American Journal of Clinical Hypnosis* 1 (1958): 3–8.

Hilgard, E.R. "Dissociation and Theories of Hypnosis." In *Contemporary Hypnosis Research,* edited by E. Fromm and M.R. Nash, 69–101. New York: Guilford Press, 1992.

Hull, C.L. *Hypnosis and Suggestibility: An Experimental Approach.* New York: Appleton-Century, 1933.

James, W. *Principles of Psychology.* Vols. 1–2. New York: Holt, 1890.

Janet, P. *L'automatisme psychologique* [The Psychological Automatism]. Paris: Felix Alcan, 1889.

Kirsch, I., S.J. Lynn, and J.W. Rhue. "Introduction to Clinical Hypnosis." In *Handbook of Clinical Hypnosis,* edited by S.J. Lynn, J.W. Rhue, and I. Kirsch, 1–22. Washington, DC: American Psychological Association, 1933.

Krippner, S., and Friedman, H. "Hypnotic-Like Indigenous Healing Practices: Cross-Cultural Perspectives for Western Hypnosis Researchers and Practitioners." *Psychological Hypnosis* 18 (2009): 4–7.

Lazarus, Jeffrey E., and Susan K. Klein. "No Pharmacological Treatment of Tics in Tourette Syndrome Adding Videotape Training to Self-Hypnosis." *Journal of Developmental and Behavioral Pediatrics* 31, no. 6 (July/August 2010): 498–504.

Leskowitz, E., ed. *Transpersonal Hypnosis.* Boca Raton, FL: CRC Press, 1999.

*I*

---

## IMMUNE SYSTEM/LYMPHATIC SYSTEM

The natural world is an exceptionally hostile place, with pathogenic and parasitic organisms waiting to exploit any weakness in an organism. Fungi, bacteria, parasitic worms, protistans, and viruses abound in the natural world. The concept of survival of the fittest extends from the lowest life forms to the complex environments of primates. In order to survive, all organisms must possess some mechanism of combating invaders. Humans are no exception to this rule. They are in a biological arms race with the microscopic world. Luckily, humankind possesses one of the most elaborate defensive systems on the planet—the lymphatic system, commonly known as the immune system.

The primary task of defending the approximately 100 trillion cells of the body against this onslaught of invaders rests with the lymphatic system. While other systems do provide some protection, such as the acids of the stomach and the structure of the skin, it is the job of the lymphatic system to initiate an immune response against invading pathogens. The lymphatic system is the system of the body that is responsible for the immune response. This tiered system of defense utilizes physical barriers, such as the skin, and general defense mechanisms, such as the white blood cells. But perhaps the most significant weapon in its arsenal is the specific defense system. In this aspect of the immune response, specialized cells called lymphocytes detect specific invaders (such as fungi, bacteria, and viruses) and eliminate them from the body. This response can be directed against both free pathogens in the body or against cells that have become infected. As an added protection, the specific response has the ability to "remember" an infection, practically ensuring that you will never be infected by the same organism or virus twice.

The lymphatic system does have other roles in the body. First, it acts as a second circulatory system. The lymphatic system is responsible for returning the fluid from the tissues of the body, called interstitial fluid, to the circulatory system. In this regard, the lymphatic system helps regulate water balance, ensuring

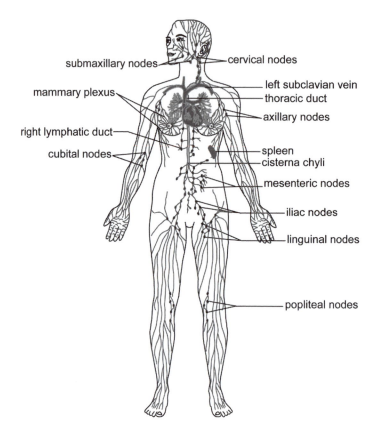

submaxillary nodes

cervical nodes

left subclavian vein

thoracic duct

mammary plexus

axillary nodes

right lymphatic duct

cubital nodes

spleen

cisterna chyli

mesenteric nodes

iliac nodes

linguinal nodes

popliteal nodes

This illustration shows the primary groups of lymph nodes and the lymph vessel system. The right and left subclavian veins return lymph to the body's blood supply. (Sandy Windelspecht)

not only that the tissues have proper fluids, but that excess fluids do not accumulate in the extremities. The second—often overlooked—role is that of a transport system. The lymphatic system moves fat-soluble nutrients from the digestive system to the circulatory system using a special class of molecules called the lipoproteins.

Unlike other body systems, such as the digestive system and endocrine system, the lymphatic system does not have a large number of organs dedicated to the role of immune response. While there are some, such as the thymus and spleen, the majority of the lymphatic system consists of small ducts, minor glands, and specialized cells located in other body systems, which will be discussed in this entry.

**Chemicals and Cells** The lymphatic system is a complex group of cells, tissues, and organs that are widely dispersed throughout the human body. The lymphatic system has three primary functions. First, its cells are primarily responsible for the immune response of the body. For this reason, the lymphatic system is frequently called the immune system. Most people are familiar with the immune system as it provides resistance to disease. Modern diseases such as acquired immune deficiency syndrome (AIDS) and sudden acute respiratory syndrome (SARS) greatly challenge the capabilities of our immune system.

Second, the vessels of the lymphatic system actually represent a separate circulatory system in the human body. Unlike the cardiovascular circulatory system, the lymphatic system does not directly supply nutrients or oxygen to the tissues of the body, but rather is primarily involved in the return of fluids from the tissues. Finally, the lymphatic system is involved in the transport of select nutrients from the digestive system to the circulatory system.

These initial sections of this entry provide an overview of the molecules, cellular components, and chemical signals of the lymphatic system. The focus is primarily on those aspects that are associated with the immune response, although some transport molecules are also discussed. The interaction of these cells, signals, and molecules to create an immune response will be covered later.

### Subcellular Components

*Complement Proteins*   As the name suggests, these proteins complement or assist in the function of the immune response. These are nonspecific components of the lymphatic system, meaning that they do not recognize specific types of pathogens entering the body, but instead target any form of invading bacteria or fungus. From an evolutionary perspective, complement proteins probably represent the simplest and oldest form of immune system. Forms of complement proteins are found in all animals. There are approximately 20 different types of complement proteins in humans; collectively, they are called the complement system.

Complement proteins move throughout the circulatory system in an inactive form, commonly called a zymogen. The mechanism by which they are activated is dependent upon the class of the complement protein. Although complement proteins are found in the circulatory system, they are considered to be part of the lymphatic system due to their association with the immune response.

The complement proteins may either target invading fungal and bacterial cells directly, or they may be recruited by antibodies or other cells of the immune system. The proteins have a variety of functions. Some classes are involved with attacking the membrane of the invading pathogen causing it to lyse, or break. Other classes interact with the antibodies secreted by the B lymphocytes. This is often called the classical pathway, because it is the most common mechanism of complement system activation. Once activated by an antibody, the complement proteins form a pore in the membrane of the invading cell, causing it to lyse.

Some complement proteins act as molecular flags. This class sticks to the surface of the pathogen, but rather than causing the membrane to rupture, these proteins signal macrophages and other phagocytic cells of the immune system to envelop the invading cell and destroy it. Other classes of complement proteins are involved in the inflammatory response or in activating enzymes in the blood.

The complement proteins that directly lyse the membrane of the pathogen do so by what is called the alternative pathway. In this case, the inactive proteins are activated by some component of the bacterial or fungal cell wall. Once activated, the proteins congregate on the invading cell and form a pore through the membrane, disrupting the membrane barrier of the cell and causing it to lyse.

While complement proteins may appear to be an effective mechanism of immune response, they lack the ability to target specific types of cells that are invading the body. The task of targeting specific invaders falls to the cells of the immune system.

***Chylomicrons and Lipoproteins*** One aspect of the lymphatic system that is not involved in the immune response is the transport of fat-soluble material from the digestive tract. This includes not only triglycerides, but also the fat-soluble vitamins. These hydrophobic molecules are packaged within the small intestine into spherical structures called lipoproteins.

Lipoproteins are a combination of fats and proteins. Following enzymatic digestion in the lumen (cavity) of the small intestine, fatty acids are reassembled into triglycerides in the epithelial cells of the small intestine. They are then packaged into chylomicrons. Chylomicrons represent one form of lipoprotein that is manufactured within the lining of the small intestine. Due to their size and hydrophobic characteristics, chylomicrons cannot pass into the capillaries within the villi of the small intestine, and thus are unable to be transported to the liver in the same manner as the majority of nutrients. Instead, they enter into the lacteals of the digestive tract.

Once in the lacteals of the intestines, the chylomicrons utilize the lymphatic system to bypass the liver and travel to the heart via the thoracic duct, where they enter into the bloodstream. At this point the vitamins and energy-rich nutrients within the chylomicron are removed by the tissues, and the chylomicron becomes an empty shell. The other lipoproteins, such as low-density lipoproteins (LDLs) and high-density lipoproteins (HDLs), are manufactured by liver tissue and do not enter the lymphatic system.

***Antimicrobial Proteins*** The surface cells of the body, called the epithelia, are most often the first to experience an attack by an invading organism. For this reason, many of the body's surfaces secrete antimicrobial proteins or enzymes. An enzyme is a chemical compound (usually a protein) that accelerates a chemical reaction. Although enzymes are most often thought of in association with the digestive or nervous systems, in fact they are active in all of the systems of the body.

The surfaces of the eyes and mouth, because they are moist environments and warmer areas of the body, represent an ideal location for a microbial attack. At these locations, the body secretes an enzyme called lysozyme in the saliva and tears. Lysozyme acts by degrading the cell walls of invading bacteria. Because animal cells lack cell walls, they are not disturbed by the presence of the enzyme.

This is not the only example of antimicrobial compounds in the body. Technically, the protease enzymes of the stomach may be considered a part of the immune response, because, in cooperation with the hydrochloric acid of the stomach, they inhibit the activity of pathogenic organisms. In the small intestine, specialized cells called Paneth cells secrete an antimicrobial compound called cryptidin. Even the bacteria located within the large intestine assist with patrolling against incoming pathogens. *Escherichia coli* (commonly called just *E. coli*), frequently considered to be a pathogen itself, helps protect the large intestine by secreting a chemical called colicin that prevents growth of pathogenic organisms.

These antimicrobial systems are not designed to completely prevent an attack by a pathogenic organism. Instead, like the complement proteins, the antimicrobial substances noted in this section act to slow the growth of an invader and give the specific defense mechanisms (lymphocytes) time to prepare. In this regard, antimicrobial systems are very effective in their mode of action.

*Lymphatic Fluid*   The fluid content of the lymphatic system is actually derived from the circulatory system. In the circulatory system, the capillaries represent the location where gas and nutrient exchange is most likely to occur with the surrounding tissue. Capillaries are fragile structures, whose walls are typically only one cell thick. However, these cells, called endothelial cells, do not form a solid structure, like that of a hose. Instead, there are small pores between the cells that form the lining of the capillaries.

These pores are too small to allow the cells and plasma proteins of the circulatory system to pass, but large enough to allow a free exchange of fluid with the surrounding tissues. This fluid represents the medium through which nutrients and gases may be exchanged. The fluid, called interstitial fluid, bathes most tissues of the body. Cells typically deposit waste in the interstitial fluid for pickup by the circulatory system, and receive nutrients and gases to conduct their metabolic processes.

The majority of this fluid is reabsorbed back into the capillaries. However, this process is only about 85 percent effective. Each day, about 3.17 quarts (3 liters) of fluid is not reabsorbed back into the capillaries, but instead remains in the tissue. This amount may not sound significant, but in an average adult, there is only 5.28 quarts (5 liters) of blood. It would seem that the loss of fluid from the capillaries would represent a severe challenge for the circulatory system, and the organism as a whole.

The lymphatic system makes up the difference by recycling the interstitial fluid and returning it back to the circulatory system. In most people, the lymphatic system returns around 3.17 quarts (3 liters) of fluid daily. In other words, the output of the circulatory system to the tissues is matched by the input of interstitial fluid from the lymphatic system.

Lymphatic fluid does not contain red blood cells, and in general lacks any pigmentation. However, despite its lack of color, there are plenty of ions, molecules, and cells in lymphatic fluid. These include ions such as sodium (Na+) and potassium (K+), chylomicrons, and a host of cells associated with the immune response.

One of the human body systems' most important—and difficult—jobs is to protect the body against the myriad of organisms that threaten its health and homeostasis. While each of the human body systems has its own defense mechanisms, the duty to protect the body against dangerous invaders falls primarily to the lymphatic system. This system contains specialized cells called lymphocytes that detect threatening organisms and put into motion an immune response that eliminates them from the body. The immune response also protects the rest of the body against free pathogens and cells that might already have been infected. In addition, this response mechanism actually remembers the infection for future defense purposes; if the invading organism enters the body again, protection will be in place.

Unlike other systems in the human body, there are only a few primary and secondary organs in the lymphatic system. The bone marrow and thymus are the primary organs, while the secondary organs include the spleen, tonsils, adenoid, Peyer's patches, and appendix.

*Julie McDowell and Michael Windelspecht*

*See also* Acquired Immune Deficiency Syndrome (AIDS).

### References

Abrahams, Peter, ed. *How the Body Works.* London: Amber Books, 2009.

American Academy of Allergy, Asthma and Immunology. www.aaaai.org.

American Academy of Otolaryngology. www.entnet.org.

"Did You Know . . . Facts about the Human Body." Health News. www.healthnews.com.

"Interesting Facts about the Human Body." Random Facts. http://facts.randomhistory.com/ 2009/03/02_human-body.html.

Lyman, Dale. *Anatomy DeMystified.* New York: McGraw-Hill, 2004.

McDowell, Julie, and Michael Windelspecht. *The Lymphatic System.* Westport, CT: Greenwood, 2004.

"Medical References." University of Maryland Medical Center. www.umm.edu/medref/.

Mertz, Leslie. *The Circulatory System.* Westport, CT: Greenwood, 2004.

"National Cholesterol Education Program." National Heart Lung and Blood Institute. www.nhlbi.nih.gov/chd/.

National Institute of Allergy and Infectious Diseases. www.niaid.nih.gov.

"Spinal Cord Research." Christopher and Dana Reeve Foundation. www.christopherreeve. org/site/c.ddJFKRNoFiG/b.4343879/k.D323/Research.htm.

Watson, Stephanie. *The Endocrine System.* Westport, CT: Greenwood, 2004.

Windelspecht, Michael. *The Digestive System.* Westport, CT: Greenwood, 2004.

## IMMUNIZATIONS. *See* VACCINATIONS

## INFLUENZA

According to the U.S. Centers for Disease Control and Prevention (CDC) ("Seasonal Influenza [Flu]"), influenza, also called *flu,* "is a contagious respiratory illness caused by influenza viruses. It can cause mild to severe illness, and at times can lead to death." Some people also refer to the "stomach flu," which is not truly influenza, but instead more properly called viral gastroenteritis, which the Centers for Disease Control and Prevention calls "an infection caused by a variety of viruses that results in vomiting or diarrhea" ("Viral Gastroenteritis").

In 1918, a strain of influenza known as the Spanish flu raced across the world, infecting and killing millions of people. Although few people today remember the pandemic or recall even learning about the event in school, some scientists have studied influenza with intensity and can now distinctly outline its path through time. Although the 1918 pandemic is considered a part of the world's collective history now, influenza continues to have significant impact as a disease, with impressive global consequences. In its seasonal outbreaks, it can affect 10–20 percent of the total world population. Annual epidemics in developed countries are thought to result in 3–5 million cases of severe illness and 250,000–500,000 deaths each year. Data from the tropical and developing countries are limited with regard to accurate reporting, but the disease is known to have high attack rates and can cause considerable morbidity and mortality in these parts of the world. Thus, the study of the influenza, and the virus that causes it, continues with great interest.

In considering influenza, it is important to understand the terminology used to describe its disease manifestations with regard to populations. An outbreak refers to the occurrence of a large number of cases of a disease in a short period of time. Outbreaks of influenza are common and occur yearly in many places. An

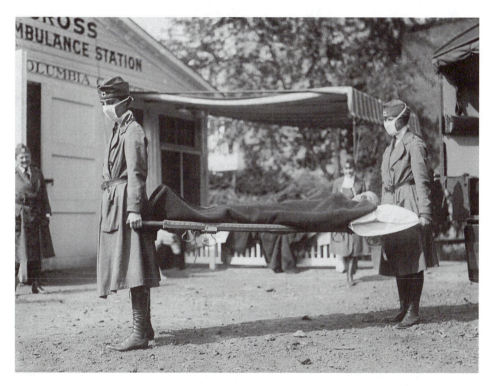

Demonstration at a Red Cross emergency station during the influenza epidemic of 1918. (Library of Congress)

epidemic refers to an outbreak that is confined to one location, such as a city or a country. Unfortunately, epidemics remain somewhat unpredictable with regard to the timing of onset and the severity of illness. Certain features make influenza epidemics more likely, including the following:

Winter months attributable to cold weather, crowding of people (usually to escape the cold), and high humidity;

Origination of the outbreak in either Eastern or Southern Hemisphere countries, with later spread to Europe and North America;

Occurrence of a variant virus with antigenic changes from previously recognized strains;

Presence of human cross-reacting antibody, acquired during previous infection, is low in the population, with regard to both the percentage of people positive for the antibody and the level of antibody present in positive individuals.

During a typical influenza epidemic, attack rates are estimated to be 10–20 percent, but, in certain populations, it can reach 40–50 percent. In temperate climates, epidemics tend to occur almost exclusively in winter months (October to April in the Northern Hemisphere and May to September in the Southern Hemisphere). Isolated cases, or even outbreaks, of influenza A have been reported during the warm weather months. In the tropics, influenza can be seen year-round. Summertime epidemics of influenza have occurred on cruise ships in both the Northern and Southern Hemispheres. Airline travel has also been linked to influenza outbreaks.

In most epidemics, a single strain of influenza will dominate, and other respiratory viruses decrease in frequency. Influenza A epidemics typically begin rather abruptly, peak over a two- to three-week period, and then last for two to three months in total. Usually, children are the first to suffer (often with an illness characterized by fever and respiratory symptoms). Increases in adult infections (with typical flulike symptoms) soon follow. Later manifestations of epidemics include absenteeism from school and work. Influenza B epidemics are generally less extensive and are associated with milder disease than those caused by influenza A. Often, the outbreaks of influenza B are reported in schools, military camps, chronic-care facilities, and nursing homes; it has also caused at least one identified outbreak on a cruise ship.

On occasion, two different strains of influenza circulate simultaneously. In addition, epidemics of influenza may occur during outbreaks of other respiratory viruses, such as adenovirus or respiratory syncytial virus. In some years, the end of an influenza epidemic is characterized by a brief spike in cases attributable to an entirely new strain of influenza. These mini-outbreaks are known as a "herald wave," and they give scientists a clue as to the likely dominant strain of the flu for the next season.

For an outbreak to be labeled a pandemic, several conditions must be satisfied: (1) after arising in a specific geographical area, the outbreak of infection spreads throughout the world; (2) a high percentage of individuals are infected, which then results in an increased death rate; and (3) the infection is caused by a new influenza A serotype, which is not related to the viruses that circulated immediately before and did not arise via mutation of the preceding viruses. Some characteristics of pandemics include the following:

- Extremely rapid transmission with concurrent outbreaks throughout the globe;
- The occurrence of disease outside the usual seasonality (including summer months);
- High attack rates in all age groups, with increased risk for complications and death in healthy young adults not generally affected by seasonal influenza;
- More severe symptoms in affected populations;
- High likelihood of increased mortality rates;
- Multiple waves of disease immediately before and after the main outbreak.

There are ongoing arguments in the medical and historical literature regarding the number of pandemics that have actually occurred as a result of influenza. Most references agree that there have been at least three in the last century.

The descriptions of the previous influenza pandemics are oftentimes disturbing, but understanding them to the fullest extent possible is necessary if preparation for a future pandemic is to be adequate. In addition to the great numbers of illnesses and deaths caused by influenza across the globe, the pandemics have had devastating consequences on social and economic circumstances in many countries.

The Spanish flu, 1918, was the most lethal outbreak of influenza ever and killed an estimated 20–50 million people worldwide. The spread of the virus was facilitated by the movement of troops involved in World War I. Second and third waves of infection occurred, with the latter waves being more deadly than the first. The influenza strain was ultimately identified as H1N1.

The Asian flu, 1957, was a pandemic that started in the Yunan Province of China in February. After causing many to become ill in China during March, it spread to Hong Kong, Singapore, Taiwan, and then Japan. Infection spread to India, Australia, and Indonesia in May; to Pakistan, Europe, North America, and the Middle East in June; to South Africa, South America, New Zealand, and the Pacific Islands in July; and to Central, West, and East Africa, Eastern Europe, and the Caribbean in August. Interestingly, a large conference held in Iowa served as a major landline for infection. Eighteen hundred young adults from 43 states and several foreign countries attended the conference; 200 of the attendees fell ill with influenza. These individuals then returned home and facilitated spread of the infection elsewhere.

Another landline was identified from Russia to Scandinavia and Eastern Europe; otherwise, the infection appears to have spread by sea travel. Within six months, the infection was worldwide. A second wave of infection occurred in early 1958, with regions in Europe, North America, Russia, and Japan involved. In some countries, the second wave was more severe. In total, the pandemic affected 40–50 percent of the world's population, with 25–30 percent showing signs or symptoms of the disease. The mortality rate was estimated to be 1 in 4,000; most deaths were in the very young and the very old. The strain was identified as H2N2, a subtype never before seen in the human population.

The Hong Kong flu, in 1968, was a pandemic that killed thousands of people worldwide (estimates suggest 700,000–1,000,000), including 34,000 in the United States. It began in Hong Kong in the summer months, traveled to Vietnam and Singapore, and eventually on to India, the Philippines, Australia, and Europe. The virus traveled to the United States in September but peaked in December and January 1969 with regard to mortality. Additional waves in 1969 and 1970 were also deadly and included cases in Japan, Africa, and South America. The decreased death rate compared with previous pandemics was thought to be multifactorial: possible partial immunity attributable to similarities to the 1957 Asian flu strain, better medical care, and availability of antibiotics to combat secondary bacterial infections. The strain was identified as H3N2, a virus subtype still in circulation today.

Experts agree that another influenza pandemic is inevitable and possibly imminent. In 2003, a World Health Organization (WHO) report by the Secretariat on Influenza projected that, if a new pandemic occurs, it will result, in industrialized countries alone, in 57–132 million outpatient health care visits, 1.0–2.3 million hospital admissions, and 280,000–650,000 deaths in less than two years. In developing countries, the impact is likely to be even more substantial. More recent estimates suggest that the appearance of a pandemic influenza virus could cause close to 3 million deaths in the United States and more than 100 million deaths worldwide.

More recently, after early outbreaks in North America in April 2009, a new H1N1 influenza virus spread around the world. The WHO declared a pandemic in June 2009, at which point a total of 74 countries and territories had reported laboratory-confirmed infections according to the WHO. This new virus led to patterns of death and illness not normally seen in influenza infections and caused the deaths of young people, including those who were otherwise healthy. Pregnant women, younger children, and people with chronic lung conditions appeared to be at a higher risk for complications and severe illness.

Although there were fears that the virus would mutate into a more lethal form, that did not occur and there were fewer deaths than originally predicted. After the pandemic was declared over, critics suggested the WHO had exaggerated its dangers. The WHO and the CDC declared the outbreak a pandemic in June 2009 and declared it over in April 2010. The WHO later examined its handling of the pandemic following continued criticism that drug companies influenced officials to spend money unnecessarily on stockpiles of H1N1 vaccines. The results found no evidence to support allegations that WHO declared a pandemic to boost pharmaceutical industry profits. Also, officials noted influenza viruses are unstable and can change rapidly due to mutations making it difficult to predict severity. The report stated that WHO and other health authorities' decisions were influenced by the severity of past pandemics, and simply erred on the side of caution ("International Response"). The CDC estimated that between 43 million and 89 million cases of H1N1 actually occurred during the pandemic, which resulted in up to 403,000 hospitalizations and possibly 18,300 deaths ("Updated CDC Estimates").

In addition to these statistics, other issues come to mind when considering a future pandemic, namely, the inability of health care systems to meet the demands cast on them during such an outbreak (e.g., there will likely be shortages of medical personnel, lack of respirators for all needy patients, inadequate isolation wards to limit spread of the disease, and too few hospital beds and other equipment for the numbers afflicted by the disease) and the worry that treatment will be delayed enough to clearly affect the death rates (e.g., vaccines may be unavailable in the early phase of a pandemic, with concurrent shortages of effective antiviral drugs in early weeks and months of the outbreak).

Despite the fact that an illness suggestive of influenza has existed for centuries, it was not until the 1930s that medical researchers, such as Richard Shope and Christopher H. Andrewes, were able to identify its viral cause. In spite of considerable medical advancements since that time, influenza continues to affect thousands of humans annually, and men, women, and children still die of flu-related complications each year. A curative treatment is not yet available, and prevention with annual vaccination remains based, to a large extent, on an educated guess. Perhaps most concerning of all is the fact that the virus has been responsible for some of the most devastating pandemics in history and is liable to cause another such event in the near future.

As a virus, influenza is simple with regard to its structure but entirely successful in achieving its goal: replication. Consisting of an inner genome, surrounded by an envelope covered in glycoprotein spikes, the influenza virus is not considered to be a living organism. However, it can easily infect a host, use the victim's own cell machinery to synthesize its proteins, and, with impressive rapidity, make new viral particles. In triggering the immune system and subsequently making its host ill, the new virions are expelled in air droplets with a cough or a sneeze. Usually, the new influenza viruses find other unsuspecting hosts to infect, and the process begins once again.

It is actually the simplicity of the influenza virus that allows its perpetual existence. The viral genome, which encodes for only eight proteins, is composed of an RNA backbone, held together with ribose sugars and phosphates. Lacking a proofreader, RNA viruses are subject to considerable mutation. In the case of influenza, the mutations are enough to cause antigenic drift, a seasonal variation in the HA and NA glycoprotein spikes projecting from the surface of the viral particles. This not only limits the ability to accurately determine what viral strains will predominate each season but also minimizes the chance that the human antibodies produced during previous infection will allow full protection against invasion of the virus in the future. Thus, humans (and other animals) are subject to annual, seasonal attacks of influenza and have suffered from disease outbreaks at least since the time of Hippocrates.

Even more worrisome, however, is the ability of influenza to undergo antigenic shift, a reassortment of viral components from both human and avian sources, allowing production of an entirely new strain of influenza that might have the unrecognizable HA or NA components from the bird genome with the transmission tendencies of the human virus. Thus, a novel influenza strain can spread unchecked, with absolutely no historical immunity to stand in its way. It is this phenomenon that likely led to most of the previous pandemics of the 20th century. The exception to this is the 1918 pandemic, which may have been caused by a purely avian strain of influenza that adapted to humans. Amazingly, medical researchers have been able to evacuate, isolate, and identify the influenza strain of 1918 from preserved autopsy specimens and from tissue obtained from victims buried in Alaska's permafrost. Now known as H1N1, the strain has been shown to have considerable lethality because of various factors such as enhanced replication capacity, high affinity for human respiratory epithelial cells, and mediation of the human immune response.

In most seasonal outbreaks of influenza, the great majority of cases tend to be uncomplicated. Occasionally, more severe manifestations of primary viral pneumonia or secondary bacterial pneumonia occur. More rarely still, extra-pulmonary manifestations are identified. Most health care providers are able to identify patients with influenza by conducting a health history and physical examination. In addition, laboratory testing with rapid antigen tests, serology, or viral culture can confirm the suspected diagnosis of influenza.

Once identified, patients with influenza can be offered supportive care, or, possibly, antiviral treatment (if symptoms have been present less than 48 hours at the time of diagnosis). Prevention of influenza is accomplished with both selective use of antiviral medications and vigilant seasonal immunization.

Currently, much attention is focused on the novel subtypes of influenza A that have more recently been identified, particularly H5N1. This avian influenza strain, initially identified in a human outbreak in Hong Kong in 1997, remains in circulation today. Although it has not yet shown strong human-to-human transmission, it continues to mutate, to cause isolated outbreaks, and to maintain an impressive lethality for its victims. It is just such an influenza strain that causes worry for a future, potentially devastating pandemic. If mutations or reassortment of H5N1 allow more ready spread between human hosts, an outbreak could rapidly spread across the globe among the current population without any hope of an antibody response. It is not difficult to imagine the consequences: high attack rates, severe morbidity and mortality, overwhelmed medical services, shortages of health care providers, political nightmares, and disruption of already fragile economies. Thus, aggressive monitoring of avian influenza strains continues through the efforts of the WHO, along with more than 50 countries and various international partners. Pandemic preparation is well underway, as are ongoing vaccine research and production. With such preemptive surveillance and proactive pandemic preparation, it is hoped that an event reminiscent of the 1918 outbreak can be averted or at least minimized.

The biography of influenza is rich with historical documentation, scientific discoveries, heroic adventures, unfortunate fatalities, and untiring research. Despite this attempt to convey its story in full, it is not likely to end here. Influenza's biography will continue to evolve along with humankind, and the manner in which the virus and humans will exist together remains to be seen.

*Roni K. Devlin*

*See also* Immune System/Lymphatic System; Pandemics; Virus; World Health Organization (WHO).

### References

Andrewes, C. H. "Fifty Years with Viruses." *Annual Review of Microbiology* 27 (1973): 1–14.

Barry, J. M. *The Great Influenza: The Epic Story of the Deadliest Plague in History.* New York: Viking, 2004.

Bureau of Public Affairs Fact Sheet. *U.S. Government Support to Combat Avian and Pandemic Influenza: An Update.* 2007. www.state.gov/r/pa/scp/86190.htm.

Centers for Disease Control and Prevention. "Seasonal Influenza (Flu)." www.cdc.gov/flu/.

Centers for Disease Control and Prevention. "Updated CDC Estimates of 2009 H1N1 Influenza Cases, Hospitalizations and Deaths in the United States, April 2009–April 10, 2010." May 14, 2010. www.cdc.gov/h1n1/estimates_2009_h1n1.htm.

Centers for Disease Control and Prevention. "Viral Gastroenteritis." www.cdc.gov/ncidod/dvrd/revb/gastro/faq.htm.

Devlin, Roni K. *Influenza.* Santa Barbara, CA: Greenwood, 2008.

Lynn, Jonathan. "WHO to Review Its Handling of H1N1 Flu Pandemic." *Reuters.* January 12, 2010. www.reuters.com.

National Institute of Allergy and Infectious Diseases. *Flu (Influenza): Timeline of Human Flu Pandemics.* 2007. www.niaid.nih.gov/topics/flu/research/pandemic/pages/timelinehuman pandemics.aspx.

U.S. Department of Health and Human Services. *Pandemic Flu.* 2006. www.pandemicflu.gov/.

World Health Organization. *Influenza: Report by the Secretariat.* 2003. www.who.int/gb/ebwha/pdf_files/WHA56/ea5623.pdf.

World Health Organization. "International Response to the Influenza Pandemic: WHO Responds to the Critics." June 10, 2010. www.who.int/csr/disease/swineflu/notes/briefing_20100610/en.

## INHALANTS

Inhalants are substances that have a chemical or volatile nature, leading to intoxication when inhaled into the lungs. These are readily available, and among the most common and insidious substances that we know to be abused. There are several general types of substances used as inhalants, whose chemical vapors can be inhaled for psychoactive (or mind-altering) effects. These include the categories of volatile substances—liquid solvents that vaporize at room temperature;

cleaning fluids—industrial or household products; fuels—including propane and gasoline; aerosols—sprays containing propellants and solvents; gases—found in household or commercial products; nitrites—a special class of inhalants abused primarily as sexual enhancement; and medical anesthetics.

People often do not think of these kinds of products as drugs—these common products have other uses and were never intended to be misused in this way. According to a recent 2009 study, these everyday substances may include such ordinary household products as gasoline, various glues, paint thinner, nail polish, nail polish remover, and spray paint. Other products misused include rubber cement, airplane glue, aerosol whipping cream and hairspray, and correction fluid. This kind of substance use and abuse is a worldwide problem, since the substances are so readily available and relatively inexpensive. In 2008 some 2 million Americans, age 12 and older, had abused inhalants according to the National Institute on Drug Abuse (NIDA). Those statistics were part of the Substance Abuse and Mental Health Services Administration (SAMHSA) National Survey on Drug Use and Health.

A minority of substances used as inhalants have medicinal purposes, such as nitrous oxide (a dental anesthetic) or amyl nitrite (which expands blood vessels, resulting in lowering of blood pressure). However, the majority of common substances mentioned above have no medicinal purpose. The abuse of these household products can be viewed as "recreational."

As mentioned in the *Diagnostic and Statistical Manual of Mental Disorders,* 4th edition, text revision (*DSM–IV–TR*; American Psychiatric Association, 2000), inhalant abuse is defined using the same listing of criteria identified for all other substance use disorders. In other words, abuse has one or more maladaptive patterns of use, resulting in clinically significant impairment or distress. This includes (1) recurrent failure to fulfill major role obligations; (2) recurrent use in physically hazardous situations; (3) recurrent substance-related legal problems; and (4) continued use despite persistent or recurrent social or interpersonal problems due to use. One marked exception is that a characteristic withdrawal symptom is not included in the *DSM–IV–TR* abuse criteria.

Inhalants are not regulated according to the Controlled Substances Act of 1970 (CSA), which serves as the foundation for the U.S. government's legal battle against drugs of abuse. Moreover, patterns of inhalant abuse are difficult to track, since there is lack of agreement of a national classification of inhalants. However, recent studies and trends in abuse and addiction have caused many state legislatures to place restrictions on the sale of many of these everyday household products to minors. As of 2000, according to the National Conference of State Legislatures, 38 states had "adopted laws preventing the sale, use, and/or distribution to minors of various products commonly abused as inhalants." In addition, many states have fines, incarceration, or mandatory treatment in place for those selling, distributing, using, or possessing inhalants.

Inhalant intoxication and abuse comes in different formats. In certain cases, the abuser inhales vapors directly from containers or bottles originally packaged by the manufacturer (called "sniffing" or "snorting"). Other abusers pour a small portion into a plastic bag and inhale a concentrated amount (called "bagging"). Still others use rags or bandannas soaked in fluids and held over the mouth (called "huffing"). Abusers can be called "glueys" or "huffers." Among the street names or slang for what can be "huffed" are glue, air gas, sniff, huff, boppers or poppers, discorama, hardware, snotballs, and laughing gas.

Short-term effects related to inhalant abuse include but are not limited to:

- Loss of inhibitions;
- Drowsiness;
- Initial feelings of well-being and relaxation;
- Flulike symptoms;
- Reckless behavior;
- Blurred vision;
- Unpleasant breath;
- Nosebleeds and sores around the mouth and nose.

Short-term effects of inhalants are felt immediately, since the chemical vapor enters the bloodstream directly from the lungs. Inhalants are depressants, so they slow down brain function and the activity of the central nervous system. This affects physical, mental, and emotional activity and responses. Common chemicals contained in these substances are fat-soluble, so the chemicals remain stored in the lungs, brain, heart, liver, and stomach lining for an extended period of time. This means that abuse often has long-term and lasting consequences. For example, the hippocampus—a region of the brain controlling memory—can be and often is affected by inhalant abuse. Abusers may lose the ability to learn new things, or even have a difficult time carrying on simple conversations. These short-term difficulties can be permanent.

Inhalants provide a sudden "high," but can also lead to sudden oxygen deficiency, or hypoxia. This may lead to brain damage or even death. Inhalation of aerosol items can be especially dangerous: these devices can generate very high concentrations of inhaled chemicals. Any use of any type of inhalant can also cause Sudden Sniffing Death Syndrome, or SSDS. Even a single session of inhalant use can induce the potential of dying from SSDS. This condition involves serious cardiac arrhythmia, which happens during or immediately following repeated inhalation. Repeated and high concentrations of inhalants also can cause death from suffocation, since the user may lose consciousness and stop breathing.

One special use of inhalants is seen as a "party drug," common to the nightclub scene. Amyl nitrite is typical of this sort of inhalant, and is made available in ampules ("poppers"). These are held to the nostrils for quick inhalation, specifically to enhance sexual arousal or stimulation. This type of drug—nitrites—are chemicals that cause vasodilation, and so have some legitimate health use, and are still used in certain medical procedures today. However, some variations of these nitrites have been banned from prescription use since the 1990s. They remain popular—in an illegal or nonprescribed form—among a certain segment of teens and young adults. The potential of SSDS remains with this form of inhalants, as well.

Heavy or frequent inhalant abuse often causes serious physical and psychological health problems. As described by the New Zealand Drug Foundation ("Inhalants and Solvents"), long-term effects may include but are not limited to:

- Weight loss;
- Muscle spasms or tremors;
- Constant thirst;
- Facial sores;
- Memory loss;
- Personality changes;
- Irritability;
- Seizures;
- Constant irregular heartbeat;
- Problems with breathing;
- Brain and nerve damage;
- Stupor or coma.

If the abuser continues to use, some of the above damage becomes irreversible. In fact, chronic inhalant abuse has come to be associated with neurological damage. Cognitive changes and abnormalities can be permanent, and can range from mild cognitive impairment to severe dementia.

Inhalants are one of the most easily obtained substances, so children and adolescents are among those most likely to abuse them. According to the NIDA, adolescents can abuse different products at different ages. For example, users ages 12–15 are likely to abuse glue, shoe polish, spray paints, gasoline, and lighter fluid. Inhalant abusers can be identified by such markers as organic solvent odors on their breath or clothes. In addition, concerned loved ones may possibly find spray paint canisters or solvent containers stashed nearby, along with the "huffing" materials such as stained rags or plastic bags.

Different classes of users (e.g., street children, school-aged children from certain geographic regions, or indigenous people-groups) are particularly prone to initial inhalant abuse. Young people involved with the juvenile system and those with exposure to the criminal justice system have been noted to be disproportionately affected by this kind of product abuse. Generally speaking, living in unhappy situations, with family-of-origin and/or school problems, poverty, child abuse and other forms of abusive behavior all are highly associated with inhalant abuse, according to a number of NIDA and other research studies (National Institute on Drug Abuse, "Inhalants").

Nitrous oxide—one of the few medically relevant inhalants, commonly used for minor dental or outpatient procedures—has long been known to be abused widely among health professionals or their staff members. Similar to nitrous oxide are other anesthetics: ether, chloroform, and halothane. This is one kind of inhalant that is not as readily available to the general public, although if someone has connections or enough money, it can be obtained without a prescription by mail order, Internet, or fraudulent or illegal means.

There are specific laws on record in states across the country prohibiting the use or sale of inhalants, citing the particular chemical compounds that induce intoxication. For example, the state of Illinois has drug statutes that have been active since January 1997, stipulating that use of such chemicals ("in any manner changing, distorting or disturbing the auditory, visual or mental processes") is legally deemed "an intoxicated condition." These drug statutes are particularly stringent when it comes to the sale or delivery of such inhalants to young people under the age of 18.

If users do decide to suddenly stop inhalant use, withdrawal symptoms can appear. These often include anxiety, depression, loss of appetite, irritation, aggressive behavior, dizziness, nausea, and a high level of craving. These withdrawal symptoms sometimes resemble alcohol withdrawal. Inpatient drug and alcohol detoxification units have some familiarity with inhalants, more so than the typical hospital emergency department (ED). The point can be made that certain hospital EDs would have more understanding about inhalants, given their proximity to vulnerable subpopulations. However, the better option would be to provide an abuser who wanted to stop his use with knowledgeable medical and clinical help.

*Elizabeth Jones*

*See also* Addiction; Drugs, Recreational.

## References

American Psychiatric Association. *Diagnostic and Statistical Manual of Mental Disorders.* 4th ed., text rev. Washington, DC: American Psychiatric Association, 2000.

Balster, R.L., S.L. Cruz, M.O. Howard, C.A. Dell, and L.B. Cottler. "Classification of Abused Inhalants." *Addiction* 104, no. 6 (2009): 878–82.

Hanson, G.R., P.J. Venturelli, and A.E. Fleckenstein. "Inhalants." *Drugs and Society.* 9th ed. Ch. 14, 418–29; "Appendix B, Drugs of Use and Abuse," 570–75. Burlington, MA: Jones and Bartlett, 2006.

Illinois Drug Statutes, Criminal Offenses (720 ILCS 690/1-2) Use of Intoxicating Compounds Act. Enacted January 1997.

National Conference of State Legislatures. Unpublished information on inhalant legislation through June 2000.

National Institute on Drug Abuse. *NIDA InfoFacts.* "Inhalants." Updated March 2010, http://drugabuse.gov/infofacts.

New Zealand Drug Foundation. "Inhalants and Solvents." www.nzdf.org.nz/inhalants-solvents.

Perron, B.E., M.O. Howard, M.G. Vaughn, and C.S. Jarman. "Inhalant Withdrawal as a Clinically Significant Feature of Inhalant Dependence Disorder." *Medical Hypotheses* 73 (2009): 935–37.

Van Dusen, V., and A.R. Spies. "An Overview and Update of the Controlled Substances Act of 1970." *Pharmacy Times,* February 1, 2007. www.pharmacytimes.com/print.php?url=2007-02-6309.

## INSOMNIA

Imagine this scenario. You go to the doctor complaining of a chronic throbbing pain in your temples and across your forehead. The doctor pauses a minute, then says, "You have a headache" and writes you a prescription for aspirin. The aspirin may alleviate the pain, but it does not address the underlying cause of the headache. Sleep medicine pioneer Dr. William Dement suggests that this headache scenario is similar to a diagnosis of insomnia. "Insomnia is simply some sort of difficulty sleeping" (Dement, 1999).

In fact, Dement (1999) asserts that insomnia is itself a symptom rather than a disorder. Kovacevic-Ristanovic and Kuzniar also define insomnia as "a complaint (symptom) related to all conditions that lead to a perception of inadequate, disturbed, insufficient or non-restorative sleep (despite an adequate opportunity to sleep), accompanied by daytime consequences of inadequate sleep" (Kovacevic-Ristanovic & Kuzniar, 2009).

In order to better understand insomnia, it is helpful to understand how the sleep process works. The sleep-wake cycle is regulated by what is commonly called the "biological clock." More precise than a well-crafted Swiss timepiece, the human biological clock regulates our varying degrees of alertness and drowsiness with remarkable consistency. We remain awake and alert as a result of our biological clock through a process called clock-dependent alerting (Dement, 1999). While we remain awake, we accumulate something else critical to our knowledge of sleep—sleep debt (Dement, 1999). "Our understanding of both clock-dependent alerting and sleep debt had provided the pillars for a very simple and elegant model of what governs why we are awake during the day and sleep at night" (Dement, 1999).

In fact, clock-dependent alerting and the tendency to sleep resulting from accumulated sleep debt combine to form a homeostatic process that Dement (1999) called the opponent-process model. The level of stimulation required to stay awake is balanced against the need for sleep. These two processes interact dynamically throughout the day. "The main reason that we can sleep through the night is that we have accumulated sufficient sleep debt during the day so that the unopposed homeostatic sleep process is free to operate all night long" (Dement, 1999). Insomnia occurs when some biological, psychological, or environmental stimulus disrupts the interaction of this process. The operation of clock-dependent alerting becomes particularly salient in circadian rhythm–related sleep disorders.

Between 33 and 50 percent of the adult population report symptoms of insomnia, while 10–15 percent report symptoms that are distressing or result in impairment (Schutte-Rodin et al., 2008). Those more at risk are older, female, have some other medical or psychiatric problem, or have a job involving shift work (Schutte-Rodin et al., 2008). Those with medical or psychiatric problems appear to be at greatest risk, with those diagnosed with either chronic pain disorders or a psychiatric disorder "having insomnia rates as high as 50 to 75%" (Schutte-Rodin et al., 2008, p. 490).

Most simply, insomnia may be subdivided into transient and chronic (Dement, 1999). Transient insomnia is episodic and short-lived, lasting from a single night to a couple of weeks, while chronic insomnia can last weeks, months, or years. Schenck refers to multiple episodes of transient insomnia as "intermittent insomnia" (Schenck, 2007). Transient insomnia may occur for any number of situational reasons, including changes in routine that disrupt sleep rhythms such as shift work or jet lag, a sleeping environment not conducive to sleep, like a spouse or roommate who snores, or even worry about not sleeping (Schenck, 2007). Excitement or anticipation of a positive event can also disturb sleep.

According to the American Academy of Sleep Medicine (2005), there are 11 sleep disorders that may be categorized as insomnias, some of which will be considered. Many overlap and may be considered together. The first is called inadequate sleep hygiene. "The essential feature of inadequate sleep hygiene is an insomnia associated with daily living activities that are inconsistent with the maintenance of good quality sleep and full daytime alertness" (American Academy of Sleep Medicine, 2005). The activities may be subdivided into those activities that increase mental, physical, or emotional arousal too close to bedtime, and activities that inhibit consistent sleep scheduling, including excessive napping, irregular bedtimes and rising times, or using the bed for nonsleep-related activities, like reading, watching television, and so forth.

Adjustment insomnia, also known as acute insomnia, occurs when an identifiable stressor is significant enough to disrupt sleep. "Specific examples include changes or disputes in interpersonal relationships, occupational stress, personal losses, bereavement, diagnosis of a new medical condition, visiting or moving to a new location, or physical changes to the usual sleep environment" (American Academy of Sleep Medicine, 2005). Adjustment insomnia may also occur with positive stressors, like a work promotion or personal achievement. Once the external stressor is resolved, the insomnia is expected to resolve as well.

Psychophysiologic insomnia develops from the negative interaction between heightened physiological arousal and conditioned responses to the arousal that inhibits sleep. "Arousal may be physiological, cognitive, or emotional, and characterized by muscle tension, 'racing thoughts,' or heightened awareness of the environment" (Schutte-Rodin et al., 2008, p. 496). These distressing physiological symptoms become paired with learned associations to the environment that prevent sleep. Imagine the troubled sleeper who lays awake exhausted but unable to sleep. She stares at the alarm clock and dwells on the importance of getting to sleep. The sense of urgency heightens her physiological arousal, which inhibits sleep onset.

This sets up a vicious cycle wherein a baseline condition of heightened tension is exacerbated by worry about not sleeping. The result is similar to what made Pavlov's dogs salivate at the sound of a bell. The patient begins associating her insomnia with her sleeping environment—her bedroom, her nighttime routine, and so forth. Whereas once setting the alarm clock was a neutral stimulus, it becomes a conditioned stimulus that provokes a conditioned response of anxiety about not sleeping, which in turn heightens the person's state of physiological arousal and perpetuates the insomnia.

Idiopathic insomnia is a rare type of insomnia believed to begin at birth resulting from dysfunction in either the brain's arousal system or those systems associated with inducing or maintaining sleep. "One hallmark of idiopathic insomnia is the absence of any factors associated with the onset or persistence of the condition, including psychosocial stressors, other sleep and medical disorders, or medications" (American Academy of Sleep Medicine, 2005). The severity of the disorder determines the psychological health of the patient; patients with mild to moderate idiopathic insomnia exhibit normal psychological levels of functioning and appear to cope successfully when not overfocused on their sleep loss.

Sleep state misperception, otherwise known as paradoxical insomnia, involves the patient's perception of suffering from insomnia when objective measures of sleep reveal otherwise. In other words, they are getting good sleep but believe they are insomniacs. Objective sleep states can be measured in sleep disorder centers by recording brain waves during sleep, otherwise known as a polysomnograph. In one laboratory study, patients with sleep state misperception complained of insomnia but showed no objective sleep disturbance (Salin-Pascual et al., 1992). When compared with patients with objective insomnia and healthy controls, patients with sleep state misperception were not significantly different from controls on total time asleep, time before falling asleep, amount of wakefulness during sleep, and number of awakenings during sleep. By comparison, patients with objective insomnia were significantly different on all of those variables when compared with both the patients with sleep state misperception and healthy controls.

Insomnias due to other factors may be categorized as insomnia due to mental disorder, insomnia due to a drug or substance, and insomnia due to a medical condition. Sleep disturbances are characteristic of both major depressive disorder and bipolar disorder. Anxiety and stress-related mental disorders may also provoke insomnia. Drugs or substances can run the gamut from prescription medication, recreational drugs including alcohol and caffeine, food, or environmental toxins. Insomnia due to a medical condition should involve a cause-effect relationship where the medical condition causes insomnia, not where insomnia and the medical condition co-occur but are independent from one another (Schutte-Rodin et al., 2008).

In general, strategies for treating adjustment, pyschophysiologic, idiopathic, and paradoxical insomnias may be grouped into three categories: (1) sleep hygiene education; (2) cognitive-behavioral interventions; and (3) medication. Education for good sleep hygiene "includes setting a fixed hour for retiring each night, eliminating daytime naps, avoiding caffeine-containing beverages or anxiety-producing activities at night, and assuring that the bedroom is quiet, dark, and comfortable" (Kovacevic-Ristanovic & Kuzniar, 2009). There are a variety of cognitive-behavioral interventions that are successful in treating insomnia, including progressive relaxation training, controlling arousal-provoking stimuli, and two types of paradoxical intention: attempting to stay awake, and sleep state restriction, which involves a prescribed amount of hours the patient is permitted to sleep (Dement, 1999; Schutte-Rodin et al., 2008).

Medications typically used in treating insomnia include a short- to intermediate-acting primary sedating medication like Ambien, sedating antidepressants, and, when the patient does not respond to either of those or a combination thereof, use of anti-epilepsy medications or atypical antipsychotics. Over-the-counter sleep aids and herbal supplements are not subject to appropriate clinical drug trials or regulation for purity by the Food and Drug Administration and many physicians discourage their use (Dement, 1999; Schutte-Rodin et al., 2008).

Breathing-related sleep disorders would also meet Dement's definition for insomnia, that which includes any difficulty sleeping. Of those, obstructive sleep apnea appears to be the most prevalent. Dement (1999) asserts that 40 percent of the population suffers from some form of sleep apnea, half of which are serious enough to warrant medical attention. During episodes of sleep apnea, the sleeper's throat collapses, blocking the airway and depriving the sleeper of oxygen, much like a pillow over the face. "At this breathless moment, the immediate future holds only two possibilities: death or waking up to breath" (Dement, 1999). As the sleeper suffocates, the brain becomes increasingly alarmed with the dramatic loss of oxygen and reacts; the sleeper struggles awake with a loud exhalation of breath that resembles a giant snore and is often accompanied by vocalizations.

These micro-awakenings can occur hundreds of times during the night. People suffering from obstructive sleep apnea are often loud snorers and complain of as many of the symptoms as others who suffer from insomnia, but additional symptoms include complaints of dry mouth, headache, and uncontrollable sleep attacks where the patient falls asleep in sedentary situations, while driving, and even while carrying on conversations (American Academy of Sleep Medicine, 2005). Severe cases can lead to significant impairment in social and occupational functioning. Obstructive sleep apnea may be successfully treated through the use of continuous positive air pressure, or CPAP, which occurs through the use of a machine that is calibrated to open the patient's airway sufficiently enough to permit normal respiration. There are a variety of models, but generally CPAP machines force air through the nasal passages with an apparatus that either fits over the face or is fitted against the nostrils.

Movement-related sleep disorders also cause difficulty sleeping. One of these, Restless Leg Syndrome (RLS), "is the third-most-commonly reported sleep disorder, and is one of the most common causes of severe insomnia" (Schenck, 2007). RLS is characterized by abnormal, uncomfortable sensations in the legs that compel the patient to move them in order alleviate the feelings. Patients often describe these sensations as "creeping," "crawling," or "tingling" (Schenck, 2007). These sensations occur prior to sleep or when the patient is relaxing. Additionally, they can occur during sleep, compelling the patient to wake long enough to alleviate the symptoms through movement. One patient described how her symptoms presented during the night: "Meanwhile, my patient husband lost sleep because I kicked him all throughout the night. He told me I spooned up against him and 'jackhammered' his back with both my knees—rapidly and repeatedly, often throughout the night" (Schenck, 2007). Treatment of RLS typically involves the use of medication.

Another source of insomnia comes from disruptions to the circadian rhythms that coordinate sleep and wakefulness. One such example is delayed sleep phase disorder. A patient suffering from delayed sleep phase disorder will be unable to fall asleep at the conventional or socially acceptable times, delaying her sleep by at least two hours (American Academy of Sleep Medicine, 2005). Similarly, her preferred wake-up time would be later in the morning than would be otherwise conventional. Those required to wake at the conventional time would begin their day with a significant sleep debt and exhibit excessive daytime sleepiness (Kovacevic-Ristanovic & Kuzniar, 2009). A similar such sleep disorder is advanced sleep phase disorder, which involves a disruption of the circadian rhythm wherein the patient becomes ready for sleep much earlier in the evening than is otherwise conventional and prefers to wake up much earlier in the morning than is otherwise conventional; complaints involve excessive late afternoon or early evening sleepiness and early morning insomnia (American Academy of Sleep Medicine, 2005). Both sleep disorders may respond successfully to phototherapy; bright light exposure during the early morning may alleviate delayed sleep phase disorder, while bright light exposure during the evening may alleviate advanced sleep phase disorder (Dement, 1999).

It would seem counterintuitive to think that something as simple and natural as sleep would be so elusive for some, but those who suffer from insomnia and the excessive daytime fatigue that accompanies it know only too well its grave consequences. It is one thing to fall asleep at the movies; it is altogether different to fall asleep while driving a car or operating machinery. Except in rare cases, insomnia is a treatable symptom and those who suffer from it may, with the correct diagnosis and treatment, regain the healthful effects of a good night's sleep.

*Kevin J. Eames*

*See also* Bipolar Disorder; Depression.

## References

American Academy of Sleep Medicine. *International Classification of Sleep Disorders, Revised: Diagnostic and Coding Manual.* Westchester, IL: American Academy of Sleep Medicine, 2001.

American Academy of Sleep Medicine. *International Classification of Sleep Disorders, 2nd edition: Diagnostic and Coding Manual.* Westchester, IL: American Academy of Sleep Medicine, 2005.

American Psychiatric Association. *Diagnostic and Statistical Manual of Mental Disorders.* 4th ed. Washington, DC: American Psychiatric Association, 1994.

Dement, W.C. *The Promise of Sleep.* New York: Delacorte Press, 1999.

Kovacevic-Ristanovic, R., and T.J. Kuzniar. "Sleep Disorders." In *Clinical Adult Neurology,* edited by J. Corey-Bloom and R.B. David, 167–84. New York: Demos Medical, 2009.

Salin-Pascual, R.J., T.A. Roehrs, L.A. Merlotti, F. Zorick, and T. Rother. "Long-Term Study of Sleep of Insomnia Patients with Sleep State Misperception and Other Insomnia Patients." *American Journal of Psychiatry* 149, no. 7 (1992): 904–8.

Schenck, C.H. *Sleep.* New York: Avery, 2007.

Schutte-Rodin, S., L. Broch, D. Buysee, C. Dorsey, and M. Sateia. "Clinical Guideline for the Evaluation and Management of Chronic Insomnia in Adults." *Journal of Clinical Sleep Medicine* 4, no. 5 (2008): 487–504.

# INSTITUTE OF MEDICINE (IOM)

The Institute of Medicine (IOM) represents the health care arm of the National Academies, which along with the IOM, refers to the National Academy of Sciences, National Academy of Engineering, and the National Research Council. Together these private, nonprofit organizations strive to provide the U.S. government with sound independent policy guidance regarding science, technology, and medicine.

The National Academy of Sciences was established by President Abraham Lincoln in 1863 to serve in an advisory capacity to the U.S. government. Over time scientific matters became more varied and complex, which meant the work of these three organizations ultimately became more important. The research council was chartered in 1916, and more recently the academy of engineering in 1964, and the IOM in 1970.

Election to membership in the academies is one of the highest honors a scientist or engineer can receive. IOM members are among the most distinguished leaders in the health care professions; the natural, social, and behavioral sciences; law; administration; engineering; and the humanities. They volunteer their time in service to the nation. Their collective knowledge and expertise aid in informing public opinion and the advancement of medicine.

To accomplish its mission of improving health, the IOM draws on these diverse specialists and a wide array of stakeholders to provide independent, objective counsel on health-related issues. They assist the public and private sectors in making educated health decisions.

Often the studies, and other activities, conducted by the IOM are done in response to congressional orders, but others begin as requests from federal agencies and independent organizations. All study reports and policy documents produced by the IOM are authored by a committee of experts and then undergo peer review by anonymous experts who did not participate in the development of the original research. The evidence-based findings, widely distributed and disseminated, have an impact on the best ways to ensure public wellness. This can directly and indirectly affect the health behaviors of the consumer health user and the general U.S. population.

In one study on tobacco control, the IOM cautioned that children of parents who smoke were nearly twice as likely to start smoking compared to children in households where the parents did not smoke; in another, IOM experts called for uniform certification of personal protective technologies to better shield employees from injury or danger in their workplace. On a broader scale, environmental disasters such as the 2010 Gulf of Mexico oil spill also involved the institute. A review of the health effects associated with the oil spill and setting research priorities for assessing those effects has become part of its agenda. Epilepsy, with more than 40 types, afflicts 1 in 100 adults and 1 in 20 children and has major consequences for all aspects of public health. It is another example of the medical diseases or conditions studied by the IOM for its impact on a population's health and quality of life.

The Institute of Medicine's work touches every American and his overall health. Its role will remain important as approaches to health care and medical science continue to evolve.

*Dianne L. Needham*

*See also* U.S. Department of Health and Human Services (HHS).

### References

Institute of Medicine. www.iom.edu/.
Institute of Medicine. "Certifying Personal Protective Technologies: Improving Worker Safety." www.iom.edu/Reports/2010/Certifying-Personal-Protective-Technologies-Improving-Worker-Safety.aspx.
Institute of Medicine. "Ending the Tobacco Problem: A Blueprint for the Nation." May 2007. www.iom.edu/~/media/Files/Report%20Files/2007/Ending-the-Tobacco-Problem-A-Blueprint-for-the-Nation/Tobaccoreportbriefgeneral.pdf.
Institute of Medicine. "The Public Health Dimensions of the Epilepsies." www.iom.edu/Activities/Disease/Epilepsy.aspx.
Institute of Medicine. "Review of the Federal Response to the Health Effects Associated with the Gulf of Mexico Oil Spill." Fall 2010. www.iom.edu/Activities/PublicHealth/FedResponseOilSpill.aspx.
National Academies of Science. www.nationalacademies.org/.

## IRRADIATION

As the distance our food travels from field to table increases, scientists and consumers are asking with more urgency how we can keep our food supply safe. The Centers for Disease Control and Prevention (CDC) estimate that every year, more than 76 million people become ill from something they have eaten, and of these, some 5,000 die from a variety of foodborne diseases (CDC, 2009). The government and nuclear industry suggest food can be treated with irradiation to improve its safety. However, this decades-old idea still raises strong emotions, and—as with any controversial issue—there are two sides to the argument with two vastly different opinions on what it means for our health.

**What Is Irradiation?**   Food irradiation is a way to preserve food and extend its shelf life by exposing that food, either prepackaged or in bulk, to very high-energy, invisible light waves or radiation. Supporters compare the irradiation of food to the pasteurization of milk, using the phrase "cold pasteurization" to describe the process. Like pasteurization, irradiation kills a number of harmful bacteria, but not all, which means foods can be reinfected if not handled properly. Critics of irradiation argue that it is nothing like pasteurization. They challenge the food industry to instead reduce harmful bacteria by cleaning up the process of food handling itself. Critics fear that irradiation may do more harm than good to the very people it is designed to protect.

There are three basic types of energy used for irradiation: X-rays, electron beams, and gamma rays. The majority of irradiated meat is processed using elec-

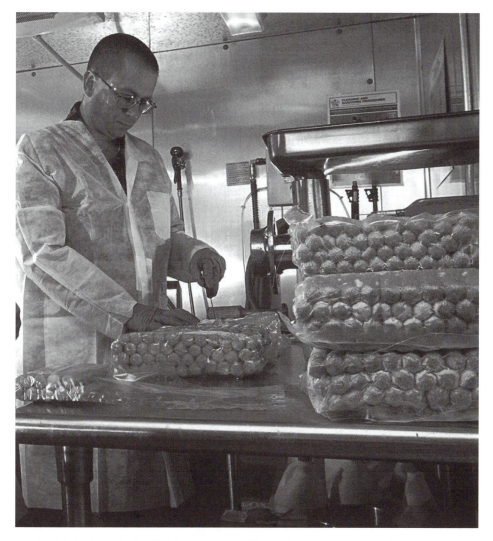

A microbiologist with the U.S. Department of Agriculture vacuum-seals hot dogs in preparation for irradiation. Food irradiation is a safety technology that uses ionizing radiation to kill disease-causing organisms in such foods as raw meat, raw poultry, and fresh produce. (U.S. Department of Agriculture)

tron beam or gamma ray technology. Gamma rays are produced by cobalt-60 or cesium-137—radioactive substances, called radioisotopes, that continuously emit dangerous rays when not submerged in water. A cobalt-based irradiator consists of a rack of radioactive rods, and requires a substantial amount of space to house the 15-foot-deep pool of water needed to absorb and neutralize the gamma rays when the rods are not in use.

Conveyor belts carry the food around the radioactive rack so the rays can penetrate all sides. The rays can penetrate food to a greater depth than electron beams, so irradiation treatment times vary: fresh strawberries might take 5 minutes, whereas frozen meat would need up to 20 minutes of treatment time (Goldstein & Goldstein, 2002). Like cobalt-60 irradiators, cesium-137 irradiators are stored in pools of water when not in use. They use fuel from decommissioned nuclear weapons and other radioactive waste. Cesium is water-soluble, making it very dangerous in the event of an accident, and it remains radioactive for hundreds of years, making it expensive to store.

Electron beam, or e-beam, irradiators lack penetrating power, but they do deliver faster and higher doses of radiation than gamma ray irradiators. They can only penetrate up to four inches, making them suitable for flat products such as hamburger patties. Food packaged in cartons is usually too thick to be processed with this method. The electron beams are not from radioactive sources, so they do not create radioactive waste; however, they do generate ionizing changes in foods. Ionizing radiation works by damaging the DNA of disease-causing bacteria such as *Salmonella* and *E. coli;* it either kills the microorganisms or genetically alters them so they can't reproduce. Whereas higher doses damage molecules in the food, lower doses damage only microorganisms and insects. Another positive aspect of e-beams is that the energy produced can be adjusted or turned off, making them safer for the environment and for workers.

The development of X-ray technology for irradiation is a blend of the other two techniques. X-rays penetrate like gamma rays, but are nonradioactive like electron beams. Produced by machines more powerful than those used in hospitals or dental offices, X-rays used in food irradiation penetrate well but have a slower processing speed. This means that larger volumes can be irradiated with X-ray systems, but that the process takes longer to accomplish.

Whichever method is used, food is irradiated at one of three dose levels—a dose being the amount of radiation absorbed by the food. The dose is based on the intensity of the radiation used and on the length of time it is applied. In the early days of the technology, doses were measured in rads—short for "radiation absorbed dose." However, the U.S. Food and Drug Administration (FDA) later switched from the rad to the gray (Gy), which is equal to 100 rads. A kilogray (kGy) is equal to 1,000 Gy. For example, to kill *Salmonella* bacteria, chicken receives from 1 to 10 kGy while a single chest X-ray gives a dose of only half a milliGray—many million times less radiation than is delivered to the chicken (FDA, *Federal Register* 51, 1986).

Over the years, the FDA has approved irradiation treatment for various types of food at low, medium, or high dose levels. Fresh bagged and loose iceberg lettuce and spinach was approved for ionized radiation in August 2008 after it had earlier been approved to kill bugs at lower doses in 2006. A low dose is up to 1 kGy, and is applied to control insects in grains, stop potatoes from sprouting, control trichinae in pork, and delay decay in fruits and vegetables. Medium doses, from 1 to 10 kGy, are used to neutralize *Salmonella, E. coli, Campylobacter,* and *Shigella* in meat, poultry, and fish, as well as to delay the growth of mold on strawberries and other fruits.

The highest doses, above 10 kGy, can kill microorganisms and insects in spices, and commercially sterilize foods to the same degree as canning. These highest doses are used for special hospital diets given to immune-compromised patients. Hospitals and other medical facilities routinely use radiation to sterilize equipment. This began in the mid-1960s, when a division of Johnson & Johnson sterilized sutures using radiation. Today, the United States has more than 40 licensed irradiation facilities, and most are used to sterilize medical and pharmaceutical supplies as well as other consumer products such as bandages, baby-bottle nipples, and cosmetic raw materials.

It is important to note that irradiation does not kill viruses, the bacteria that cause botulism, or the prions thought to cause mad cow disease (also known as bovine spongiform encephalopathy). It also does not eliminate the possibility of cross-contamination, especially of meat. Irradiated meat can still become contaminated if handled improperly, so consumers need to follow the same cooking and handling methods as with regular meat. For this reason, opponents question the benefit of food irradiation. They argue that no real need exists if people follow traditional food safety rules, and especially if the food industry significantly improves how food is handled during processing.

**Early Radiation**    French physicist Antoine-Henri Becquerel was the first scientist to harness radiant energy or radiation. For his part in the discovery of the radioactivity of uranium salts, Becquerel shared the 1903 Nobel Prize in physics with Marie and Pierre Curie. Marie Curie was Becquerel's graduate student at the time, and was involved in an intensive study of radiation for her doctoral thesis. Curie was the first woman to win the Nobel Prize, and one of the few scientists to win it twice.

It was American biologist Samuel Prescott who linked radiation with food safety in 1904. A professor of biology at the Massachusetts Institute of Technology (MIT), Prescott initiated studies on the effect of gamma rays from radium on bacteria, and demonstrated that the rays could kill bacteria in food. However, the lack of suitable radiation sources and their high cost hindered his research. That same year, he founded the Boston Biochemical Laboratory so he could continue his work on the problems of bacteria in preserved food.

It was 50 years later that commercial irradiation of food finally kicked into high gear. On December 8, 1953, President Dwight Eisenhower stood before the United Nations General Assembly and gave his "Atoms for Peace" address. The Atoms for Peace program, spearheaded by the U.S. Atomic Energy Commission, aimed to use atomic energy for peaceful purposes. Eisenhower also formed the National Food Irradiation Program, which launched research projects on food irradiation sponsored by both the Atomic Energy Commission and the U.S. Army. The army then conducted a series of experiments with fruits, vegetables, dairy products, fish, and meats, with an eye toward providing sterile foods that it could substitute for canned or frozen meals for soldiers, particularly in combat situations.

The nuclear age brought with it large sources of radiation materials, but consumers were afraid of anything suggesting nuclear exposure after seeing the effects of the explosions at Hiroshima and Nagasaki. Americans also connected the concept of radiation with nuclear power plants and medical X-rays, both caution-filled technologies that constantly guard against unnecessary exposure. To this day, discussion of food irradiation elicits a very emotional response from opponents of the technology, based on these same fears.

When U.S. consumers reacted negatively to the early introduction of gamma irradiation for treating food, American lawmakers decided to maintain tight control of the developing technology—especially because, up to that point, it had been completely funded by the government. In crafting the 1958 Food, Drug, and Cosmetic Act, Congress defined food irradiation as an additive rather than a process. This decision was intended to guarantee continued oversight and testing by the Food and Drug Administration (FDA) as manufacturers became involved in irradiation and rolled out new products.

Defining irradiated foods as additives also ensured that those foods and their packaging would need FDA approval. Moreover, if animal products were involved, approval from the U.S. Department of Agriculture (USDA) was necessary as well. FDA regulations still require manufacturers seeking approval for irradiation products to file a food additive petition with either agency after gathering data to demonstrate safety. USDA regulations also mandate that workers be trained in the safe operation of irradiation equipment. Manufacturers who choose to irradiate meat or meat products need to comply with USDA Food Safety and Inspection Service (FSIS) and FDA requirements, as well as with regulations from the Nuclear Regulatory Commission, the Environmental Protection Agency, the Occupational Safety and Health Administration, the Department of Transportation, and state and local governments.

Even with oversight from so many government agencies, the question of safety testing remains a controversial issue and a battleground between supporters and opponents of irradiation technology. The 1958 act called on the government to set up safe conditions of use and parameters that irradiated food must meet. However, beginning in the 1960s, when the first petition for the treatment of food with radiation was submitted to the FDA, the agency failed to decide on test procedures to establish a reasonable certainty of no harm. Following decades of debate, the final statute did not come until April 1986, and did not prescribe what safety tests should be performed, instead leaving that determination to the "discretion of scientists" (Pauli & Takeguchi, 1986).

In 1963, the FDA approved irradiation of wheat, flour, and canned bacon using cobalt-60 gamma rays, largely on the basis of early research by the U.S. Army. Other products quickly followed, including wheat and wheat products irradiated to control insect infestation. A few weeks later, the FDA again approved irradiation of canned bacon, this time using electron beam radiation at 45 to 56 kGy. The following year, the FDA amended the regulation to include irradiation of white potatoes to inhibit sprout development using cobalt-60 at 50 to 100 Gy.

**Labels and Packaging**   Other changes were made to the regulation, detailing radiation types and doses for a growing list of products, but it wasn't until 1965 that the USDA issued a regulation requiring the labeling of irradiated foods. This new regulation required that the phrase "Processed by ionizing radiation" appear on the labels. It was the first explicit government labeling requirement (Pauli

& Takeguchi, 1986). The regulations were amended several times, with the final statement, effective on March 2, 1967, remaining in place until April 18, 1986 (Pauli & Takeguchi, 1986). The labeling regulations required various statements, including "Treated with ionizing radiation" on retail packages of low-dose-treated foods; "Treated with ionizing radiation—do not irradiate again" on wholesale packages of bulk shipments of low-dose-treated foods; and "Processed by ionizing radiation" on foods treated with high-dose gamma ray, electron beam, and X-ray radiation. Manufacturers were allowed to replace the term *ionizing radiation* with *gamma-radiation, electron radiation,* or *X-radiation,* as appropriate.

All foods must be completely packaged before being irradiated, so several petitions for packaging materials were submitted for approval to the FDA beginning in 1965. The regulations were amended several more times as the agency worked to establish clear rules in a rapidly developing technology. However, the FDA continued to wrestle in particular with the issue of how to test irradiated foods for safety.

Historically, the FDA has used feeding studies to determine the safety of a food additive. By the spring of 1967, there was growing concern that petitions for irradiated foods were not meeting the agency's safety standards and were failing to win approval. That year, the FDA's Bureau of Science conducted a seminar for government scientists and administrators to improve the quality of petitions in the hope of increasing the petition approval rate. The report issued from that seminar by the associate director of the Bureau of Science addressed key questions, including, "What is the significance of radiation-induced mutations in microorganisms?"; "What is a sound basis for extrapolation of data from one product to another, from one species to another, or from one level of exposure to another?"; and "What is the significance of the destruction of vitamins?" (FDA, *Federal Register* 33, 1968).

Those questions were not immediately answered due to the growing concern over the quality of safety data. The situation came to a head in 1968, when the FDA rejected a petition for radiation-sterilized ham that relied on many of the same reports submitted in the original, successful petition for radiation-sterilized bacon in 1963. In a move that received little media attention, the agency revoked the regulations for high-dose gamma ray, electron beam, and X-ray radiation processing of canned bacon in October 1968. The FDA reported noticeable problems in animal studies that raised doubts about the safety of irradiated bacon, listing "significant adverse effects on reproduction in animals fed irradiated bacon, increased death rates in rats and reduced red blood cell counts in dogs and rats." The report added, "Indications were also present that animals on the irradiated diets may show a higher incidence in the development of cataracts and tumors than animals on control diets" (FDA, *Federal Register* 33, 1968).

However, even with these concerns about irradiated bacon, another decade passed before the FDA decided to revisit its policies on testing. In 1979, the agency established the Bureau of Foods Irradiated Food Committee (BFIFC) to make recommendations for establishing toxicological testing that would adequately assess the safety of irradiated foods. This time the first questions the committee tackled concerned what exactly should be tested, and what the difference was between an irradiated and a nonirradiated food. The committee focused on any products formed during the irradiation process and eventually concluded that 10 percent of the products of the process were substances not normally present in nonirradiated food. The BFIFC used the term *unique radiolytic products* (URPs) to describe these substances introduced into food by irradiation.

The committee suggested that URPs would be formed in minute amounts if products were treated at doses below 1 kGy. Based on this assumption, the BFIFC concluded that this small quantity of URPs would be diluted in a large amount of food. It therefore waived the requirement for animal feeding tests, holding that the tests would not provide any significant findings and would be a waste of time and taxpayer dollars. Additionally, the BFIFC recommended that foods comprising no more than 0.01 percent of the daily diet, and irradiated at 50 kGy or less, be considered safe for human consumption without toxicological testing (Pauli & Takeguchi, 1986).

When critics brought up the irradiated bacon study results, the agency responded that the numbers of animals examined in those studies was too small, and that the studies were of too poor a quality to have any statistical significance. The FDA agreed with the BFIFC conclusion, and ruled that adequate safety was demonstrated without the toxicological testing. The FDA adopted the BFIFC recommendations on March 27, 1981 (FDA, *Federal Register* 46, 1981). Later that year, the FDA's Bureau of Foods stepped in and gathered a second team of scientists, called the Irradiated Foods Task Group, to review all the available data and to put to rest any lingering safety concerns.

The goal of this task group was to compile and summarize any toxicology data available at the time, and to identify patterns and report any adverse findings. Its final report was in agreement with the BFIFC and the FDA that any toxicological testing of irradiated foods was too insensitive to accurately measure problems, given the low concentrations of URPs in irradiated foods. There was no discussion of potential problems associated with any cumulative effects. The task group determined that although toxicological data could be helpful in evaluating the safety of irradiated foods, it was not scientifically necessary. Instead, chemical formulas were created and used to predict the amounts of irradiated food a person might eat and what effect that food would have on overall human health.

At the same time, the FDA continued to approve irradiation requests. In 1983, approval was granted to use irradiation to kill insects and control microorganisms in a specific list of herbs, spices, and seasonings. In 1985, the FDA approved irradiation of pork to control trichinosis. In 1986, approval was given for irradiation to control insects and inhibit mold growth and ripening in a number of fruits, vegetables, and grains. In 1990, poultry was added to the list—although irradiation only reduces and does not eliminate all bacteria, so irradiated poultry still requires refrigeration. The FDA approved irradiation of red meat in 1997, with a dose of 4.5 kGy for uncooked, refrigerated meat and 7 kGy for frozen meat and meat products.

Although no comprehensive information exists on the total amount of food currently irradiated in the United States, industry experts estimate the amount of food being irradiated has remained steady since 2000 when ground beef and imported fruits were included. Since 2000, poultry is no longer being irradiated according to a February 2010 report released by the Government Accountability Office (GAO), which stated the amount of irradiated ground beef in the United States has also declined (GAO, 2010).

The same GAO report described the increased use of irradiation for fruits and spices in the United States, although no exact figures were available since the spice industry does not track information on the exact quantity of spices currently being irradiated. According to the GAO some 88 million pounds of spices were irradiated in 2008. At the same time many spice processors have stopped using ethylene oxide, a gas identified by the Environmental Protection Agency (EPA) as a probable human carcinogen, to alternative treatments. From 2007 through April 2009, some 9.5 million pounds of imported fruit were irradiated according to Animal and Plant Health Inspection Service (APHIS) officials. The fruit included guavas from Mexico and mangoes from India. In addition some 7 to 8 million pounds of purple sweet potatoes and other fruits grown in Hawaii were irradiated to eliminate pests.

**Opponents**   Despite widespread support of irradiation from government, industry officials, and scientists, critics call food irradiation an untested experiment on American consumers. They argue that there is a lack of testing and an attempt by the government to disregard any tests showing adverse effects.

One of the most vocal opponents of food irradiation is the watchdog organization Public Citizen. This group was founded by consumer advocate Ralph Nader, and has been in operation since 1971. Public Citizen has charged the FDA with ignoring studies indicating that food irradiation may be dangerous, especially in light of the test results that caused the agency to revoke approval of irradiated canned bacon. The organization's chief fear concerns the unknown effects of eating irradiated food over time. It argues that irradiation creates toxic substances in the food. For example, critics point to a 1986 FDA statement identifying detectable quantities of hydrogen peroxide, organic peroxides, and hydroperoxides formed during irradiation of foods. These peroxides are the result of free radical chemical exchanges between oxygen and the radiolytic products from the carbohydrates, fats, oils, and water in food. The FDA considered the potential carcinogenicity of hydrogen peroxide created during irradiation, and concluded that there was no specific evidence that it would damage healthy cells before it was neutralized by natural enzymes or antioxidants in the food.

Public Citizen and other opponents also note that *Clostridium botulinum* spores may survive irradiation and produce botulinum toxin in food. Consumers would not notice the toxins, because irradiation prevents typical signs of spoilage. The FDA identified this as a legitimate concern in its April 1986 rules. The agency found that irradiation below 1 kGy will destroy only a few spoilage bacteria, and will not change the essential spoilage patterns of the food. In other words, the food will continue to rot even after it is irradiated, and that decay should alert consumers to the potential for other toxins.

Public Citizen and others have additionally suggested that irradiation may create potentially harmful radiation-resistant bacteria or viral mutants. Although the

FDA admitted that mutants are produced during the irradiation of food, it labeled them "essentially the same as those that occur naturally" (FDA, *Federal Register* 51, 1986). Government scientists acknowledged that radiation may increase the frequency of mutations, and the FDA reported that this effect on the rate at which mutations occur is the only meaningful impact of irradiation on mutations. However, the FDA ruled that this was not a significant problem.

Other opponents of irradiation have claimed that the FDA has not addressed the destruction of vitamins and other important nutrients during radiation treatments. The Organic Consumers Association (OCA), a nonprofit public interest group, was formed in 1998 as part of a backlash against proposed changes to USDA organic food regulations. In addition to calling for a global moratorium on genetically modified foods, the association has been a vocal critic of irradiation. The OCA estimates that irradiated foods can lose up to 80 percent of important vitamins, including vitamins A, C, E, and B. It claims that different foods lose different vitamins, and that the loss increases with the radiation dose and with the storage time of each food.

Another strong anti-irradiation advocate is Food and Water Watch, a national environmental organization based in Vermont. This group suggests that the government is approaching the issue of foodborne illness from the wrong direction. It advocates an immediate cleanup in the current system of food production, especially in slaughterhouse facilities, factory farms, and large-scale vegetable and fruit production sites.

Food and Water Watch warns that the cost of irradiating the U.S. food supply would dramatically raise food prices for consumers. It estimates that in order to irradiate the 8 billion pounds of hamburger Americans eat every year, the industry would have to build "80 multi-million dollar irradiation facilities" (Food and Water Watch, "Irradiation"). When the costs of transportation and handling are added, Food and Water Watch calculates that consumers would see a jump of up to one dollar per pound in the price of ground beef, in contrast with the USDA estimate that the price per pound would increase by only a few cents.

**Supporters**   The International Food Information Council (IFIC) is a key player on the other side of the debate over irradiated food. The IFIC was created to communicate science-based information on food safety and nutrition to government officials, educators, journalists, nutrition and health professionals, and others who work with consumers. The council is financed thanks to a number of companies in the food, beverage, and agricultural industries.

The International Irradiation Association (IIA) is another group focused on supporting the growth of food irradiation. The IIA was developed in 2003 to improve communication between irradiation industry members and special interest groups. Members include companies with an interest in every aspect of radiation technology, among them Johnson & Johnson, E-Beam Services, and China Biotech Corporation.

The American Dietetic Association boasts more than 68,000 members and is also among the country's strongest supporters of food irradiation. As an advocate organization for the public on food and nutrition issues, the ADA strongly encourages its members to support the availability of irradiated foods, and has worked to make educational resources available to consumers on local, national, and international levels.

**International Issues**    Worldwide, about 50 countries have approved some 60 products to be irradiated. In May 2010 Indonesian officials with the National Nuclear Energy Agency announced their intention to consider the use of irradiation technology. Officials with the agency explained that testing of irradiated products began following the earthquake in Padang, West Sumatra, in 2009 when food was needed for the victims. The country has two irradiator facilities.

The United States, South Africa, the Netherlands, Thailand, and France are among the leaders in adopting irradiation technology (Amin, 2006). Whereas food irradiation has been used for decades in the United States, the technology has been slow to find support in many parts of Europe, especially the United Kingdom. The British Food Standards Agency (FSA) was set up as an independent government department in 2000 to protect the public's health and consumer interests in relation to food. In 2007, it recommended no changes to its current permitted uses of irradiated food.

There are seven categories of irradiated food permitted in the United Kingdom, including fruit, vegetables, cereals, bulbs and tubers, spices and condiments, fish and shellfish, and poultry. As of 2009 the FSA website reported only one license for the irradiation of herbs and spices had been granted. All items must be labeled "irradiated" or "treated with ionizing radiation." Imported irradiated food is only allowed in the United Kingdom if it was treated in an authorized plant and accompanied by full documentation relating to that treatment.

From the beginning, European governments showed little interest in financing the research needed to advance radiation technology in their countries. In an early effort to move development forward the International Atomic Energy Association (IAEA) established a Joint Expert Committee on Food Irradiation (JECFI) that joined with the United Nations Food and Agriculture Organization (FAO) as well as the World Health Organization (WHO). Beginning in 1964, this alphabet soup of organizations—the IAEA, FAO, and WHO—held a series of meetings to assess the quality and safety of irradiated foods. From those meetings came a series of reports, which concluded that all irradiated foods were safe to eat.

In 1997, the Joint FAO/IAEA/WHO Study Group on High Dose Irradiation released its final report, which stated, "food irradiated to any dose appropriate to achieve the intended technological objective is both safe to consume and nutritionally adequate." It added that "no upper dose limit need be imposed, and . . . irradiated foods are deemed wholesome throughout the technologically useful dose range from below 10 kGy to envisioned doses above 10 kGy" (WHO, 1997). The study group's overall objective was to standardize the EU member states' national laws on irradiation, and each member state was directed to implement legislation laid down in the group's directives. But doubts continued, and so did the debate.

The United Kingdom took labeling regulations a step further in 2000, removing an exemption that allowed small amounts of irradiated foods in compound ingredients to remain unlabeled. The change means that any foods containing irradiated ingredients must now be labeled as such. Concerns were later heightened in Europe when research raised questions about substances known as 2-alkylcyclobutanones (ACBs)—byproducts created when fat in foods such as ground beef is irradiated. A 2003 study by Germany's Federal Research Centre for Nutrition suggested that 2-ABCs may promote colon cancer. This prompted the European Commission (EC) to place a moratorium on many irradiated foods. However, the EC will allow the approval of other irradiated foods in the future if all EU countries reach a consensus on which foods to allow. In the United States, the FDA had already approved the use of irradiation for a variety of foods, including meat, poultry, and eggs, before the German study was published in *Nutrition and Cancer* in December 2002 (Raul, 2002). Although the German researchers warned against using the study results to discredit irradiation of meat, they also called for more scrutiny of 2-ACBs.

In direct contrast to the UK regulation, the United States requires labels on all irradiated foods except compound food products with irradiated ingredients. For example, potato soup made with irradiated potatoes, onions, and spices does not need to be labeled as irradiated, because the ingredients are not irradiated after they are combined. However, if irradiated potatoes are sold separately after they are irradiated, they must be labeled and carry the irradiation symbol. This parallels the differences in labeling requirements for genetically modified organisms (GMOs) in the United States and Europe. In Europe, foods containing any GMOs require labels, whereas in America, combined foods that use GMOs are not labeled. Americans who wish to avoid irradiated foods or genetically modified foods should select organically processed foods.

That may change, however, in light of a 2007 FDA proposal to modify the way irradiated food is labeled. The measure would allow manufacturers to petition the agency to forego a label entirely if the irradiation makes no material changes to the nutritional or functional properties of the food, or to use other terms for irradiation, such as cold pasteurization. The FDA continues to review the proposal with no stated timetable for a final decision.

**The Future of Irradiation**   According to supporters of food irradiation technology, the most important reason to continue development is to make the nation's food supply safe. Other factors that support development include improved living standards for people around the world, and an end to food shortages for a growing world population. Critics of irradiation argue that consumers, already facing rising food prices, would feel a bigger financial pinch if additional, expensive irradiation facilities were constructed.

Overall, both sides do agree that food irradiation supports the global trend of centralized mass production and distribution of foods worldwide—a trend that raises the price tag for individual consumers as oil prices climb and global warming increases. Prolonged shelf life means foods can be transported over greater distances. This brings food to isolated or impoverished areas, but also increases fuel consumption and pollution. The use of irradiation is largely unacceptable to European consumers. Americans, on the other hand, have shown some reluctance to purchase irradiated food when it is labeled as such, but otherwise have adopted a "don't ask, don't tell" attitude. Are irradiated foods safe to eat or a dangerous experiment using American consumers? After more than 50 years, it still depends on whom you ask.

*Sharon Zoumbaris*

*See also* Food and Drug Administration (FDA); Food-borne Illness; Food Safety; Genetically Modified Organisms (GMOs); U.S. Department of Agriculture (USDA).

## References

Amin, Ahmed El. "Irradiation Regulation Remains Inconsistent Worldwide." *Food Naviga tor.com.* February 15, 2006. www.foodnavigator.com/news/printNewsBis.asp?id=65836.

Centers for Disease Control and Prevention, Food Safety Office. Updated January 19, 2009. www.cdc.gov/foodsafety.

Food and Drug Administration. "Food Additives Intended for Use in Processing of Canned Bacon: Proposed Revocations." *Federal Register* 33, no. 166 (August 24, 1968): 12055.

Food and Drug Administration. "Irradiation in the Production, Processing and Handling of Food." *Federal Register* 51, no. 75 (April 18, 1986): 13376.

Food and Drug Administration. "Policy for Irradiated Foods: Advance Notice of Proposed Procedures for the Regulation of Irradiated Foods for Human Consumption." *Federal Register* 46, no. 59 (March 27, 1981): 18992.

Food and Water Watch. "Irradiation: Expensive, Ineffective, and Impractical." www.foodand waterwatch.org/food/foodirradiation/irradiation-facts.

Goldstein, Myrna Chandler, and Mark A. Goldstein. *Controversies in Food and Nutrition.* Westport, CT: Greenwood Press, 2002, 29.

Government Accountability Office (GAO). "Food Irradiation: FDA Could Improve Its Documentation and Communication of Key Decisions on Food Irradiation Petitions." GAO-10-309R (February 16, 2010).

Pauli, George H., and Clyde A. Takeguchi. "Irradiation of Foods: An FDA Perspective." *Food Reviews International* 2, no. 1 (1986): 90. www.cfsan.fad.gov/~acrobat/irrahist.pdf.

Raul, Francis, Francine Gosse, Henry Delincee, Andrea Hartwig, Eric Marchioni, Michel Miesch, Dalal Werner, and Dominique Burnouf. "Food-Borne Radiolytic Compounds (2-Alkylcyclobutanones) May Promote Experimental Colon Carcinogenesis." *Nutrition and Cancer* 44, no. 2 (December 2002): 188–91.

World Health Organization. "High-Dose Irradiation: Wholesomeness of Food Irradiated with Doses above 10 kGy." Report of a Joint FAO/IAEA/WHO Study Group, Geneva, September 15–20, 1997. Technical Report Series, no. 890: 161. www.who.int/foodsafety/ publications/fs_management/irradiation/en/.

# *K*

## KAVA

Rising health care costs in the United States and side effects of certain prescription drugs have created a growing interest in alternative medicines. But how can American consumers be certain which herbal supplements really work? That depends on whose research you believe. The use of kava to treat anxiety is a perfect example of a supplement some believe is effective while others see it as a serious health risk.

What is kava? Kava comes from a tall shrub that grows in the islands of the Pacific Ocean. Its scientific name is *Piper methysticum,* and common names include kava, kava kava, awa, and kava pepper. The root and underground stem are used to prepare everything from drinks, capsules, or extracts to tablets and topical solutions. It is primarily used to treat anxiety, insomnia, and menopausal symptoms but has also been used for toothache, urinary tract infections, colds, canker sores, menstrual cramps, and seizures.

Even though the U.S. Food and Drug Administration (FDA) does not approve of its use, the FDA does not have the authority to inspect or regulate supplements or natural remedies like it does prescription drugs. The FDA issued a warning in 2002, telling consumers that kava supplements had been linked to a risk of severe liver damage. Studies on kava funded by the National Center for Complementary and Alternative Medicine were suspended at that time.

Despite the U.S. warning and bans by other countries including Germany and the United Kingdom, kava remains a popular supplement in the United States. The bans were prompted by the deaths of patients in Europe who had used kava. The debate over kava pills prompted the World Health Organization to launch its own study, and its findings, released in 2007, raised questions about the use of stems and leaves of the plants rather than the traditional use of the roots and questioned if this could have been a factor in the problems experienced by the European patients. Additionally, the WHO report called for quality control and a change in the manufacturing process. The ban on the sale of pills was finally lifted in October 2008 and the international trade in kava has resumed.

The term *kava* is used for both the plant and the beverage made from the root. The word refers to the bitter taste of the beverage, which has been both a social and ceremonial drink in the South Pacific for generations. The root of the plant is pounded or chewed and water added to produce a drink in countries from Fiji, several Polynesian areas, Tonga to many other Pacific Island countries. The soothing, relaxing qualities of the drink first attracted pharmaceutical manufacturers in the 1980s when the market for herbal alternatives was growing at a rapid pace. Kava's popularity grew alongside St. John's Wort, gingko, and ephedra. Kava ranked ninth in U.S. retail sales in 2000.

The FDA issued its warning after reports from Europe showed kava might cause damage to the liver, including hepatitis, cirrhosis, or liver failure. Reports also surfaced in the United States of kava-related liver damage, including the case of a healthy woman who required a liver transplant. Then in 2004 when the FDA banned ephedra, Consumers Union named a "Dirty Dozen" of what it considered dangerous supplements still on the market. Kava was on that list along with aristolochic acid, which is believed to be a potent carcinogen linked to kidney failure.

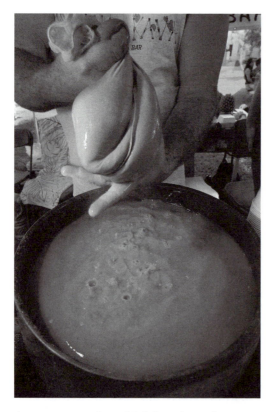

A man prepares kava drink from kava plant root, during a festival in Hawaii, October 7, 2006. (AP/Wide World Photos)

The dietary supplement industry responded to the warnings and bans on kava by hiring a professional toxicologist to evaluate the potential for liver damage from kava consumption. Its report cautioned that kava should not be taken with prescription drugs associated with liver damage, by those with preexisting liver disease or compromised liver function, and should not be taken along with alcohol. However, the reported added that "there is no clear evidence that the liver damage reported in the U.S. and Europe was caused by the consumption of kava" (Cass, 2002).

In fact, kava has a long tradition of safe use in the South Pacific, even at considerably higher doses than those suspected of causing problems in Europe. With its discovery by the pharmaceutical companies it has also become a major cash crop for many Pacific Island nations. Early side effects reported by frequent consumers of the beverage were nothing more serious than scaly skin and bloodshot eyes. The Pacific kava trade was hurt by the 2002 ban; however, since the restrictions were lifted in 2008 trade has resumed. Sales of kava are increasing, and new markets are opening including a handful of kava cafés that have opened in the United States. One café in St. Petersburg, Florida, is located across the street from the St. Petersburg High School and attracts a large number of student customers. In an interview with the *St. Petersburg Times,* the owners of the café were reassuring about potential problems for high school students who drink the kava. "Teenagers can drink kava, just like they drink coffee or tea," according to Laurent Olivier, the café owner (Matus, 2009).

Still, critics of kava continue to voice concerns about it. The September 2010 edition of the popular consumer magazine, *Consumer Reports,* released an updated list of "Dirty Dozen" supplements including kava, aconite, bitter orange, chaparral, colloidal silver, coltsfoot, comfrey, country mallow, germanium, greater celandine, lobelia, and yohimbe. To create its list the magazine worked with the Natural Medicines Comprehensive Database, an independent research group to identify the ingredients most linked to serious adverse events by clinical research or case reports. Other factors influencing which ones made the final list included whether the ingredients were effective for their advertised uses and how available they were to consumers.

The report also identified supplements considered to be both safe and effective: calcium, cranberry, fish oil, glucosamine sulfate, lactase, lactobacillus, psyllium, pygenum, and vitamin D. In response to the *CR* report, the Natural Products Association (NPA) in Washington, DC, said the supplement industry has an enviable safety record and called the *CR* investigation far from a balanced or accurate representation of the supplement industry or the laws that regulate it. The debate continues and consumers considering kava or any supplements should talk to their primary care provider about any natural remedy. Both prescription drugs and natural supplements can change the way medicines work together. Vitamins and certain foods may also interact with different products and in some cases might cause harmful side effects.

*Sharon Zoumbaris*

*See also* Dietary Supplements; Ephedra/Ephedrine; Food and Drug Administration (FDA); Vitamins.

## References

Cass, Hyla. "New FDA Kava Warnings: How Safe Is It?" *Integrative Medicine: Natural Solutions for Mind, Body and Spirit.* April 2, 2002. www.cassmd.com/library/kava.warnings.html.

"Consumer Reports Publishes 'Dirty Dozen' List: Magazine Widely Publicizes 12 Problem Supplement Ingredients, Industry Responds." *Nutraceuticals World* 13, no. 7 (September 2010): 14.

Gelles, Jeff. "How to Learn about Product Warnings." *Philadelphia Inquirer,* January 18, 2009. www.philly.com/philly/living/20090118_how_to_learn_about_product_warnings.html.

Matus, Ron. "Kava Bar Percolates across from School: The Bitter Brew Is Described as Relaxing." *St. Petersburg Times,* December 6, 2009, 19.

National Center for Complementary and Alternative Medicine. "Herbs at a Glance: Kava." www.nccam.nih.gov/health/kava.

Natural Medicines Comprehensive Database. www.naturaldatabase.com.

Pollock, Nancy J. "Sustainability of the Kava Trade." *The Contemporary Pacific* 21, no. 2 (Fall 2009): 265.

U.S. Food and Drug Administration, Center for Food Safety and Applied Nutrition. "Consumer Advisory: Kava-Containing Dietary Supplements May Be Associated with Severe Liver Injury." March 25, 2002. www.cfsan.fad.gov/~dms/addskava.html.

World Health Organization. *Assessment of the Risk of Hepatotoxicity with Kava Products.* Carbondale, CO: WHO Press, 2007.

## KELLOGG, JOHN HARVEY

By virtue of his name, physician John Harvey Kellogg is automatically equated with cornflakes and breakfast cereal. However, he was also an influential spokesman for vegetarianism, an early inventor of soy-based meat substitutes, the director of a health sanitarium, and a surgeon. Throughout his life he wrote extensively and lectured on the importance of a healthy diet, exercise, and natural remedies to treat illness. Kellogg, in his own way, changed America's eating habits and was an early visionary who saw the relationship between personal habits and physical well-being.

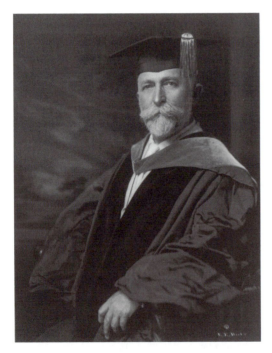

John Kellogg spent his lifetime promoting healthy eating and exercise through his work as a doctor and as founder of a holistic sanitarium in Battle Creek, Michigan. (Library of Congress)

**Early Days** Kellogg was born on February 26, 1852, in a rural part of Livingston County, Michigan. He was the fourth of eight surviving children of John Preston Kellogg and his wife, Ann Janette Kellogg. He was a toddler when his family relocated to Battle Creek, Michigan, after his parents joined the newly formed Seventh-Day Adventist Church, which was headquartered in Battle Creek. The Seventh-Day Adventist Church is the largest American religious denomination to endorse vegetarianism. In Battle Creek, the senior Kellogg joined others to found the Western Reform Institute, a church-affiliated health clinic that specialized in hydrotherapy and vegetarianism.

After finishing his medical training John Kellogg eventually took over the institute and renamed it the Battle Creek Sanitarium. His nutritional theory was centered on a meatless diet along with sparing use of eggs, refined sugar, milk, or cheese and complete abstinence from alcohol, tea, coffee, tobacco, and chocolate. He called his health regimen "biological living," and stressed that for good health individuals also needed regular exercise, fresh air and sunshine, good posture, sensible clothing, and plenty of water, as much as 8 to 10 glasses daily. He was also a strong believer in the value of a daily enema to keep the intestines clean and disease-free. Kellogg served as the director of the sanitarium, popularly known as "The San," for more than 50 years.

At its peak of popularity the facility had 700 beds and was host to some of the country's most famous and powerful people. In all, more than 200,000 patients received treatment including John D. Rockefeller, J.C. Penney, Henry Ford, and Harvey Firestone. The facility employed more than 1,000 people including 20 full-time doctors and 300 nurses and bath attendants (Davis, 2004). The building was six stories high with a lobby the size of a football field and indoor swimming pools. It was in every respect a luxury hotel and spa whose director, Kellogg, dressed in white from head to toe for what he described as health reasons.

In his efforts to invent healthy foods for his patients Kellogg worked with his brother Will on a slow-baked cereal biscuit they eventually called granola. They continued to try different recipes and also developed a method of roasting wheat and corn flakes that became a popular cereal. The Kelloggs experimented with nut butters for their patients with poor teeth, so they could enjoy the health benefits of nuts in their diet. Peanuts were the least expensive nut at the time and peanut butter quickly became a favorite at The San, and across the nation.

**Business or Health?**   However, John was not interested in business; he was interested in reforming American eating and health habits. His brother Will, on the other hand, was more of a businessman and wanted to keep pace with the fierce competition that had developed among cereal companies. An ex-patient of the sanitarium named C.W. Post had started his cereal company based on his own granola biscuits and a cereal-based drink he called Postum. In fact, the Kelloggs were not the first to market dry cereal. In 1893 Henry Perky of Colorado invented a machine that shredded wheat, which he sold commercially under the name Shredded Wheat.

Kellogg and his brother Will incorporated the Toasted Corn Flake Company in 1906 with John as majority stockholder. He shared stock with sanitarium doctors, but Will wanted more say in how things were run and he began to buy up stock until he owned a majority of shares. Will renamed the company, using the Kellogg name and setting off a battle between the brothers, filled with lawsuits and bad feelings that lasted most of their lives. For years John had stressed healthy living as a religious duty of all Seventh-Day Adventists and he had studied the writings of early health reformers including Sylvester Graham. At the same time Will, in an effort to improve the popularity of their cereal, added sugar to the recipe and used advertising to market products as convenient and delicious rather than healthy.

Both brothers had little schooling as boys due to their church's view of Christ's second coming. His parents believed church officials who named the date Christ would reappear. That prediction made school seem unnecessary to Kellogg's parents. The Seventh-Day Adventists evolved from an early religious sect known as the "Millerites," who were well known for predicting the exact day of Christ's return. The newer group also focused on the second coming and believed the health of their community was the best way to prepare for Christ's return.

**Medical Training**   Kellogg's entry into medical school was also directly tied to the interests of his church. In 1872 Kellogg had just entered a teacher training program at Michigan State Normal College. At the same time Adventist church leaders had grown increasingly critical and distrustful of conventional medicine. The church moved to develop its own professionally trained doctors who would share their religious views. It selected several promising young male Adventists, including Kellogg, to attend a medical training course in New Jersey. Kellogg now began to consider a career in medicine.

Kellogg enrolled in the Bellevue Hospital College in New York to pursue a degree in medicine. He had just completed his undergraduate work. When he graduated in 1875, Kellogg returned to Battle Creek and was offered the position of administrator of the institute. He married Ella Eaton of New York in 1879. The two did not have children but throughout their marriage they served as foster parents to more than 40 children, several of whom they adopted.

Kellogg was interested in the science of nutrition. He served on the Michigan State Board of Health from 1878 to 1891 and again from 1911 to 1917. He also traveled to Europe to study surgical techniques and over the years performed thousands of operations. During his trips to Europe he observed the use of herbs for treatment of various health problems. In France he saw firsthand the laxative qualities of psyllium and brought some seeds to the Battle Creek clinic and introduced them to the patients.

Psyllium is a grain that grows on a stalk and resembles wheat. The outer portion of the seed is edible and has been used as a remedy for everything from bladder ailments, colds, kidney ailments, and diarrhea to constipation. It has been an ingredient for decades in the laxative Metamucil. In 2008 research results showed it is useful in lowering cholesterol levels and it decreases the risk of coronary heart disease (Bazzano, 2008).

Kellogg and his brother also introduced soybean products to patients at his clinic. The brothers invented products that replaced milk and meat with soy. However, Americans for the most part did not embrace soy in their diets until the 1960s and 1970s. It was almost 20 years before soy was endorsed by the Food and Drug Administration (FDA) in 1999 and the American Heart Association in 2000 as a healthy protein alternative. Soybeans are unique in that they supply all the essential amino acids the human body requires, unlike other plant foods.

After decades as the sanitarium director Kellogg faced criticism from the church over some of his decisions. For example, his admission policy was seen as catering to the rich and powerful rather than the common man or the church faithful. In 1906 the church excommunicated Kellogg and severed its ties with the sanitarium. Kellogg finally closed the doors of the sanitarium at the beginning of the 1930s due in part to the effects of the Great Depression. He moved to Florida and renovated a hotel that had been donated by a previous patient at The San. Kellogg managed the Miami–Battle Creek Sanitarium for several years until his death at age 91.

*Sharon Zoumbaris*

*See also* Graham, Sylvester; Soy; Vegetarians.

## References

Anderson, James W., Michael H. Davidson, Lawrence Blonde, W. Virgil Brown, Wl. James Howard, Henry Ginsberg, Lisa D. Allgood, and Kurt W. Weingand. "Long-Term Cholesterol-Lowering Effects of Psyllium as an Adjunct to Diet Therapy in the Treatment of Hypercholesterolemia." *American Journal of Clinical Nutrition* 71, no. 6 (June 2000): 1433–38.

"Battle of the Cornflakes." *History Today* 56, no. 2 (2006): 58.

Bazzano, Lydia A. "Effects of Soluble Dietary Fiber on Low-Density Lipoprotein Cholesterol and Coronary Heart Disease Risk." *Current Atherosclerosis Reports* 10, no. 6 (December 2008): 473.

"Can a Familiar Laxative Also Boost Bone and Heart Health?" *Environmental Nutrition* 33, no. 1 (January 15, 2010): 3.

Davis, Ivan. "Biologic Living and Rhetorical Pathology: The Case of John Harvey Kellogg and Fred Newton Scott." *Michigan Academician* 36, no. 13 (Fall 2004): 247.

"John Harvey Kellogg." *Encyclopedia of World Biography.* Vol. 21. Detroit: Gale, 2001.

"Kellogg, John Harvey." *Merriam-Webster's Biographical Dictionary.* Springfield, MA: Merriam-Webster, 1995, 3B19.

"Psyllium Is a Rich Source of Fiber." *Better Nutrition for Today's Living* 53, no. 11 (November 1991): 10.

Schneider, Louise E. "John Harvey Kellogg." In *Nutrition and Well-Being A to Z,* edited by Delores C.S. James. New York: Macmillan Reference USA, 2004.

Smith, Andrew F. "John Harvey Kellogg." In *Encyclopedia of Food and Culture,* edited by Solomon H. Katz. New York: Charles Scribner's Sons, 2003.

## KETOSIS

Ketones or ketone bodies are created by the liver when it converts fats into chemicals for the body to use as fuel. Ketosis is an abnormal increase of ketone bodies in the bloodstream, triggered by starvation or by a low- to no-carbohydrate diet. Turning off the carbohydrate supply to the body forces it into ketosis and forces the body to turn to fat for energy. During digestion the liver converts carbohydrates into the simple sugar glucose, an important fuel for most body functions. Proteins replace themselves as needed and any excess protein also becomes glucose.

Ketosis occurs during this shortage of carbohydrates for fuel, which triggers the production of large amounts of ketone bodies to compensate for the lack of glucose. Problems develop because the tissue in the brain and in the muscles used for rapid movement cannot use ketone bodies as efficiently as they use glucose for fuel. Critics of low-carbohydrate diets suggest the lack of carbs forces the brain to use ketones for its fuel. This change in fuel slows thinking and reaction times. The brain's need for carbohydrates is one of the reasons the American Dietetic Association recommends 100 grams of carbohydrates per day to avoid ketosis.

The symptoms of ketosis include unpleasant or bad breath odor, nausea, dehydration, constipation, and diarrhea and decreased appetite. Severe and prolonged ketosis may lead to kidney disease, gallstones, gout, or cardiac complications. Advocates of high-protein, low-carbohydrate diets, such as the Scarsdale Medical Diet and the Atkins Nutritional Approach, acknowledge that dieters following their eating programs will experience ketosis. However, they claim the condition can enhance the effectiveness of a low-carbohydrate diet. Supporters of low-carbohydrate diets say research has shown the long-term use of a ketogenic diet is safe. One study, published in 2004, concluded that a low-carb diet resulted in successful weight loss along with a significant decrease in the level of triglycerides, total cholesterol, LDL or "bad" cholesterol, and glucose and a significant increase in the level of HDL or "good" cholesterol in those patients involved in the study (Dashti et al., 2004).

According to the U.S. Department of Agriculture, a number of factors contribute to weight loss for people who choose to follow a low-carbohydrate diet. They include water weight loss, decreased appetite, and the unpleasant symptoms of ketosis along with the elimination of carbohydrates as a food group, which creates a corresponding decrease in calorie consumption. While some organizations like the American Diabetes Association and the Academy of Family Physicians have recognized "low-carb" or ketogenic diets as a suitable approach to weight loss, in contrast others, including the American Dietetic Association and the American Heart Association, continue to oppose their use due to the risks they say are associated with ketosis.

Doctors have also successfully prescribed ketogenic diets for people afflicted with epilepsy. Those ketogenic diets slow down all brain functions, making it less likely the brain will react to the triggers that set off an epileptic episode. The National Institutes of Health has studied the use of ketosis in the treatment of epilepsy and other neurological illnesses. Findings from one study of 150 children whose seizures wee poorly controlled by medication found that about one-fourth of the children had a 90 percent or better decrease in seizures with a ketogenic diet and another half of the group had a 50 percent or better decrease in their seizures (National Institute of Neurological Disorders and Stroke, "Seizures and Epilepsy"). Moreover, it reported some children could discontinue the ketogenic diet after several years and remain seizure-free. One possible side effect noted was a buildup of uric acid in the blood, which can lead to the formation of kidney stones. Researchers are not sure just how ketosis inhibits seizures and studies are continuing.

*Marjolijn Bijlefeld and Sharon Zoumbaris*

*See also* Atkins, Robert C.; Carbohydrates; Diets, Fad; MyPlate.

## References

Dashti, Hussein M., Thazhumpal C. Mathew, Talib Hussein, Sami K. Asfar, Abdulla Behbahani, Mousa A. Khoursheed, Hilal M. Al-Sayer, Yousef Y. Bo-Abbas, and Naji S. Al-Zaid. "Long-Term Effects of a Ketogenic Diet in Obese Patients." *Experimental and Clinical Cardiology* 9, no. 3 (Fall 2004): 200–205.

DiNardo, Kelly. "Ask the Nutritionist." *Shape* 24, no. 1 (September 2004): 196.

"Fad Diets." *The Nurse Practitioner* 25, no. 10 (October 2000): 1S18.

*Merriam-Webster's Medical Dictionary.* Springfield, MA: Merriam-Webster, 1995.

National Institute of Neurological Disorders and Stroke, National Institutes of Health. "Seizures and Epilepsy: Hope through Research." www.ninds.nih.gov/disorders/epilepsy/detail_epilepsy.htm#166453109.

Tarnower, Herman, and Samm Sinclair Baker. *The Complete Scarsdale Medical Diet.* New York: Rawson, Wade, 1978.

Volek, Jeff. "Low-Carb Lies." *Men's Fitness* 21, no. 3 (April 2005): 34.

# L

## LACTOSE INTOLERANCE

Food intolerances or metabolic food disorders are inborn defects in food metabolism. A very common worldwide example is lactose intolerance. Milk and dairy products contain lactose, a milk sugar. Many people lack the intestinal enzyme, β-galactosidase (also called lactase), which breaks down the lactose molecule. When this enzyme is missing, lactose remains intact as it travels through the intestine. Bacteria then begin to work on the undigested lactose when it reaches the colon. This bacterial action produces symptoms of abdominal pain, bloating, cramping, diarrhea, or intestinal gas. While some of these symptoms mimic milk allergy symptoms, milk intolerance is actually a defect in lactose digestion and *not* a "true" milk allergy.

Lactose, fructose, and gluten are responsible for most food intolerances. Lactose intolerance follows the same avoidance diet that individuals with a milk allergy follow. Avoiding milk and dairy foods is necessary to avoid symptoms and requires constant vigilance. Some individuals are able to tolerate specific amounts of milk and dairy products and remain symptom-free, whereas others cannot. Fructose intolerance and malabsorption necessitate excluding all foods containing fructose.

*Dairy-free* is a term used by food manufacturers, but it has no FDA regulation in place governing its use. This food will usually have caseinates or whey, which indicates milk protein is present. Thus, it is unsafe for anyone with a milk allergy. *Non-dairy* is a regulated ingredient term, but the regulation allows milk protein (casein) in the product. It too is not safe for anyone with a milk allergy. Some lactose-intolerant individuals can use a small amount of these products and not experience symptoms, but it depends on the individual.

Although there are some medical disorders that are speculated to be triggered by foods, research has no conclusive evidence to date that firmly links them. However, other medical disorders known as food intolerances (nonallergic food hypersensitivity) have evidence showing a connection to food triggers. Lactose intolerance is a common digestive defect worldwide and affects about 70 percent of the world population and is often confused with milk allergy. Symptoms of a milk allergy will usually occur immediately after consuming milk or milk products.

Those typical symptoms involve the immune system and include bloating, diarrhea, gas, hives, vomiting, wheezing, and the possibility of anaphylactic shock. But some of these symptoms are very similar to those of lactose intolerance. Symptoms of lactose intolerance include abdominal cramping, bloating, diarrhea, and gas. Distinguishing between the two is based on results of allergy testing, symptoms, and results of a lactose tolerance test, hydrogen breath test, and, in young children or infants, a stool acidity test.

Infants are usually born with adequate amounts of the enzyme lactase, which breaks down the milk sugar lactose that is naturally present in milk and milk products. After maturity, lactose begins to decline in the adult gastrointestinal tract. For some people, this decline is significant enough to allow lactose to pass undigested through the colon, where bacteria begin to work on it. This bacterial action produces the symptoms listed above, but lactose intolerance does not activate the immune system and can be a temporary condition. Normal gastrointestinal flora can be destroyed with antibiotic use and by some cancer treatments. When these medications or treatments are over, the normal gastrointestinal flora returns and with it, sometimes, the ability to digest lactose again.

Cow's milk is found in many dairy and processed foods (butter, cheese, cream, most margarines, and yogurt). Milk is a good source of calcium, pantothenic acid, phosphorus, riboflavin, and vitamins A and D. But enriched soy, potato, or rice milks are also good sources for calcium and vitamins A and D. Nondairy calcium-rich foods are tofu made with calcium, calcium-fortified cereals, fruit juices, and some vegetables.

Beans, meats, nuts, peas, peanuts, soy, and whole grains are good sources of pantothenic acid, phosphorus, and riboflavin. The following ingredients do *not* contain milk protein and are safe to eat (even though they "sound" risky):

Calcium lactate
Calcium stearoyl lactylate
Cocoa butter
Cream of tartar
Lactic acid
Oleoresin
Sodium lactate
Sodium stearoyl lactylate

Milk is included in many processed foods, so label reading is imperative. The term *nondairy* also does *not* mean milk-free. *Nondairy* coffee creamers, whipped toppings, imitation cheeses, soft-serve ice cream, and frozen desserts often contain casein or caseinates. Asian exotic fruit beverages frequently add milk. Many prescription drugs use lactose as a filler.

Lactose-intolerant individuals, infants with Heiner Syndrome, and those with food protein–induced enterocolitis or proctocolitis must follow a milk-free diet as well. But some lactose-intolerant individuals can remain symptom-free after eating milk and dairy products if they do not exceed a specific amount (based on individual response) of lactose or by taking lactase tablets or using Lactaid milk or Lactaid foods. Lactase tablets provide the missing enzyme needed to break down lactose when it is eaten, and Lactaid milk products are sold with the lactose already broken down.

However, caution is advised for any individual who has a mold or fungus allergy. A fungus is used to break down milk lactose, so Lactaid food products and lactase tablets may trigger an allergic reaction in susceptible individuals. Anyone with a milk allergy should avoid Lactaid milk or products because they still contain small amounts of milk protein and are, therefore, high risk.

A food allergy is defined as an exaggerated immune response triggered by a specific food, usually a protein. There are different classification systems in use when defining food allergies and hypersensitivities. In the 1960s researchers Robin Coombs and P.H.G. Gell established the most widely used allergy classification system. This classification system, called the Gell and Coombs Classification System, defines six different classes of hypersensitive reactions. Type I hypersensitivity and Type IV hypersensitivity classes define adverse food reactions (Gell and Coombs, 1968). Type I hypersensitivity reactions occur when IgE antibodies are produced and mast cells or basophils release inflammatory mediators. Type IV hypersensitivity reactions are non-IgE adverse food reactions and are known as food intolerances.

In 2001 the European Academy of Allergology and Clinical Immunology (EAACI) proposed redefining an allergy as "a hypersensitivity reaction initiated by immunologic mechanisms" (Johansson et al., 2001). The EAACI distinguishes an adverse food reaction as a food hypersensitivity. Hypersensitivity is defined as "objectively reproducible symptoms or signs, initiated by exposure to a defined stimulus at a dose tolerated by normal subjects" (Johansson et al., 2001) and is distinguished by whether IgE antibodies are produced or not. If IgE antibodies are produced, the reaction is classified as a food allergy or IgE-mediated food allergy. All other adverse food reactions, including food intolerances such as lactose intolerance and food-related medical disorders or hypersensitivities, are classified as nonallergic food hypersensitivity. Both classification systems are in use today.

Type I hypersensitivity (food allergy) defines a "true" food allergy as a reaction that stimulates the immune system to produce IgE when an allergenic food is eaten. Termed IgE-mediated food allergy, food allergies are divided into two categories: immediate hypersensitivity reactions and delayed hypersensitivity reactions. Symptoms that develop anywhere from within minutes to one to two hours after eating the offending food are called immediate hypersensitivity reactions. In delayed hypersensitivity reactions, symptoms usually do not appear until 24 to 72 hours later and occur at the cellular level of the immune system (a Th2 response). True food allergies are relatively rare and account for only a small percentage of adverse food reactions, involving a limited number of foods.

Type IV hypersensitivity (nonallergic food hypersensitivity) defines all other adverse food reactions and is usually caused by food intolerances, food chemical reactions, or food-related medical disorders. There are different types of nonallergic food hypersensitivity classifications: food intolerances (metabolic disorders), anaphylactoid reactions, and idiosyncratic reactions.

*Alice C. Richer*

*See also* Allergies, Food; Basal Metabolism; Immune System/Lymphatic System.

## References

American Academy of Allergy, Asthma and Immunology. "Food Allergy Statistics." May 2008. www.aaaai.org.

Broussard, M. "Everyone's Gone Nuts: The Exaggerated Threat of Food Allergies." *Harper's Magazine,* January 2008, Annotation: 64–65.

Food Allergy and Anaphylaxis Network. "Food Allergy Facts and Statistics." May 2008. www. foodallergy.org.

Gell, P.G.H., and R.R.A. Coombs. *Clinical Aspects of Immunology.* 2nd ed. Oxford: Blackwell, 1968.

Johansson, S.G.O., J. O'B Hourihane, J. Bousquet, C. Bruijnzeel-Koomen, S. Dreborg, T. Haahtela, M.L. Kowalski, N. Mygind, J. Ring, P. van Cauwenberge, M. van Hage-Hamsten, and B. Wüthrich. "A Revised Nomenclature for Allergy." An EAACI Position Statement from the EAACI Nomenclature Task Force. *Allergy* 56 (2001): 813–24.

Madsen, Charlotte. "Prevalence of Food Allergy: An Overview." *Proceedings of the Nutrition Society* 64 (2005): 413–17.

Melina, Vesanto, Jo Stepaniak, and Dina Aronson. *Food Allergy Survival Guide.* Summertown, Tennessee: Healthy Living, 2004.

National Digestive Diseases Information Clearinghouse. "Facts and Fallacies about Digestive Diseases." August 2008. http://digestive.niddk.nih.gov/ddiseases/pubs/facts/#ibd.

National Institute of Allergy and Infectious Diseases, National Institutes of Health. March 13–14, 2006. "Report of the NIH Expert Panel on Food Allergy Research." September 2008. www3.niaid.nih.gov/topics/foodAllergy/research/ReportFoodAllergy.

Skripak, J.M., E.C. Matsui, K. Mudd, and R.A. Wood. "The Natural History of IgE-Mediated Cow's Milk Allergy." *Journal of Allergy and Clinical Immunology* 120 (2007): 1172–77.

University of Michigan Health System. "Students with Food Allergies Often Not Prepared." *ScienceDaily.* August 2008. www.sciencedaily.com/releases/2008/08/080806081451.

U.S. Food and Drug Administration. "Evidence-Based Review System for the Scientific Evaluation of Health Claims." September 2008. CFSAN/Office of Nutrition, Labeling and Dietary Supplements. www.cfsan.fda.gov/~dms/hclmgui5.

U.S. Food and Drug Administration. "Food Allergen Labeling and Consumer Protection Act of 2004." September 2008. www.cfsan.fda.gov/~dms/alrgact.

## LIPOSUCTION

Liposuction is a surgical procedure to remove pockets of fat from the body. A narrow tube is inserted into a fat layer beneath the skin, and the fat cells are broken up and suctioned out. Typically, liposuction is used to sculpt the abdomen, hips, buttocks, thighs, knees, upper arms, chin, cheeks, and neck. Cost of the surgery ranges from about $2,000 to as high as $14,000. There is limited medical insurance coverage available for liposuction unless it is necessary to address a diagnosed medical condition.

Liposuction for years was the most common cosmetic surgery in the country according to the American Society of Aesthetic Plastic Surgeons. However, in 2009, for the second year in a row, breast augmentation numbers surpassed liposuction in the United States. Recent advances in liposuction, such as ultrasound-assisted lipoplasty (UAL), have made the procedure less painful and the recovery a little easier. However, despite its popularity, the decision to have surgery shouldn't be taken lightly.

Liposuction has distinct risks—including death. Since its introduction in 1975, liposuction technique has improved. However, there continued to be serious problems with the procedure. There were 95 deaths associated with liposuction between 1994 and 1998. The *Philadelphia Inquirer* and other Knight/Ridder newspapers printed an article detailing the death of an 18-year-old who died following surgery, apparently from a fat clot that got loose during surgery and traveled through her bloodstream to her lungs. The mother told the newspaper, "We never would have let her do it if we knew she could have died. It wasn't supposed to be a big deal."

In an April 2001 issue of *Teen People,* another mother described the agony and shock at the death of her 23-year-old daughter following liposuction. The family received a $500,000 settlement in a malpractice lawsuit against the doctor, who had reportedly damaged a vein in the young woman's leg. The resulting blood clot traveled to her lungs, and she died during a seizure the following day. "Our lawyer thought we should have gotten a much higher sum, but we didn't care. More than anything, we just wanted the public to know what had happened to our daughter," the mother wrote.

The most common causes of death associated with liposuction are pulmonary embolus, otherwise known as a blood clot in the lung; infections; injury to abdominal organs including the liver and intestines; and drug reactions and side effects of anesthesia. The dangers from anesthesia and infections have been reduced dramatically thanks to the technique known as tumescent liposuction, developed by Paris surgeon Yves-Gerard Illou, who introduced the technique in 1983. The biggest advantage of tumescent liposuction over traditional liposuction is that only local anesthesia is used making this an outpatient procedure. Blood loss is significantly reduced, there is a shorter recovery time, and the patient is able to move around soon afterward.

New technology continues to improve the procedure, making it safer and quicker, which improves outcomes for patients. Some plastic surgeons have turned to ultrasound-assisted liposuction, which uses ultrasound waves to homogenize the fat. However, the American Society of Dermatology rates ultrasound-assisted liposuction as an experimental method. Nutational infrasonic liposuction (NIL) is another new form of liposuction now approved by the FDA for U.S. consumers. Also known as TickleLipo, the procedure, popular in Europe, uses low-frequency acoustic vibration to break up the fat.

Liposuction does not remove cellulite. Nor can a physician guarantee results. Sometimes, the area where the fat was removed may look dimply, a "cottage cheese" effect. Excess skin may stay loose and sag. Fat deposits may develop in new places, and if the patient gains more than 10 pounds after surgery, the fat may come back to haunt the same area, as well.

The American Society of Plastic Surgeons, which offers a web-based clearinghouse at www.plasticsurgery.org, suggests that the best candidates "are normal-weight people with firm, elastic skin who have pockets of excess fat in certain areas. You should be physically healthy, psychologically stable and realistic in your expectations. Your age is not a major consideration; however, older patients may have diminished skin elasticity and may not achieve the same results as a younger patient with tighter skin." The site notes that the risks increase for people with medical problems, especially heart or lung disease or poor blood circulation.

The surgeons' site details the different kinds of liposuction procedures, and prospective patients should discuss the options and their expectations with their physician. It also suggests getting help at home for a day or two following surgery. Liposuction can be performed in an office-based center, an outpatient surgery center, or a hospital. Smaller procedures can be done in the doctor's office, but it is important for those considering liposuction to fully discuss the appropriate setting for their surgery especially if other procedures are being done at the same time. How long the surgery takes depends on how much fat is being removed and how many areas are being sculpted. According to www.plasticsurgery.org, following surgery, "You may still experience some pain, burning, swelling, bleeding and temporary numbness." Most people can return to work within a few days and begin to feel better in the next week or so. A noticeable difference in the way a person looks occurs about four to six weeks after surgery when the swelling has gone down, but it can take about three months for the full effect to emerge.

Scientists and doctors are also attempting to use the excess fat from liposuction and turn it into stem cells. In 2007, an international team of scientists created a breakthrough when they showed that skin cells could transform into pluripotent stem cells; those are cells that have the ability to become any other type of cell. In 2008 a team of U.S. doctors took a quart of fat from a liposuction surgery and injected the same reprogramming genes into the fat. It took just 20 days compared with an average eight weeks needed to turn skin cells into stem cells for the fat to turn into stem cells. An added bonus, the fat yielded many more stem cells. Among potential uses of the new stem cells could be to grow cardiac muscle for diseased hearts. Scientists say the benefits would include that the fat would be collected directly from the patient, eliminating the possibility of immune rejection.

*Marjolijn Bijlefeld and Sharon Zoumbaris*

*See also* Body Image; Health Insurance.

## References

Binns, Corey. "Extreme Makeover: Scientists Turn Liposuction Leftovers into Stem Cells." *Popular Science* 275, no. 6 (December 2009): 23.

"Boom (and Busts) for Plastic Surgeons." *U.S. News & World Report,* June 25, 2001, 10.

Diclementi, Deborah. "Pressure to Be Perfect: Since 1996, the Number of Teens Having Plastic Surgery Has Nearly Doubled. Is That a Healthy Choice—or a Dangerous Trend?" *Teen People,* April 1, 2001, 200.

"Dr. Daniel Ronel Is One of the First in the U.S. to Offer TickleLipo." *PRWeb Newswire.* July 1, 2010. General Reference Center Gold. http://find.galegroup.com.

Fitzgerald, Susan, and Marian Uhlman. "A Popular Surgery, a Young Life Lost." *Philadelphia Inquirer,* August 5, 2001, A1.

Gerhart, Ann. "Nipped in the Bud: More and More Young Women Choose Surgical 'Perfection.'" *Washington Post,* June 23, 1999, C1.

Henig, Robin Marantz. "The High Cost of Thinness." *New York Times Magazine,* February 28, 1988, 41.

"Liposuction Rated as Most Popular Procedure for Second Year." *Women's Health Weekly,* February 28, 2002, 11.

Patrick, Stephanie. "Doctors Pioneer Gentler Liposuction." *Dallas Business Journal* 24, no. 49 (July 20, 2001): 3. www.plasticsurgery.org.

## LIVING WILLS AND ADVANCE DIRECTIVES

Life requires preparation. So does the end of life. This explains why people create wills to ensure that their property and possessions are divided according to their wishes. Medically, people also draw wills to communicate their last wishes for medical treatment and organ donation. These living wills remove some of the difficult decisions that must be made when a person reaches the end of his life. They can reduce the emotional toll faced by loved ones who must let go of someone for whom they care deeply.

Living wills also help those who may become temporarily or permanently incapacitated and unable to make a decision about their current care. Living wills are part of a larger document called an advance directive. An advance directive allows an individual to make decisions about every possible aspect of his medical care in the event that the person cannot decide for himself. This important document is designed to give adults some measure of control over life's expected and unexpected medical situations.

Only 36 percent of Americans have a living will according to a survey released in March 2010 by FindLaw, a provider of online legal information ("Most Americans"). Many Americans believe living wills are documents only needed by older adults, but this isn't true. Legal experts suggest every adult, age 18 and older, should have a living will. After all, accidents and illness happen at any age. Once an individual is considered an adult with the ability to make important decisions about her well-being without parental approval, she too has the opportunity to make her wishes known if something should happen and she is no longer able to speak for herself. Living wills are like a legally recognized advocate for anyone.

The need for a living will has grown as medical technology has advanced. In fact, people who would have died from severe injuries or illnesses just decades ago can now be kept alive much longer thanks in many cases to modern medicine. However, even though the technology can keep an individual alive in a very diminished capacity, many families ultimately face end-of-life decisions that would be best if made earlier by that person. For example, a persistent vegetative state is a condition where an individual is unaware of herself in spite of experiencing periods of wakefulness and physiologic sleep cycles. In this condition an individual's eyes are open yet the person is permanently unconsciousness (American Hospital Association, 2005). Several high-profile legal cases showed what could happen without a living will when individuals lingered in a vegetative state for years. Legal battles have erupted between family members over the question of ending care or using extreme measures to keep a loved one alive.

Living wills and advance directives allow individuals to spell out the type of medical treatments and life-extending steps they do or do not want. These measures include being connected to ventilators to help with breathing when one cannot breathe on his own, having feeding tubes inserted when one cannot feed himself, or receiving cardiopulmonary resuscitation if the heart stops. A living will also allows individuals to choose a person to make decisions on his behalf, such as a spouse or a parent. This person is sometimes called a proxy, and the option to designate a legal advocate is called medical power of attorney (POA).

Do Not Resuscitate (DNR), these three little letters often mentioned in medical television dramas, are a choice included in a living will that is then added to a patient's chart. Once the DNR becomes known to medical personnel (Mayo Clinic, 2009), no extra measures will be taken to keep that patient alive if he stops breathing or his heart stops beating. Although a DNR is a commonsense decision, if not stipulated by the patient, it can also be a heartwrenching choice family members may be forced to make when the moment of death arrives.

When accidental injuries or death occurs, the lack of a living will may put loved ones at odds with each other over what to do for the patient. In this instance, medical decisions can again turn into legal battles that involve lawyers, courts, and even the media. For those not covered by a living will or an advance directive, it is helpful to have a designated POA who will carry out an individual's wishes when she is unable to communicate with nurses and doctors. A person also can express her wishes to family members before the unexpected can strike. Though they aren't easy topics to discuss, a direct and calm demeanor can help make conversations with loved ones go smoothly. These conversations can also reveal if family members agree with the one's wishes and could help determine if the individual needs the services of a POA (Mayo Clinic, 2009).

What specific treatments can individuals choose through living wills and advance directives? CPR is administered when the heart stops beating and is designed to "buy time" until heart function can be repaired. It involves chest compressions and rescue breathing. It can involve the use of a machine called a defibrillator, which delivers a shock to the heart in order to make the heart start beating again or to force the heart back into a regular rhythm (American Heart Association, 2011).

Mechanical ventilation delivers oxygen to the lungs and removes carbon dioxide from the body. It is delivered by a machine that does the breathing for those who cannot breathe on their own (U.S. Department of Health and Human Services, 2011). Nutrition and hydration aid give individuals nutrient-fortified substances through either a stomach tube or intravenously. Another procedure called dialysis gets rid of waste in the bloodstream when a person's kidneys stop functioning. These procedures can be refused through a living will or the will can specify how long they may be administered (Mayo Clinic, 2009).

Organ donation is an important area that receives lots of attention due to the need for donors and the number of people each year whose lives are saved by donated organs. In the United States about 3,700 transplant candidates are added to a national waiting list each month and every day approximately 77 people receive organ transplants. Unfortunately, those statistics include also the fact that 18 Americans die each day waiting for a transplant that will not take place due to a shortage of donated organs (U.S. Department of Health and Human Services, 2006).

Many people feel a responsibility to leave behind their organs upon death, knowing that it can help someone else. Others may believe that their bodies should remain intact after death, often for religious reasons. Interestingly, Belief.net asserts that all American Protestant denominations as well as the Catholic Church recognize organ donation (Easterbrook, 2001). Individuals express their wishes to donate their organs through a living will or an advance directive. There are popular misconceptions about organ donation. Some include the belief that hospitals won't work hard to save lives if they know a person is an organ donor or that age is a barrier to donation. Some believe that they cannot have an open-casket funeral if they donate their organs (Mayo Clinic, 2009).

In reality, organ donation does not prevent open-casket funerals, clinicians in hospitals are only focused on saving the lives before them and not whether the person's organs can go to someone else, and age does not prevent organ donation. For minors, parents can make the decision on behalf their child. Also, organ donation does not add cost burdens to surviving family members. Many states support organ donation as an important and worthwhile decision and include organ donation status on each state-issued driver's license, identification that most adults carry with them at all times.

Research shows that advance directives are strongly associated with dying outside of a hospital setting, important information for those who would prefer to be surrounded by family and loved ones in their final days. Information published in the *Annals of Internal Medicine* found that the presence of a living will decreased the chances of a person passing away in a hospital. Whether it was a nursing home resident or a person living in his community, people 70 years of age or older who possessed a living will had a higher probability of dying "in place." Being able to have increased control over location at the time of death may offer empowerment and comfort to many (Degenholtz, Rhee, and Arnold, 2004).

Obtaining an advance directive is easy. There are many resources available to aid those who wish to complete one. According to National Healthcare Decisions

Day, an organization as well as the name given to an observance day in the month of April, advanced care planning can have different rules from state to state and websites are available to help individuals understand what their states require. The U.S. government also supports advance directives and living wills through the Federal Patient Self-Determination Act, legislation that calls for all medical facilities that participate in the federal Medicare program to ask patients about their advance directives and provide information if a patient does not have one (National Healthcare Decisions Day, 2011).

Advance directives and living wills are legal documents and while it is not always necessary, a lawyer may be consulted about the procedures and legalities of filling out the document. Copies of the document should go to primary care physicians, family members, and an individual's designated proxy. From time to time individuals should review their choices. As individual health changes or as individuals age, some decisions may need to be reconsidered. A person can change her mind about any item included in her living will or advance directive at any time (Mayo Clinic, 2009).

*Abena Foreman-Trice*

*See also* Cardiopulmonary Resuscitation (CPR); Grief; Medical Power of Attorney; Medicare.

## References

American Heart Association. *Cardiopulmonary Resuscitation (CPR)*. 2011. www.american heart.org/presenter.jhtml?identifier=4479.

American Hospital Association. *Put It in Writing: Questions and Answers on Advance Directives*. Booklet. Chicago: American Hospital Association, 2005.

Chen, Pauline W. "Making Your Wishes Known at the End of Life." *The New York Times,* April 15, 2010. www.newyorktimes.com/2010/04/16/health/15.chen.html.

Degenholtz, Howard B., YongJoo Rhee, and Robert M. Arnold. "Brief Communication: The Relationship between Having a Living Will and Dying in Place." *Annals of Internal Medicine* 141, no. 2 (2004): 113–17.

Easterbrook, Gregg. *Organ Donation: Where Your Religion Stands.* May 2001. www.beliefnet. com/Faiths/2001/05/Organ-Donation-Where-Your-Religion-Stands.aspx.

Mayo Clinic. *Living Wills and Advance Directives for Medical Decisions.* July 2009. www.mayo clinic.com/health/living-wills/HA00014.

"Most Americans Do Not Have Living Wills, Says New Survey by FindLaw." FindLaw. com. March 9, 2010. www.findlaw.com.

National Healthcare Decisions Day. *National Healthcare Decisions Day.* 2011. www.nhdd. org/p/facts.html.

U.S. Department of Health and Human Services (NIH). "National Heart Lung and Blood Institute: What Is a Ventilator?" National Heart Lung and Blood Institute. February 2011. www.nhlbi.nih.gov/health/dci/Diseases/vent/vent_what.html.

U.S. Department of Health and Human Services (NIH). "Organ Donation and Transplantation." National Women's Health Information Center. July 2006. www.womenshealth. gov/faq/organ-donation.pdf.

## LOVE CANAL

The Love Canal was one of the first domestic environmental disasters to gain mainstream recognition in the United States. A small community known as Love Canal located in Niagara Falls, New York, was exposed to toxic chemicals that were buried directly beneath the houses, streets, and schools. In 1980 the Love Canal was declared a national emergency; it was the first time this distinction had been used for something other than a natural disaster. The incident was followed by an intensive period of activity by the federal government to define environmental protection from contamination by toxins.

The Love Canal disaster served another important purpose in bringing awareness to the health dangers of exposure to toxic chemicals. Scientific studies from the Love Canal era helped establish a connection between exposure to toxins and certain diseases. This newfound knowledge of environmentally related diseases motivated many Americans to take a closer look at pollution in their own communities and to toxins inside and outside their homes. Now many watchdog groups, community organizers, and ordinary citizens take a more active role in advocating for safe and healthy living conditions.

Due to environmental disasters like the Love Canal, a growing number of chemicals and toxins are now being evaluated for their possible role in everything from environmentally triggered illness and irritable bowel syndrome to depression. While there are no clear answers to how much chemical exposure is too much, safety standards continue to be based on short-term exposure and do not consider the cumulative effects of the chemicals in the products we use, foods we eat, and all the toxins we now interact with on a daily basis.

The Love Canal community was named after William T. Love, who began the construction of a canal in the early 20th century to connect the upper and lower Niagara Rivers and potentially generate power. This project was eventually abandoned and Love left behind a hole 3,000 feet long, up to 20 feet deep, and almost 100 feet wide (Sherrow, 2001). By the 1940s, the Hooker Chemical and Plastics Corporation established a factory near the canal and began manufacturing industrial chemicals, plastics, fertilizers, and pesticides. The company purchased the unfinished canal and used it as a dumpsite for chemical waste until 1953. It is estimated that the Hooker Company dumped more than 42 million pounds of waste into the canal; some was put inside metal containers or fiber drums, but much of the waste was free-flowing (Sherrow, 2001). There is also speculation that the U.S. Army may have used the canal as a dumpsite in the 1940s, when it was also a landfill for the city of Niagara Falls.

The Love Canal was covered with hard-packed clay (a common landfill technique used to block out water that could become a leachate) and sold to the city of Niagara Falls for only $1 in 1953 (Sherrow, 2001). The Hooker Company stipulated in the deed that the land was not suitable for development because it was filled with chemical waste products, but the city disregarded the recommendation and began construction in 1955 (Bailey, 2010). During the construction of a school on

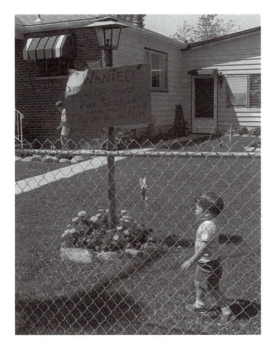

Children play in the front yard of their Love Canal home in New York on August 4, 1978. The community was built over a chemical waste dump site. (AP/Wide World Photos)

the property workers breached the clay covering and found a pit filled with chemicals. The city responded by moving the school 85 feet off to the side (Sherrow, 2001). Once the pit had been disturbed, it began to slowly leach the toxic sludge into the ground. Studies show that the waste contained benzene, a known human carcinogen that can cause blood cancers or other blood diseases (Sherrow, 2001). The waste also contained large quantities of dioxin, known to cause nerve damage, cancer, and various diseases (Sherrow, 2001).

A small working-class community had built up around the contaminated site, and by 1978 some of the worst effects of the toxic chemicals became apparent. Trees, gardens, and lawns were turning black and dying, and puddles of toxic leakage were reported all around the community in basements, on the school grounds, and in yards (Beck, 1979). Children returned from playing outside with chemical burns and rashes (Sherrow, 2001). A large percentage of residents had a high white-blood-cell count, a possible precursor of leukemia. There was an elevated rate of birth defects and miscarriages (Beck, 1979). Families also reported cases of chronic respiratory problems, allergies, and rashes (Sherrow, 2001).

Residents realized their homes were dangerous. They expected the federal government to have a swift response, but instead they had to remain in the toxic environment and wait for support. The situation made their homes worthless, and most homeowners did not have the money to move. The citizens mounted a grassroots campaign to demand the state and federal government relocate all of the families in the area. On August 5, 1979, President Carter declared Love Canal a federal disaster area. The federal government agreed to buy the homes of people who lived within two blocks of the old dumpsite. However, the residents that were left behind felt victimized and were livid. After another round of protests to the government, President Carter declared a second federal emergency on May 21, 1980, and the remaining families sold their homes to the government.

The Love Canal disaster raised contentious questions about liability for the extensive costs and damages of fixing the contaminated area. Was the state government to blame for willfully building a housing development over a known dumping site? Or was the Hooker Chemical Company at fault for improperly disposing of toxic chemicals? If the liable party could not afford the cleanup process, was the federal government responsible for providing funding? Congress ultimately answered those questions by passing the Comprehensive Environmental Response Compensation and Liability Act of 1980 (CERCLA). This became known as the Superfund Law, and it set up a $1.6 billion fund for toxic waste cleanups and emergencies (Sherrow, 2001). This law states that polluters will pay the cleanup costs if possible, but the government is responsible if the company has disbanded or cannot provide adequate funds.

The Superfund works by placing contaminated sites on the National Priorities List and dealing with the cleanup in order of severity of the threat to public health and safety. Of the 1,562 sites that have been placed on the list, only 319 have been satisfactorily treated and deleted from the list ("Superfund," 2008). The cleanup process was originally funded by a tax on chemical and oil companies, which are considered the most likely source of future contamination. However, Congress let this tax expire in 1995, which halted many planned cleanups as of 1996. Those cleanup efforts began again slowly, and money now comes directly from taxpayers after any funds are recovered from the polluting party (Sherrow, 2001).

Years after the incident was resolved the residents were still seeking a fair settlement for their suffering. The Hooker Chemical Company and the city of Niagara Falls paid a settlement of $20 million to a group of former residents. The chemical company also agreed in 1994 to pay the state of New York $98 million and in 1995 to pay the federal government $129 million for reimbursement for some of the cleanup costs. The legal process in this groundbreaking environmental case was lengthy. Modern victims of toxic contamination still turn to the Love Canal case as a precedent.

*Leslie Shafer*

*See also* Environmental Health; Environmental Protection Agency (EPA).

## References

Bailey, Ronald. "Love Canal, Three Decades Later." *Reason* 41, no. 11 (April 2010): 14. General Reference Center Gold. Gale.

Beck, Eckardt C. "The Love Canal Tragedy." *EPA Journal.* January 1979. www.epa.gov/history/topics/lovecanal/01.htm.

Houde, Julie. "Students Find Nothing to Love at Love Canal." *State News Service.* May 10, 2010. General Reference Center Gold. Gale.

Ross, Benjamin, and Steven Amter. *The Polluters: The Making of Our Chemically Altered Environment.* New York, NY: Oxford University Press, 2010.

Sherrow, Victoria. *Love Canal Toxic Waste Tragedy.* Berkeley Heights, NJ: Enslow, 2001.

"Superfund." Center for Public Integrity. 2008. http://projects.publicintegrity.org/superfund/default.aspx?act=faq.

Zechman, Marlin. "A Tragic Mess: Cleaning up an Environmental Disaster." *Risk Management* 54, no. 5 (May 2007): 28 (5). General Reference Center Gold. Gale.

## L-TRYPTOPHAN

Tryptophan is an amino acid that normally helps control the brain chemical serotonin, and affects sleep, mood, and appetite. It is most easily recognized as the ingredient in milk or turkey responsible for a sleepy feeling after a turkey dinner or a glass of warm milk at bedtime. Isolated as a nutritional supplement, it was incorporated into pills and sold in health food stores under a variety of brand names.

Unfortunately, the more than 5,000 people who became ill and the 38 who died from the genetically modified supplement L-tryptophan in 1989 are proof that supplements, even when they are labeled natural, in some cases, can also be deadly.

Once sales of the supplement began in the late 1980s, people across the country developed debilitating symptoms, including muscle weakness, pain spasms, high fevers, and rashes. The common link was L-tryptophan. The problem was eventually traced back to a batch of L-tryptophan from one of the largest chemical companies in Japan. The pills were manufactured after the company had substantially changed its production process. The company had also used genetically engineered bacteria in the production of the drug. Opponents of genetic engineering suggested that the engineered bacteria may have caused the problem. Another theory focused on a recently installed filtration system, which may have let through toxic impurities; the same toxic compounds were discovered in batches of unmodified bacteria used by other manufacturers of L-tryptophan.

As more and more people got sick and the common link was clearly established, doctors theorized that some people were more susceptible to L-tryptophan eosinophilia myalgia syndrome (EMS), as a reaction to the pure amino acid. EMS is a serious systemic illness characterized by elevations of certain white blood cells and severe muscle pain. Sadly, the Japanese batch made a reaction more likely. The company destroyed the modified bacteria.

Although L-tryptophan was banned in 1989, in March 2010 the U.S. regulatory agencies reversed that ban on its over-the-counter sale and now allow it to be sold as a dietary supplement. The United States joins other countries including Japan, the Netherlands, and the United Kingdom in once again allowing public access to L-tryptophan for treatment of depression, insomnia, and other disorders.

There are also new supplements for sale that label themselves alternatives to L-tryptophan; they are marketed as antidepressants, as sleep aids, and for weight loss. One alternative, known as 5-HTP, is the acronym for 5-hydroxytryptophan, also called 5-hydroxy-L-tryptophan. The compound is made from tryptophan, a natural amino acid found in foods. There has been some uncertainty about the effectiveness of 5-HTP and the Mayo Clinic and FDA confirmed the presence of a contaminant in 5-HTP similar to the one found in the 1989 L-tryptophan. There have been 10 reported cases of EMS associated with 5-HTP use; however, the manufacturers suggest the contaminant was not at high enough levels to cause illness (Rowland et al., 2009). The FDA suggests that anyone taking these newer products remain vigilant and watch for EMS symptoms.

What if L-tryptophan had been named a drug instead of a supplement? First, its manufacturers would have been required to perform detailed studies of possible risks. Second, the manufacturing process would have been closely regulated, and the plants would have been inspected. As a supplement, L-tryptophan faced none of those safeguards.

However, the FDA did try to take amino acids off the shelves before the L-tryptophan crisis. As early as 1976, the FDA attempted to set limits on the potency of vitamins and certain supplements. Its efforts triggered an avalanche of letters and calls protesting any changes. The reaction from the supplement industry and angry consumers was so strong that it resulted in passage of the Proxmire Amendment. Named after the bill's chief sponsor, Senator William Proxmire of Wisconsin, the legislation prohibited the FDA from putting limits on the potency of vitamins and minerals in food supplements, or, more important, from regulating them as drugs based on their potency. Congress made sure vitamins and supplements would not be regulated without clear and substantial proof of real danger.

Following the lifting of the ban on L-tryptophan the FDA urged health professionals to remain vigilant regarding signs of EMS and continues to advise consumers to be aware of drug interactions with any supplements. L-tryptophan is believed to increase serotonin levels and patients taking antidepressants should watch for signs of serotonin excess or Serotonin Syndrome, which can be life threatening. The timing of when L-tryptophan is taken can influence its effectiveness especially in relation to meals. Taking the supplement with a protein-rich meal may decrease its effectiveness while taking it on an empty stomach will increase its overall effectiveness.

*Sharon Zoumbaris*

*See also* Amino Acids; Dietary Supplements.

## References

"Clarification: 5-HTP Supplements Not Always Safer." *Family Practice News* 32, no. 23 (December 1, 2002): 12.

Gaby, Alan R. "L-tryptophan Is Back." *Original Internist* 17, no. 1 (March 2010): 47.

"Impurities in Dietary Tryptophan Products." *WHO Drug Information* 13, no. 1 (Winter 1999): 20.

Manders, Dean Wolfe. "The FDA Ban of L-Tryptophan: Politics, Profits and Prozac." *Social Policy* 26, no. 2 (Winter 1995): 55–59.

Rowland, Belinda, Samuel Uretsky, D. Pharm, and David Edward Newton. *The Gale Encyclopedia of Alternative Medicine*. 3rd ed. 4 vols. Detroit: Gale, 2009.

Smith, Jeffrey. *Genetic Roulette: The Documented Health Risks of Genetically Engineered Foods*. Fairfield, IA: Yes! Books, 2007.

Susman, Jeff. "Observations from Practice." *Journal of Family Practice* 53, no. 7 (2004): 516.

## LUPUS

Lupus is a chronic, autoimmune disease that can trigger the body to attack itself. While scientists are not sure what causes lupus, the end result is damage to many parts of the body including skin, joints, and internal organs. Also known as systemic lupus erythematosus (SLE), this chronic condition lasts a lifetime and may move between active times known as "flares" and quiet periods of remission. When a disease is labeled chronic, that means it lasts longer than six weeks and often for many years.

It is true that genetics may play a role in who gets lupus; if a family member had a similar autoimmune disease, it is more likely you might have one as well. It is estimated that between 161,000 and 322,000 adults in the United States have SLE (CDC, 2010), which is the most common type of lupus. Studies suggest that more than 16,000 new cases are diagnosed each year in the United States.

Female hormones are thought to play a role in causing lupus and more women than men have the disease. In fact, some 90 percent of those who have been diagnosed with lupus are women, most between the ages of 15 and 44 (CDC, 2010). Since hormones play a role in lupus, symptoms may appear or worsen during pregnancy due to a natural change in hormones and their production that coincides with the development of the fetus. Lupus can also be caused by certain medicines, a condition known as drug-induced lupus, which may disappear if the medicine is discontinued. Lupus symptoms can be triggered by an injury, stress, or even a simple infection like the common cold but the disease itself is not contagious and cannot be "caught" from someone else with lupus.

Lupus symptoms include pain in the joints along with swelling and redness, plus additional swelling in the face, legs, or lymph nodes in the neck or arm. There may also be fever, feelings of constant fatigue, chest pain, hair loss, a rash often in the shape of a butterfly on the face, nausea, diarrhea, and stomach pain with accompanying weight loss.

This difficult and complicated illness affects each person differently and other potential consequences of the disease range from a hardening of the arteries to kidney problems, headaches, vision problems, anemia, depression, anxiety, confusion or dizziness, and Raynaud's syndrome, which turns fingers blue or white when exposed to cold.

Scientists do not know what causes an individual's immune system to attack itself. Normally the immune system creates proteins known as antibodies that protect the body from invaders like bacteria and other germs. Autoimmune diseases occur when the immune system does not recognize the difference between healthy tissues and foreign tissues or germs. In individuals with lupus, the immune system creates antibodies but they attack and destroy healthy tissue. This causes inflammation, swelling pain, and damage in various parts of the body.

Surprisingly, even though lupus can attack any part of the body, most people with the disease find it focuses in just a few areas. For example, one person with lupus may have swollen knees and fever while another may experience a great deal of fatigue combined with fever or a rash. Someone else may have kidney trouble; lupus is different for everyone who has it.

Treatment varies just as much as the disease itself. For some patients immuno-suppressive drugs and steroids such as prednisone may provide some relief. In fact, prednisone is commonly prescribed for lupus. Other treatment options focus on learning how to manage stress and different ways to exercise that do not increase joint pain. Since there is no cure, physicians see an important focus of treatment as prevention of long-term damage to the body as they also seek to manage pain and discomfort and control the symptoms for their patient. Fortunately for many people, lupus remains a mild disease with only occasional "flares."

If the disease is severe, drug treatment is necessary and several types are considered including nonsteroidal anti-inflammatory drugs known as NSAIDs. NSAIDs are routinely used for pain relief and to reduce swelling in joints and muscles. They are most effective in cases of mild lupus. Aspirin, ibuprofen, and naproxen are examples of over-the-counter NSAIDs.

Corticosteroids are another type of medication used in lupus treatment. They are defined as synthetic versions of what the human body can already produce, and they can be helpful in treating swelling, tenderness, and pain in many parts of the body since they are known to calm the immune system. These drugs are also referred to as steroids. However, once a treatment program begins it is important not to stop taking corticosteroids all at once. Make sure to follow your doctor's instructions when starting or stopping these medicines.

Antimalarial drugs are sometimes prescribed for lupus patients to treat the rash, joint pain, or mouth sores. Finally, immunosuppressive agents are used in very severe cases of lupus, and work to suppress the immune system and stop or limit damage to vital organs. These are only used when other treatments have failed, and they can cause very serious side effects including an increased risk of cancer and infection.

The term *lupus* refers most often to SLE, which is the most common form of the disease. However, there are other types as well.

- Discoid lupus erythematosus, also called DLE, mainly affects the skin. A red rash may appear. Or, the skin on the face, scalp, or elsewhere may become scaly or change color. Sometimes DLE causes sores in the mouth or nose. A doctor will remove a small piece of the rash or sore and look at it under a microscope to tell if someone has DLE. If you have DLE, there is a small chance that you will later get SLE. There is no way to know if someone with DLE will get SLE.
- Drug-induced lupus is a lupuslike disease caused by certain prescription drugs. The symptoms of drug-induced lupus are similar to those of systemic lupus, but only rarely will any major organs be affected. Symptoms can include joint pain, muscle pain, and fever. Symptoms are mild for most people. Most of the time, the disease goes away when the medicine is stopped. More men get this type of lupus because the drugs with the highest risk of causing it are used to treat heart conditions that are more common in men; however,

not everyone who takes these drugs will develop drug-induced lupus. The drugs most commonly connected with drug-induced lupus are procainamide (Pronestyl, Procanbid) and hydralazine (Apresoline; also, hydralazine is an ingredient in Apresazide and Bidil).

- Neonatal lupus is a rare condition that affects infants of women who have lupus and is caused by certain antibodies from the mother acting upon the infant in the womb. At birth, the infant may have a skin rash, liver problems, or low blood cell counts, but these symptoms disappear completely after several months with no lasting effects. Some infants with neonatal lupus can also have a serious heart defect. With proper testing, physicians can now identify most at-risk mothers, and the infant can be treated at or before birth. Most infants of mothers with lupus are entirely healthy (U.S. Department of Health and Human Services, Office on Women's Health, 2009).

Researchers are looking at new treatments for lupus. The U.S. Food and Drug Administration (FDA) announced approval of Benlysta to treat patients with lupus in March 2011. In making its announcement of approval of this medication, the FDA noted it is the first drug developed in 50 years exclusively to treat lupus. As with any medication, it is does not treat everyone effectively. According to researchers the drug helped fewer than half the patients in the GlaxoSmithKline and Human Genome Sciences study. It also was not as effective for African Americans or people of color as a group, although some individuals did see benefits (Jackson, 2011). Trials for the medicine began in 2004 and have been extended as researchers follow the original participants in the trial to observe long-term effects.

Efforts to raise money for lupus research received a boost in 2011 from musician Julian Lennon, who was named Global Ambassador by the Lupus Foundation of America. Lennon is the son of the late Beatle, John Lennon. As Global Ambassador, Lennon will help raise awareness about World Lupus Day and Lupus Awareness Month held each May. He also plans to add his star power to fundraising for research, and he established the Lucy Vodden Research Grant Award in 2010 in memory of his childhood friend, Lucy Vodden. Vodden, who died from lupus in 2009, was a friend of Lennon's as well as the inspiration for his father John to write the well-known song "Lucy in the Sky with Diamonds," based on a drawing of Vodden by the younger Lennon. According to the LFA, Lennon has been a strong supporter of lupus research.

*Sharon Zoumbaris*

*See also* Immune System/Lymphatic System; National Institutes of Health (NIH); Steroids; Stress.

## References

Centers for Disease Control and Prevention. "Systemic Lupus Erythematosus (SLE or Lupus)," August 1, 2010, www.cdc.gov/arthritis/basics/lupus.htm.

"FDA Approves Benlysta to Treat Lupus." U.S. Food and Drug Administration. March 9, 2011. www.fda.gov.

Jackson, Harry, Jr. "New Treatment for Lupus Offers Hope for Sufferers." *St. Louis Post-Dispatch.* April 6, 2011. www.stltoday.com.

"Musician and Philanthropist Julian Lennon to Elevate the Global Profile of Lupus." Lupus Foundation of America. April 20, 2011. www.lupus.org.

U.S. Department of Health and Human Services. "Lupus." National Institute of Arthritis and Musculoskeletal and Skin Diseases. April 2009. www.niams.nih.gov/Health_Info/Lupus/shades_of_lupus.asp.

U.S. Department of Health and Human Services. "Lupus." Office on Women's Health. March 20, 2009. www.womenshealth.gov/faq/lupus.pdf.

## LYMPHATIC SYSTEM. *See* IMMUNE SYSTEM/LYMPHATIC SYSTEM

# M

## MACROBIOTICS

Macrobiotics is a diet and way of living based on the idea that we are the foods we eat, and we can achieve balance and harmony by eating the proper varieties and proportions of certain foods, especially whole grains and vegetables. Macrobiotics principles stem from the ancient Asian philosophy of yin and yang. The name comes from the Greek words *macro,* meaning great, and *bios* meaning life. Many people eat a macrobiotic diet, or variations of it, including entertainer Madonna, who swears by it, and actress Gwyneth Paltrow and actor Tom Cruise are fans of it as well.

**Early History**   George Ohsawa is credited with introducing macrobiotics to the West in 1965 with the publication of his book *Zen Macrobiotics.* He was born Yukikazu Sakurazawa, in Kyoto, Japan, in 1893. As a young man he attended a commercial high school and began to prepare for a career in business. That placement exposed him to Western culture and Western ideas. When he was 18, Sakurazawa was diagnosed with tuberculosis, which was untreatable at that time. During his illness he turned to the writings of Sagen Ishizuka, a Japanese doctor who had developed a theory of nutrition and medicine based on a traditional Asian diet. When Sakurazawa's health improved he devoted his life to writing about Ishizuka's teachings. He then went on to develop his own ideas based on Ishizuka's work and incorporated the concepts of yin and yang into his 12 principles of macrobiotics.

According to Ishizuka, health problems were caused by the imbalance of yin and yang, a concept that Sakurazawa took further when he linked yin with potassium and yang with sodium. After World War II Sakurazawa changed his name to George Ohsawa and named his philosophy "macrobiotics." In the late 1960s Ohsawa's dietary principles gained a following in the United States as a natural way to maintain health and fight disease. At that time the diet was considered mainly brown rice and was identified frequently with hippies, dropouts, and the drug culture.

**Nutritional Fears**   In 1971 the American Medical Association condemned macrobiotics, labeling it a "major public health problem" that posed a serious hazard to the health of individuals (Wells, 1978). However, Harvard nutritionist Dr. Frederick Stare went on the record supporting macrobiotics and compared it to a typical vegetarian diet in a *New York Times* interview.

According to the American Cancer Society website, the early U.S. version of macrobiotics practiced by some people involved eating mainly brown rice and water and was linked to severe nutritional deficiencies. However, the ACS has now publicly linked macrobiotic eating with a vegetarian diet and added, "A diet consisting mostly of vegetables, fruits and whole grains is associated with general health benefits and lower risk for several diseases and a macrobiotic diet, by virtue of its main components, can also achieve these benefits" ("Macrobiotic Diet"). However, the organization stops short of accepting the idea that a macrobiotic diet can prevent cancer. The National Institutes of Health's National Center for Complementary and Alternative Medicine (NCCAM) has funded a pilot study to determine whether a macrobiotic diet may prevent cancer but that research is ongoing ("Macrobiotic Diet").

**Yin and Yang**   While the macrobiotic philosophy is predominantly vegetarian, it also favors in-season and locally grown foods. Specific macrobiotic food choices are as varied as the people who practice it. Yin energy is expansive and includes leafy vegetables that grow upward such as leeks, kale, and bok choy as well as grains, beans, and seaweed. Yang energy is contractive and is associated with root vegetables that grow down such as carrots and other foods including animal products like fish and fowl. Macrobiotic followers aim for a balance of five parts yin to one part yang in their diet. Boiling vegetables in water enhances yin, and baking and roasting and exposing food to heat enhances yang.

While Ohsawa proposed 10 different diets, the general dietary recommendations suggest that 40 to 60 percent of calories each day should come from whole grains, including rice, millet, barley, wheat, rye, corn, oats, and buckwheat.

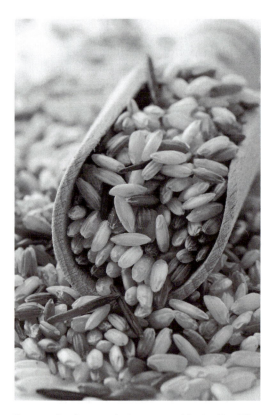

Brown rice is a staple in a macrobiotic diet. The word "macrobiotic" comes from the Greek and essentially means long life or great life. (Hlphoto/Dreamstime.com)

A classic macrobiotic eating plan would likely include the 40 to 60 percent of calories from whole grains along with 25 to 30 percent of the diet from fresh vegetables. Soybean products or seaweed might be 5 to 10 percent of the daily intake.

**New Macrobiotic Food Choices**   Food preparation is an equally important part of the macrobiotic plan, and cooking is supposed to be done only with gas or wood heat. Electric stoves and microwave ovens are to be avoided, and pots should be glass, ceramic, or stainless steel. Another important aspect is that eating should be done mindfully. That means attention is placed on eating as an activity rather than something done with little thought while watching TV or driving. Plus, food should be chewed thoroughly so it can be savored slowly, allowing for more enjoyment and less food.

Macrobiotics encourages the consumption of sea vegetables, many of which are gaining popularity in the United States. Kombu or kelp is a brown algae used as a flavoring agent in soups and stews. Wakame is a relative of kombu and must first be soaked, and then it can be sliced and also added to soups or salads. Hijiki is a black algae that should be soaked before it can be sautéed with vegetables such as corn, mushrooms, or carrots. Nori is sold in sheets and is familiar to many people as a sushi wrapping. It is rich in calcium and iron and can be crumbled or sliced into slivers and added to salads.

Scientists have confirmed that the macrobiotic focus on using vegetables at their peak and in season is healthy thanks to the antioxidants and phytochemicals in fresh vegetables. A new version of macrobiotic cooking popularized by Japanese chef Mayumi Nishimura is known as "petit macro," and according to Nishimura, it allows more flexibility in food choices. Nishimura served as the singer Madonna's private chef for seven years, ending in 2007. She lived with the singer and her family and traveled with her on worldwide tours. The chef also suggested that anyone interested in macrobiotics could try it on weekends as a start and recommends that beginners not become overly concerned about food rules.

*Sharon Zoumbaris*

*See also* National Center for Complementary and Alternative Medicine (NCCAM); Vegetarians.

## References

Barrett, S., and V. Herbert. "Questionable Cancer Therapies." www.quackwatch.org/01 QuackeryRelatedTopics/cancer.html.

Kushi, Michio. *The Cancer Prevention Diet: The Macrobiotic Approach to Preventing and Relieving Cancer.* New York: St. Martin's Griffin, 2009.

"Macrobiotic Diet." American Cancer Society. www.cancer.org.

Nishimura, Mayumi. *Mayumi's Kitchen: Macrobiotic Cooking for Body and Soul.* Tokyo: Kodansha International, 2010.

Ohsawa, George. *Zen Macrobiotics: The Art of Rejuvenation and Longevity.* Reprint. Chico, CA: George Ohsawa Macrobiotic Foundation, 1995.

Otake, Tomoko. "Macrobiotic Master Extols Joy of Cooking." *Japan Times,* February 25, 2010. www.japantimes.co.jp.

Porter, Jessica. *The Hip Chick's Guide to Macrobiotics: A Philosophy for Achieving a Radiant Mind and a Fabulous Body.* New York: Avery Trade, 2004.

Priesnitz, Wendy. "Macrobiotics for Health." *Natural Life* (January–February 2004): 18.

Spitalnick, Amy. "Mind Your Meals: Dive into a Holistic Approach to Cooking and Eating." *Vegetarian Times,* October 2008, 80.

Wells, Patricia. "Macrobiotics: A Principle Not a Diet." *New York Times,* July 19, 1978, C1–9.

## MALNUTRITION

Malnutrition is the result of not getting enough calories or nutrition to stay healthy. It can be caused by a variety of factors including an improper diet or the extreme situation of famine. In its most severe form it leads to starvation and death. Even though poverty is considered the leading cause of malnutrition around the world, people in wealthy and developed countries can also suffer from undernourishment and, more seriously, from malnutrition.

Specific deficiencies in a diet if left untreated eventually cause malnutrition as an individual's body struggles to get the nutrients it requires. Anemia is the most common diet deficiency in developed countries. Anemia is caused by iron deficiency. However, there are other less common dietary problems including vitamin A deficiency, which can cause blindness; rickets due to a lack of vitamin D or adequate sunlight; scurvy, which is the result of too little vitamin C; Crohn's disease, which is an inflammation of the digestive tract linked to the immune system; and celiac disease, which is a condition caused by a reaction to eating gluten that damages the small intestine and prevents proper absorption of food.

Malnutrition may develop over time and as it reaches the severe stage it can create problems with the heart, lungs, or kidneys. It can also lead to serious changes in the levels of chemicals found in the blood known as electrolytes. The World Health Organization (WHO) has identified malnutrition as the single most important risk factor for disease in the world. The Universal Declaration of Human Rights, established by the United Nations in 1948, identifies nutrition as a fundamental human right. Yet malnutrition remains one of the world's most prevalent health issues and brings with it long-lasting and widespread costs both in health and in dollars.

Ignorance of basic nutrition may be a factor behind undernourishment in developed nations. An exaggerated faith in vitamin pills as a substitute for fresh food, for example, can cause undernourishment if carried to extremes. Eating disorders such as anorexia or bulimia can also play a role in diet deficiencies and lead to malnutrition. Even an overreliance on processed foods can lead to undernourishment, and in the United States is also linked to growing rates of obesity.

Who is at risk for malnutrition? Infants and children are most at risk for not eating the correct calories or nutrients. Seniors or those who have decreased appetite or who are taking medicines that affect digestion and absorption of nutrients also should be aware of the possibility of undernourishment. People with eating disorders, with certain diseases including celiac, Crohn's, kidney or liver conditions, or cancer are at risk. People who abuse alcohol or drugs may also, over time, suffer from malnutrition.

Signs and symptoms of malnutrition may not appear until the later stages. Early signs include fatigue and irritability, slowed growth, and weight loss. As malnutrition progresses symptoms include bone or joint pain, muscle weakness, bloating in various body parts, brittle nails, dry and scaly skin, and hair loss, along with loss of appetite and a slowdown in the ability of wounds to heal.

Treatment depends on the initial cause of the malnutrition. Once diagnosed, the most immediate change needs to be an increase in calories and nutrients. These can be administered through small meals throughout the day if it is difficult for the individual to eat large meals. Liquid supplements are often used for increasing calories and nutrients without the intake of large quantities of food. Vitamin and mineral supplements may also be prescribed, especially if the malnutrition was caused by a health problem rather than a lack of food.

Efforts to end malnutrition around the world have been growing and various nations, including the United States, have contributed by providing food fortification, supplementation, dietary improvements, improved food access, agricultural enrichment, nutritional education, and improved sanitation and health care. The International Micronutrient Malnutrition Prevention and Control Program (IMMPACT) was established by the Centers for Disease Control and Prevention (CDC) in 2000 with the goal of eliminating deficiencies in iron, vitamin A, iodine, and folate. The IMMPACT program brings together the CDC, the WHO, the Global Alliance for Improved Nutrition (GAIN), and the Micronutrient Initiative (MI). According to the CDC, deficiencies in these four nutrients and zinc affect nearly one-third of the world's total population ("IMMPACT–International Micronutrient").

These four nutrients are among the 40 that people need to be healthy, and, unfortunately, they are often in short supply. Vitamin A is important for establishing the mucous membranes that protect the eyes. A deficiency in this vitamin causes blindness in half a million children each year ("Hidden Hunger," 2011). Zinc deficiency can create problems with brain and motor functions and is blamed for more than 400,000 deaths each year. Iron deficiency affects half of all women of child-bearing age in the world and can result in anemia, which weakens the immune system ("Hidden Hunger," 2011).

As international organizations work to reduce the incidence of malnutrition, they are also confronting its many causes. Severe droughts such as those in the summer of 2010 in Russia, Ukraine, and Kazakhstan have caused price spikes in the international wheat market due to the fact that Russia is the fourth-largest wheat exporter in the world. Russia's 2010 wheat exports were smaller by some 12 million metric tons, and Russian Prime Minister Vladimir Putin also announced a ban on grain exports as a way to secure a reserve of grain for Russian citizens and ease concerns about rising food prices in that country (Kramer, 2010). According to the United Nation's Food and Agriculture Organization (FAO), 1 billion people already suffer serious malnutrition due largely to droughts and crop failures (United Nations, 2010).

Population growth is another factor to be addressed. There are estimates that the global population will expand from its current 6.5 billion to some 9 billion by the middle of this century. That adds up to an additional 77 million people each year, growth that will put pressure on agriculture to meet the extra demand for food ("GM Foods," 2010).

The development and growth of genetically modified organisms (GMOs) has been considered as a possible solution to meeting foods needs, especially for developing nations. Genetically modified organisms (GMOs) are plants created for human or animal consumption using biotechnology instead of conventional plant breeding. The use of GM crops continues to raise concerns among European consumers, who for years have strongly blocked their use. Concern has centered on food safety, the effect of GMOs on the ecosystem, the possible loss of biodiversity, and potential corporate control of the food supply. Opponents of GMOs include the Organic Consumers Association and Greenpeace.

The European Commission (EC) continues to study the biosafety of GMOs and has invested more than $300 million in research since 1982 ("Biotechnology," 2010). A report released by the EC in December 2010 suggested that GMOS may provide opportunities to reduce malnutrition and to increase food yields, but the report cautioned that strong safeguards would be needed to control any potential risks ("A Decade," 2010). The report was a summary of 10 years of EU-funded research projects on GMOs.

There are other ways that nutrient-rich foods can improve or prevent malnutrition. As food prices climb many families, especially those in poverty, tend to switch from buying nutrient-rich fruits, vegetables, and meats to purchasing cheaper, less nutritious foods. Growth of agriculture, while no magic solution, would bring more foods to local markets and to poor people. The utilization of smaller farm and home gardens is also considered a positive way to generate income for poor families. In many developing countries women are responsible for the farm work and by growing their own food, they then create access to food to feed their children. One example of this principle at work was demonstrated by the charitable organization, Helen Keller International. In 1990 the organization encouraged home gardens in Bangladesh and provided families with information, advice, and seeds. By 2003 when the last available research was released, more than 80 percent of the families in the program had gardens and each family's intake of vitamin A from green vegetables had risen dramatically ("Hidden Hunger," 2011).

President Barack Obama demonstrated a strong commitment to global agricultural development and food security during his attendance at the G8 Summit in Italy in 2009. The countries in attendance jointly announced a new international fund, the Global Partnership for Agriculture and Food Security, during their session. The World Bank is charged with overseeing the partnership and with administering the $20 billion promised by the nations to finance initiatives that improve food security around the globe (Ho & Hanrahan, 2010).

In the United States another organization, Nourish America, has been working for nearly two decades to bring nutritional foods to America's poor and undernourished. In 2010 the program provided almost $3.5 million worth of nutritional products to more than 200,000 Americans according to its website. Nourish America was started in the 1990s by Dr. Michael Morton, his wife, author and journalist Mary Walker Morton, and other philanthropists who saw signs of malnutrition while working with mothers and their children in the nation's homeless shelters.

Nourish America currently provides daily multivitamins to more than 24,000 at-risk children at more than 130 partner sites in 32 states. Those partner sites include Head Start, Healthy Start, and WIC programs; public schools; battered women shelters; YMCA and YWCA; Boys and Girls Clubs; and other community-based and faith-based organizations that serve seniors, children, and teens. The United States will also continue to partner with other international organizations to provide emergency and humanitarian food assistance in response to natural disasters and to find solutions to food insecurity and malnutrition around the world.

*Sharon Zoumbaris*

*See also* Anorexia Nervosa; Bulimia Nervosa; Head Start and Healthy Start; Vitamins.

## References

"Biotechnology: Fifty Research Projects Analyse Safety of GMOs." *Europe Agri* (2010): 285357.

"A Decade of EU-Funded GMO Research (2001–2010)." European Commission. June 17, 2010. http://ec.europa.eu/research/biosociety/pdf/a_decade_of_eu-funded_gmo_research.pdf.

Food and Agriculture Organization of the United Nations. "The Spectrum of Malnutrition." *United Nations.* 2010. www.fao.org/worldfoodsummit/english/fsheets/malnutrition.pdf.

"GM Foods: Genetic Manipulation or Global Malnutrition? GM Food Is the Subject of the Second in the SCI's Series of Public Lectures." *Chemistry and Industry* (November 22, 2010): 33.

"Hidden Hunger: Agriculture and Nutrition." *The Economist (US)* (March 26, 2011): 69.

Ho, Melissa D., and Charles E. Hanrahan. "International Food Aid Programs." *Congressional Research Service (CRS) Reports and Issue Briefs* (February 2010).

"I AM Enlightened Nutrition Partners with Nourish America to Battle Malnutrition." *PR Newswire,* March 11, 2011. General Reference Center Gold.

"IMMPACT–International Micronutrient Malnutrition Prevention and Control Program." Centers for Disease Control and Prevention. www.cdc.gov/immpact/index.html.

Kramer, Andrew E. "Drought in Russia Ripples beyond the Wheat Fields." *New York Times,* August 27, 2010. www.nytimes.com.

Nourish America. www.nourishamerica.org.

Wandera, Stephen, and Eve Mashoo. "Experts Raise Red Flag on Malnutrition Levels." *Africa News Service,* March 25, 2011. General Reference Center Gold.

## MAMMOGRAPHY

Breast cancer is the most common cancer in women. According to recent figures from the Centers for Disease Control and Prevention (CDC), more than 200,000 U.S. women are diagnosed with breast cancer and more than 40,000 die each year ("Fast Facts"). One important weapon in the battle against the disease is the use of mammography. The test, known as a mammogram, screens the breast using x-ray technology, to find cancer before it is discovered during a self-exam of the breast or a clinical exam by a doctor or nurse. There are two types of mammograms, a screening mammogram for women who have no known problem and a diagnostic mammogram that is used to evaluate a patient or as a follow-up to earlier x-rays that showed an abnormality.

Studies show that regular mammograms can increase a woman's chances of discovering early stage breast cancer when it is more likely to be curable. However, in 2009, the United States Preventive Services Task Force, an independent panel of experts appointed by the Department of Health and Human Services to examine health questions, recommended less frequent mammograms for women and recommended that women start breast cancer screening later in life at age 50 rather than age 40. Their recommendations did not include the small group of women with unusual risk factors for breast cancer. The best advice for any women is to check with their physician and consider individual risk factors. The test can also be helpful for men, who also get breast cancer. In men, the cancer can occur at any age but is most common in men between the ages of 60 and 70 years. Still, male breast cancer is uncommon, for every 100 cases of breast cancer, less than one is diagnosed in men ("Fast Facts"). The American Cancer Society, American College of Surgeons, American Medical Association, and the American College of Radiology all recommend annual mammograms for women past the page of 40 and as requested by their physicians for men.

New technology in mammography now includes the use of magnetic resonance imaging (MRI), ultrasound, and digital imaging. While these technologies improve the quality of the breast image and improve the actual diagnosis, they have not replaced traditional or standard mammography as the best way to spot breast cancer. In fact, according to the results of a trial funded by the National Cancer Institute, led by investigators at the University of North Carolina at Chapel Hill, digital mammography was neither better nor worse than standard mammography in finding breast cancers except in the cases of women with dense breasts when digital was superior.

According to researchers, a chief advantage of digital mammography is that radiologists can fine-tune the images to make any abnormalities more noticeable. No matter which type of equipment is used, both digital and standard mammography equipment must be certified by the U.S. Food and Drug Administration (FDA) according to the Mammography Quality Standards Act (MQSA). The MQSA took effect October 1, 1994, and called for FDA certification of all mammography equipment and facilities, including hospitals, outpatient clinics, doctors' offices, or other clinics.

A screening mammogram is conducted by having a woman stand and face the mammography machine. She must wear a hospital gown or other covering so that she can expose each breast, which is then placed on a plastic or metal film holder approximately the size of a placemat. The technician lowers the machine until the breast is compressed as flat as possible between the film holder and a paddle or rectangle, again the same size of a placemat. The compression lasts for seconds as the x-rays are taken. While compression is uncomfortable, it is necessary to provide the best view of breast tissue, especially in the case of dense breast tissue. Screening mammograms find some 85 percent of breast cancers.

The radiologist then examines the x-rays to determine the appearance of the breasts and creates a report with the details. A mammogram with no abnormalities receives a rating of BIRADS1, based on the Breast Imaging Reporting and Data System (BIRADS), created by the American College of Radiology. A BIRADS2 is benign or noncancerous if one or more abnormalities were found but are variations of normal. The rating system extends to BIRADS5, which means an abnormality has been found that appears highly suggestive of cancer and a biopsy is recommended.

Since the biggest risk factors for developing breast cancer are age or a positive family history of the disease, guidelines recommend an annual screening mammogram for every woman at age 40 and younger for those women with more risk factors. According to the American Cancer Society one in eight women in the United States will develop breast cancer so education about yearly mammograms and monthly breast self-examination may make a difference. An early diagnosis may mean successful treatment while an end-stage diagnosis may reveal little can be done for the patient.

*Sharon Zoumbaris*

*See also* Cancer; Centers for Disease Control and Prevention (CDC).

## References

American Cancer Society (ACS). www.cancer.org.

"Digital Mammography Better for Some Women." *Staying Healthy from the Faculty of Harvard Medical School.* August 21, 2006.

"Fast Facts." Centers for Disease Control and Prevention (CDC). 2010. www.cdc.gov/cancer.breast/basic_info/fast_facts.htm.

"Mammography in Women over Forty Catches Disease Earlier." *Women's Health Weekly,* August 14, 2003, 14.

National Cancer Institute. Office of Cancer Communications. NCI/Cancer Information Service. http://cancernet.nci.nih.gov.

Smith, Robert A., Debbie Saslow, Kimberly Andrews Sawyer, Wylie Burke, and Mary E. Costanza. "American Cancer Society Guidelines for Breast Cancer Screening: Update 2003." *Cancer* (May–June 2003): 141–70.

U.S. Cancer Statistics Working Group. "United States Cancer Statistics: 1999–2007 Incidence and Mortality Web-Based Report." Department of Health and Human Services, Centers for Disease Control and Prevention, and National Cancer Institute. 2010. http://apps.nccd.cdc.gov/uscs/.

## MANAGED CARE

The term *managed care* has grown out of other terms in the U.S. health care system, such as *health maintenance organizations (HMOs)* and before that *prepaid group practices (PPGP)*. The term *managed care* today refers to health insurance plans that contract with health care providers and medical facilities to offer care for members, often at reduced costs for what the care would cost if a person had no health insurance. Of course, most providers now offer discounted arrangements to all types of health insurance plans, so that aspect of managed care is less unique than it was a few decades ago.

Generally, within a managed care system, there are specific providers who make up the plan's network. Often, the best financial coverage for an individual patient in a managed care plan occurs if the person uses providers within the network. While in the past some managed care plans would not provide any coverage if a person did not use a network provider, now in many cases, there is some coverage of the costs of the care with a higher proportion of the costs left to be paid by the individual if he goes outside of the network providers. How much of the care the plan will pay depends on each individual network's rules.

In simplistic terms, more restrictive managed care plans generally cost the consumer less to purchase, even if the plan is part of health insurance coverage offered through work whereas more flexible plans cost more. In the past, one way to examine different types of managed care plans was to contrast health maintenance organization (HMOs), preferred provider organizations (PPOs), and point of service plans (POSs). Generally, health maintenance organizations usually only pay for care within the network and a person often must choose a primary care doctor who coordinates most care and is also in the network. Preferred provider organizations (PPOs) usually pay more if a person decides to obtain care within the network, but will still pay a portion of care if a person uses providers outside of the network. Point of service pans (POSs) plans often let an individual choose between an HMO and a PPO each time he needs care.

The term *managed care* also refers to a variety of techniques intended to reduce the cost of providing health benefits and improve the quality of care as well as to the systems of financing and delivering health care to enrollees. The central principle when using the term in this way is an organized effort to involve both insurers and providers of health care, along with the incorporation of financial incentives and specified administrative structures to reach a goal to provide appropriate, cost-efficient health care of good quality.

In its early origins, the beginnings of what we now call managed care had a focus on ways to deliver care more efficiently, at a lower cost, and with more emphasis on coverage of preventive care services than was true for most existing health care services at that time. Some of the ways to accomplish this were through different economic incentives for physicians, which in some managed care plans included having physicians paid on a salaried basis (in many Kaiser Permanente managed care plans, especially those in California); selective contracting with providers and hospitals to lower costs; and more intensive management of high-cost health care problems. In addition, the coverage of preventive services was another way, over a number of years, to help patients focus on wellness rather than just sickness care and to potentially lower costs of care in the long run by using less expensive preventive approaches to discover and treat health problems before they became more serious and expensive.

**History**   The earliest origins of *PPGPs,* when the term emphasized that care was provided through a group of doctors working together with a prepaid type of insurance arrangement, began under Henry Kaiser. This form of organization provided health care for workers during the building of the Hoover Dam in the late 1930s and continued during World War II. This was a way to provide health care coverage to workers, often in more isolated geographic locations or newer locations in the West, who were involved with ship building and steel mills as part of the war effort. After the war ended, the plan was opened to the public as Kaiser Permanente and became one of the largest systems of its type. By 1966, approximately 20 percent of all Americans in prepaid care were enrolled in Kaiser Permanente (Kronenfeld, 2002).

The term *HMO* was initially used in 1974, as part of a piece of legislation supported by President Richard Nixon. Politicians and policy experts became interested in encouraging more Americans to join these groups for their health insurance coverage, and federal legislation was passed that encouraged the growth of such groups as part of an effort to control rising health care costs. In the federal legislation, the prepaid aspects of the plans were emphasized along with the inclusion of preventive care and the idea that the services provided would help people to maintain their health, giving rise to the term *health maintenance organization.* At this time, many of the early groups had been nonprofit, such as Kaiser Permanente, but for-profit HMOs were also being encouraged. Alain Enthoven pushed the concept of "managed competition," which became the dominant approach by the 1990s (Enthoven, 1993).

By the 1990s, the term *managed care* replaced the term *HMO* as a broader way to describe the mechanisms used to deliver health care. By then, a number of managed care options were offered by large, for-profit health insurance companies such as Cigna. While the Kaiser Permanente original model included salaried physicians and ownership of its own hospitals, the coverage expanded to some states outside of the West where ownership of hospitals was not included. Many of the Cigna plans included salaried physicians as a way to control the costs and provide incentives for physicians concerning the amount of care delivered. However, Cigna plans contracted for care with a variety of local hospitals.

In many states, Blue Cross/Blue Shield plans also began to offer managed care options, generally with groups of private physicians and hospitals contracted to provide services. Growth in managed care started to accelerate at this time. In 1976 only 2.8 percent of the population of the United States was in managed care, and by 1990 some 13 percent of the U.S. population was in some form of managed care. That figure grew to 30 percent in 2000. This growth also reflected important geographical variation, ranging from around 22 percent managed care participation in the South up to 42 percent in the West (Eberhardt, Ingram, and Makuc, 2001).

**Comparison of Care**   One of the major questions concerning managed care has been whether the quality of care patients receive is the same as the care received by patients not under managed care. It has been widely accepted that older-style, not-for-profit managed care plans deliver high-quality care, generally for less money than traditional care. A more important question since the growth of for-profit managed care companies has been whether quality of care varies between investor-owed and not-for-profit plans. One important study demonstrated that investor-owned plans had lower quality across 14 different measures of quality of care (Himmelstein et al., 1999). Quality scores were better for staff and group model HMOs, such as Kaiser Permanente.

**Future of Managed Care**   For the past decade, there has been discussion about a managed care backlash and the end of managed care (Robinson, 2001; Mechanic, 2001). Some experts have argued that unrealistic expectations were placed on managed care, especially the idea that it could result in major cost containment. Often, this has occurred only when tight constraints were placed on patients and doctors over use of outside referrals or use of more expensive approaches to treat care. Patients, however, have reacted negatively to such restrictions, and in the past decade more PPOs and POS plans with fewer restrictions have become commonplace. Mechanic (2001) argued that Americans are uncomfortable with the idea of having their health care rationed, and have viewed managed care as a mechanism for rationing. Patients want to be able to trust their physicians and not doubt whether the physician is looking out for the best interests of the patient versus the financial interest of the plan. For these reasons, the *managed care* term was not used much in the recent debate over health care reform led by President Obama. Managed care approaches are still part of the health care delivery options in the United States, but often of the broader, more open type.

*Jennie Jacobs Kronenfeld*

*See also* Health Insurance; Health Savings Account (HSA).

### References

Eberhardt, M.S., D.D. Ingram, and D.M. Makuc. *Urban and Rural Health Charts, Health USA, 2001*. Hyattsville, MD: National Center for Health Statistics, 2001.

Enthoven, Alain C. "The History and Principle of Managed Competition." *Health Affairs* Supplement (March 1993): 22–48.

Himmelstein, D.U., S. Woolhandler, L. Hellender, and S.M. Wolfe. "Quality of Care in Investor Owned v. Not-for-Profit HMO." *Journal of the American Medical Association* 282 (1999): 159–63.

Kronenfeld, Jennie Jacobs. *Health Care Policy: Issues and Trends*. Westport, CT: Praeger, 2002.

Mechanic, David. "The Managed Care Backlash: Perceptions and Rhetoric in Health Care Policy and the Potential for Health Care Reform." *Milbank Quarterly* 79 (2001): 35–54.

Robinson, J. "The End of Managed Care." *Journal of the American Medical Association* 285 (2001): 2622–28.

**MANIC-DEPRESSIVE DISORDER.** *See* **BIPOLAR DISORDER**

**MARIJUANA.** *See* **MEDICAL MARIJUANA; SMOKING**

## MAYO CLINIC

The Mayo Clinic is one of the premier health facilities in the world with campuses in Rochester, Minnesota; Jacksonville, Florida; and Scottsdale, Arizona. The clinic offers patient care, research, and a graduate school medical education program that provides hundreds of medical residencies and fellowships. According to the Mayo Clinic's website, the Mayo Clinic mission remains the same today as when the institution began: to inspire hope and contribute to health and well-being by providing the best care to every patient through integrated clinical practice, education, and research (Mayo Clinic, 2011).

The physicians, scientists, and researchers from the Mayo Clinic continue to share their expertise through online articles, books, and a free online newsletter. Web content from the clinic is also provided through RSS feeds, which are a new technology for distributing web content through a subscription. Those subscribers then receive an alert when new and updated topics are published. The clinic also announced a publishing agreement in 2009 with Oxford University Press.

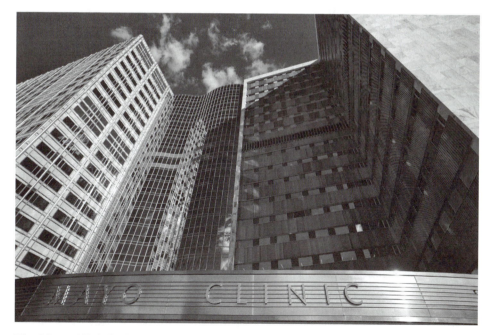

The Mayo Clinic building, located in Rochester, Minnesota, includes the medical facility, and also provides space for research and educational activities. (Pictureguy66/Dreams time.com)

The collaboration will result in jointly published medical reference books and textbooks authored by Mayo Clinic physicians and researchers.

The institution has come a long way from its early beginnings as St. Mary's Hospital in 1889. The hospital, run by the Roman Catholic Sisters of St. Francis of Rochester, was first known for its surgical expertise thanks to the Mayo brothers and their staff. William J. Mayo (1861–1939) and Charles H. Mayo (1865–1939), the two surgeons, were determined to create an institution that would showcase their humanitarian ideals and promote cooperation, collaboration, and information sharing among their colleagues in medicine. As the clinic grew in size, it attracted the leading medical practitioners of the day and steadily increased its growing specialty areas. By 1915 the institution included an educational branch known as the Mayo Foundation for Education and Research through which the brothers sought to train new generations of doctors in their joint venture with the University of Minnesota.

The goal of the clinic from its earliest days was to treat patients on the premises and also to provide information that could be used by doctors throughout the United States and the world who might be treating patients with similar conditions. In its years of early development, the clinic specialized in surgery, and its areas of expertise quickly expanded to include anesthesia, physiotherapy, social services, dietetics, and nursing education. Today, the Mayo School of Health Sciences offers 96 programs representing more than 57 health science careers. The clinic was named a "Best Hospital" by the 2010 *U.S. News & World Report* for the 21st straight year as part of the magazine's annual "Best Hospitals" issue.

In fact, the Mayo Clinic ranked second overall among the top medical facilities in the country, and remained among the top three hospitals in 10 of their specialties, putting them just 2 points below first-place Johns Hopkins Hospital in Baltimore in the 2010 *U.S. News & World Report* annual honor roll. The Mayo Clinic was the most highly regarded for its treatment of diabetes and endocrinology, kidney disorders, and gastroenterology. Other premier hospitals on the list include Massachusetts General Hospital, ranked third overall, Cleveland Clinic, ranked fourth, and Ronald Reagan UCLA Medical Center in Los Angeles, ranked fifth overall.

The brothers incorporated the clinic in 1919 under the Mayo Properties Association in order to ensure its continued success after their deaths. In fact, both William and Charles had retired to neighboring houses in Tucson, Arizona, when in the spring of 1939 William was diagnosed with stomach cancer. He returned to the clinic for surgery and Charles traveled to Rochester to help with his recuperation. While William was recovering, Charles took a trip to Chicago where he had studied medicine at the Chicago Medical School, later known as Northwestern University Medical School. While in Chicago he developed pneumonia and died in May 1939. William's surgery was ultimately not successful, and he died two months later in July 1939.

The current Mayo Clinic cares for more than half a million people each year according to statistics for 2009. The Mayo Health System directly reaches more than 70 communities in the upper Midwest. With almost 4,000 staff doctors and researchers and another 3,000 residents, fellows, and students, the total staff for the Mayo Clinic campuses includes more than 55,000 employees.

Through its medical education program the Mayo Clinic remains at the cutting edge of research in a wide range of medical specialties. The doctoral and master's programs focus on seven biomedical subspecialties, and the 248 medical residencies and fellowships offered represent virtually all medical specialties offered in medicine today. Total revenue for 2009 was more than $7 million ("Mayo Clinic Facts—2009"). The institution is funded through contributions, grants, and endowments as well as government, foundation, and industry funding sources.

William and Charles Mayo were visionaries in the field of medicine and sought to create a unique institution to treat people with dignity. Both men were recognized for their medical talents throughout their careers. Charles was named president of the American Medical Association in 1906 and in 1915 served as a professor of surgery for the University of Minnesota. William was named to the university's Board of Regents in 1907. The brothers remained active on the board of the Mayo Clinic until their deaths. Due to their efforts and the continuing work of its staff, the Mayo Clinic remains a respected facility that balances the needs of patients for humane and effective treatment with the needs of doctors to share professional experience and information in research and education.

*Sharon Zoumbaris*

*See also* Primary Care Physicians.

### References

Brink, Susan. "America's Best Hospitals." *U.S. News & World Report,* August 12, 1996, 52.

Comarow, Avery. "Best Hospitals 2010–11: The Honor Roll." *U.S. News & World Report.* July 14, 2010. www.health.usnews.com/health-news/best-hospitals/articles/2010.

"Honor Roll for 2010." Mayo Clinic. www.mayoclinic.org/feature-articles/honor-roll-2010.html.

"Mayo Clinic Enters into Publishing Agreement with Oxford University Press, Inc." Mayo Clinic. www.mayoclinic.org/new2009-rst/5539.html.

"Mayo Clinic Facts—2009." Mayo Clinic. www.mayoclinic.org.

Roberts, Kate. *Minnesota 150: The People, Places and Things That Shape Our State.* St. Paul: Minnesota Historical Society Press, 2007.

## MEDICAID

Medicaid is a U.S. government-sponsored health program for low-income families and individuals that pays their health care costs when they lack access to private health insurance. Medicaid and Medicare are similar-sounding government health care programs, but they are quite different. While Medicaid serves low-income Americans, Medicare is strictly for senior citizens above the age of 65 and younger people with certain disabilities as well as all people with end-stage renal disease. There are strict income criteria for anyone to receive Medicaid and those restrictions vary from state to state. Medicaid also covers a wider range of health care services than Medicare. In contrast, Medicare is available to all U.S. citizens over the age of 65 regardless of their income if they have paid taxes into the Social Security fund. Medicare covers hospital bills in Part A, medical insurance in Part B, and prescription drugs in Part D.

Medicaid became law in 1965 along with Medicare under Title XIX of the Social Security Act. Different groups of Americans are covered under Medicaid but even within these groups certain criteria must be met. Those include age, if someone is pregnant, disabled, or blind, along with requirements for income and resources such as bank accounts, real estate, and whether that person is a U.S. citizen or a lawfully admitted immigrant. In fact, some Americans are eligible for both Medicaid and Medicare. Children are eligible for coverage based on their status even if their parent is not eligible. Also, if a child lives with someone other than her parent, she may be eligible based on her own need rather than on her guardian's eligibility.

The Obama administration announced plans for an additional $206 billion in bonus Medicaid payments to some 15 states if they could sign up eligible children who had previously failed to enroll. The payments, which were established when the Children's Health Insurance Program (CHIP) was reauthorized in 2009, will target some of the estimated 4.7 million children who may be eligible for Medicaid coverage, but whose parents or guardians fail to apply for them.

Each state administers its own Medicaid program and the federal Centers for Medicare and Medicaid Services (CMS) monitors each of those state-run programs and establishes requirements for eligibility standards, service delivery, quality, and funding. Some states have their own name for their program such as MassHealth in Massachusetts, Medi-Cal in California, and TennCare in Tennessee. While state participation in Medicaid has been voluntary, all 50 states have participated since 1982. States provide up to half of the funding for their Medicaid programs, but they must follow federal guidelines in order to receive matching funds and grants from the federal government.

There are two basic types of Medicaid coverage, a community coverage that assists individuals who have little or no medical insurance and the nursing home coverage that pays all of the costs of nursing homes for eligible people once that individual's resources have been exhausted. Medicaid is the largest source of funding for medical and health-related services for Americans with a limited income, and as the baby boomer generation continues to age, nursing home coverage has become the fastest-growing aspect of Medicaid payments.

Another area where Medicaid coverage has escalated rapidly is in the treatment of autism spectrum disorders (ASDs) in state Medicaid programs. A three-year study by Penn State College of Medicine researchers found that dollars spent on treatment for autism was higher than in any other mental disorder and total health care expenditures for ASDs grew by 32 percent from the year 2000 to 2003 when the study was conducted ("Rapid Rise," 2010). The researchers recommended that states ensure adequate resources to provide adequate care for what they called a particularly vulnerable population.

However, problems have been associated with Medicaid reimbursement amounts for many years. Participation in Medicaid is optional for doctors and nursing homes so many do not participate in the program because the reimbursement rates are low. A report released in the summer of 2010 showed that emergency room visits to U.S. hospitals had increased more than 23 percent in the decade from 1997 to 2007, a figure double what researchers had anticipated based on population growth (Tang et al., 2010). Researchers from the University of California at San Francisco suggested those low reimbursement rates to doctors who care for Medicaid patients may be the key factor behind the increase.

According to Dr. Ning Tang, lead author of the UCSF study, physicians are refusing to accept new patients with Medicaid due to big differences in reimbursement rates. This in turn has pushed those individuals to hospital emergency rooms for everything from ear infections to heart disease. Statistics from the report showed that emergency room visit rates for adults with private insurance and those on Medicare showed no significant change while visit rates for Medicaid patients specifically accounted for the large increase. Researchers suggest this may show that Medicaid patients might not have adequate access to outpatient care. The study also noted that the number of U.S. emergency departments went down by 5 percent during the 10 years the statistics were collected, further shrinking health care access for adults with Medicaid (Tang et al., 2010).

With the 2010 Patient Protection and Affordable Care Act poised to increase coverage to an estimated 16 million Americans by expanding eligibility to the Medicaid program in 2013, researchers suggest there may not be enough doctors or services available to meet projected health care needs. This may be compounded by the 2010 law, which specifically requires states to expand eligibility for Medicaid recipients to all adults who make 133 percent of the federal poverty line by 2014. Medicaid administrators on the state level are looking for additional assistance as they prepare for this large increase in program enrollees while they deal with ongoing budget cuts, furloughs for state workers, and pay cuts as part of an overall effort to balance state budgets. Since the federal government only provides 50 percent of the funding for the programs, states will have to work hard to meet these new financial obligations.

The need to contain Medicaid costs is considered one of the most difficult budget issues facing legislators on the state and federal level. The complexity of the system, the variety of benefit packages available in different states, and the large amount of paperwork required make it vulnerable to billing fraud and other abuses. According to an annual report released by the Centers for Medicare and Medicaid Services (CMS), spending on Medicaid reached more than $339 billion in 2008, and growth is expected to average about 8 percent over the next 10 years, reaching some $674 billion by 2017 ("Medicaid"). That growth rate is more than double the 4.8 percent growth projected in the general economy. So federal and state governments are cracking down on Medicaid waste and overspending as a way to try and ease budget problems.

The amount of money lost to fraud, waste, and abuse is significant if recent figures are accurate; up to $700 billion was reportedly wasted in the U.S. health care system, not limited to federal health care programs; the majority of it due to unnecessary care, fraud, and administrative inefficiency (Waltz, 2010). Congress has also increased funding for a joint HHS–Justice Department antifraud task force known as HEAT (Health care fraud prevention and Enforcement Action Team). On December 20, 2010, the Justice Department announced a $280 million settlement with a pharmaceutical manufacturer who offered customers one price and then falsely reported inflated prices to the lists the government uses when calculating how much to pay for the drugs. This allowed the buyers to pocket the difference between the real price of the drug and the inflated price paid by the government (Waltz, 2010).

The HEAT program started in 2007 and has expanded its operations from two locations to seven metropolitan areas: Los Angeles, Miami, Detroit, Houston, Baton Rouge, Tampa, and Brooklyn. The task force has also charged more than 500 defendants through civil enforcements and has been instrumental in the return of some $441 million in federal Medicaid money back to the government ("Fight against Fraud"). The HEAT website lists activities per month and links to additional information about indictments, pleas, or sentencing. Increased enforcement has been a cornerstone of the administration of President Barack Obama, who in remarks to a joint session of Congress in 2009 suggested much of the health care reform plan could be paid for through savings from the waste or abuse that exists in the current health care system (Waltz, 2010).

One avenue to solving Medicaid budget issues is through changes like a new federal rule passed in November 2008 that allows states to charge premiums and higher copayments to Medicaid participants. The rule will limit financial losses from the program by allowing states to save more $1 billion and the federal government to save approximately $1.4 billion (Sack, 2010).

Unfortunately, the burden of paying for those premiums and copays will fall squarely on the low-income people Medicaid serves. Government estimates suggest Medicaid recipients will pay more than $1 billion over five years beginning in 2008 (Pear, 2008). Additionally, savings would come from a reduced use of services by Medicaid recipients since many of those individuals may find even a modest increase will price a doctor's visit or prescription refill out of their reach. The rules do allow states to set up a sliding scale for deciding premium and copayment amounts. However, groups such as AARP and American Academy of Pediatrics have criticized the rule change, saying the higher fees will make it more difficult for low-income children and seniors to get the health care they need (Pear, 2008). According to recent figures, Medicaid enrollment topped 50 million in 2009, up 2.4 million from 2008, with half the increase among children (Sack, 2010).

*Sharon Zoumbaris*

*See also* Autism; Health Insurance; Medicare.

## References

Colliver, Victoria. "Big Jump in Visits to Emergency Room Seen." *San Francisco Chronicle,* August 11, 2010, C1.

"Fight against Fraud Too Weak, Lawmakers Say." *CQ Healthbeat.* December 23, 2010. General Reference Center Gold.

McCarthy, Meghan. "State Medicaid Directors Scramble to Navigate Expansion." *Congress Daily AM.* July 16, 2010.

"Medicaid." Centers for Medicare and Medicaid Services. U.S. Department of Health and Human Services. http://cms.hhs.gov.

"Medicaid Spending Surging." *Inside Healthcare* 4, no. 11 (November 2008): 5.

Pear, Robert. "New Medicaid Rules Allow States to Set Premiums and Higher Co-Payments." *New York Times,* November 27, 2008. www.nytimes.com.

"Rapid Rise in Medicaid Expenditures for Autism Spectrum Disorder Treatment." *Mental Health Weekly Digest,* November 8, 2010, 29.

Sack, Kevin. "Bonuses to Reward States for Insuring More Kids." *Houston Chronicle,* December 27, 2010, 6.

Tang, Ning, John Stein, Renee Y. Hsia, Judith H. Maselli, and Ralph Gonzales. "Trends and Characteristics of US Emergency Department Visits, 1997–2007." *Journal of the American Medical Association* 304, no. 6 (August 11, 2010): 664–70.

Waltz, Judith A. "The HEAT Is On: Prepare Now for Enhanced Government Health Care Enforcement Efforts." *Journal of Health Care Compliance* 12, no. 2 (March–April 2010): 13.

# MEDICAL MARIJUANA

The debate to legalize marijuana has been raging for many years, and will continue as long as there are Americans who want to use it recreationally and for medical purposes. Although the federal government bans marijuana use of any kind, certain states sidestepped that roadblock and have allowed its limited use under the umbrella of "medical marijuana."

The word *medical* implies something used in medicine to treat a disease state, whereas *marijuana* (*Cannabis sativa*) remains classified as an *illegal* herb in most of the states in the United States, with the exception of those few where the term *medical marijuana* now protects and justifies its legal availability on the retail market.

Cannabis is an herb whose use dates back as far as 2737 BCE, as first noted in Chinese documents. In 1937, Cannabis use was criminalized in the United States despite the objection of the American Medical Association as expressed to Congress during its debate on marijuana use. At issue, the Drug Enforcement Agency (DEA) listed marijuana as a Schedule I substance, which means it has no acceptable medical use.

More than 60 years later, on March 17, 1999, a group of 11 scientists commissioned by the Institute of Medicine (IOM) to report on marijuana stated that the herb was useful for an even longer list of conditions, including wasting away due to acquired immune deficiency syndrome (AIDS), nausea and vomiting due to anticancer medications, and the pain and muscle spasms associated with multiple sclerosis. However, the argument over whether to classify marijuana as "a panacea" or "a pariah" remained under debate.

Marijuana contains more than 460 active substances and more than 60 specific chemicals known as *cannabinoids,* with the principal active constituent being Delta (9)-tetrahydrocannabinol (THC), available commercially as a medication in the United States. Unfortunately, THC is normally given orally even though when commercially made it appears its effect on nausea and vomiting, pain, and appetite loss is greater when the herb itself is smoked. Marijuana specifically, and cannabinoids as a group, possess anti-inflammatory, pain relief or analgesic effect, antioxidant, and protective effects on the nervous system cells.

The cannabinoids are known to be "neuro-modulators." That is, they have the ability to modulate the functions of the nervous system, oftentimes in a therapeutic way. This idea of nervous system protection goes against the popular belief that smoking marijuana causes damage to the nervous system. In fact, the majority of studies done on schizophrenic patients who smoked marijuana confirmed the positive effect marijuana had on the nervous system; patients who smoked marijuana demonstrated better cognitive functions than similar patients who did not inhale the herb.

The use of marijuana can also produce numerous positive outcomes in conditions such as Alzheimer's disease, Parkinson's disease, diabetes, cerebral ischemia, nausea and vomiting, and rheumatoid arthritis. Many of these positive outcomes from marijuana can be attributed to another major active constituent in the herb, cannabidiol. Researchers suggest a combination of cannabidiol and THC taken orally by patients with a variety of conditions that cause chronic pain can yield improvement in their pain management as well as in their quality of sleep.

A good number of case reports exist in medical literature on the use of marijuana and its relation to cancer. THC, for example, has been shown in various research studies to either inhibit or potentiate tumor growth (Preet, Ganju, and Groopman, 2008). The determining factor that governs this dual activity is the type of tumor involved. Overall, it appears that substances in marijuana have the ability to damage the DNA material, and by doing so damage tumor development.

Certain segments of the population, such as HIV patients, are more likely to smoke it to control symptoms such as nausea and muscle pain. Patients suffering from spinal cord injuries also reported marijuana use was effective in blocking the pain sensation they felt. However, not all studies on marijuana and cognition agree that a positive effect exists, as some reported a definite decline in the cognitive ability with its use. This combination of positive and negative effects provides strong arguments for supporters and opponents.

In fact, supporters of medical marijuana suggest the general public may be even more accepting of medical marijuana than are physicians. In the United States, marijuana is the number one illicit drug abused, especially among young adults and teens (Budney, Vandrey, and Stanger, 2010). Studies have shown that smoking marijuana for recreational use may also be associated with failure to complete a college education among young people.

Smoking marijuana also causes impairment of motor skills, regardless of how it might affect the cognitive ability of individuals. Other significant adverse events associated with cannabinoids inhalation reported in the literature included dizziness, vomiting, urinary tract infections, and relapse in multiple sclerosis.

The objection to marijuana use is often based on moral/ethical, political, and/or scientific ground. Recreational use of marijuana can lead to addiction, which requires medical intervention. Fortunately, current effective psychosocial treatments to deal with this addiction are available. However, pharmacotherapies are still lacking. Opponents of marijuana warn that repeated use can lead to a potentially greater abuse of other more serious recreational drugs.

Even if there is continued support in the general public for legalizing marijuana, politically it is a topic that many politicians shy away from due to the belief it might "send the wrong message" of support. Overall, the issue of marijuana remains politically charged as both sides hold strong opinions about its legalization, one more reason the question of its fate remains undecided. Should it be decriminalized by an act of Congress, by voters through the ballots, or by the FDA through scientific rigors? No one definitive answer has emerged. At this point, the general consensus among law enforcement officials and legislators is that drug dealers have to be stopped from making marijuana available until further decisions are reached, whether those decisions are based on scientific or moral indicators.

Currently, some 13 states have legalized marijuana on a limited therapeutic basis, increasing the conflict between state laws and federal laws governing the issue. If states assume their laws are constitutionally based, until the Supreme Court rules on the "legalization" issue, the conflicts will remain unresolved. As of January 2011 in California, the laws state that possession of one ounce or less (28.5 g) of marijuana is considered an "infraction," resulting with no criminal record. However, federal law enforcement agencies can charge an individual having a small amount of marijuana (less than one ounce) as possession with "intent to sell," which is a felony.

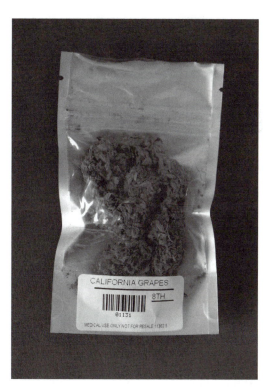

Smoking marijuana carries high risk for developing lung cancer independent from cancer caused by smoking cigarettes (Aldington et al., 2008). Also, smoking marijuana among relatively young individuals (less than 60 years of age) was found to be associated with an increased risk for developing bladder cancer. In a no dose-dependent fashion, smoking marijuana at least once a month increased the risk for developing malignant primary adult-onset glioma. In certain cases, the cannabinoids in marijuana acted as *protective* agents against the development of cancer. This was evident in the case of head and neck squamous cell carcinoma development where it was shown that moderate

One-eighth of an ounce of California grapes medical marijuana in a bar-coded bag. (Eric Broder Van Dyke/Dreamstime.com)

marijuana use was associated with a *reduced* risk of developing this cancer type (Liang et al., 2009).

One potential development of future anticancer agents is related in part to our understanding of the "endocannabinoids system." Several endogenous substances have been identified in this system with the capability to bind to cannabis receptors. These substances are known as "endocannabinoids" and they are widely distributed in various organs and the immune system, as cannabinoids receptors are now well characterized and identified. Two cannabinoids receptor types identified so far are CB1 and CB2. The CB1 receptors are mainly found in the central nervous system and peripheral tissues whereas the CB2 types are found in the peripheral and immune tissues. Researchers have also located the presence of CB2 in brain tissues as well. Activation of CB1 receptors produces psychoactive effects, but not the same as the CB2 receptors. Therefore, agents that can activate selectively the CB2 receptors have become the target of clinical investigations of many agents.

Two important chemicals that have been identified in the endocannabinoids system are the anandamide and 2-arachidonoylglycerol. They play important regulatory functions governing food intake, reproduction, the immune system, and behavioral activities (e.g., "social play" type). Disruptions in the endocannabinoids functions are associated with obesity and metabolic syndromes, and perhaps are linked to the development of migraine headaches as well.

Moreover, levels of endocannabinoids present in the brain are also associated with mood disorders such as schizophrenia, depression, and anxiety. Perhaps the most interesting aspect about these endogenous compounds is that they play a major role in blocking pain signaling, similar to that of the cannabinoids action found in marijuana in blocking pain sensation. It is believed that this analgesic (pain-killing) effect of the endocannabinoids is in part due to their anti-inflammatory actions.

The presence of cannabis receptors naturally present in mammalian tissues and the potential applications of activating (or blocking) these receptors by chemical agents have become the target of intense research for a multitude of clinical applications. Once again it does raise the question of whether this plant is really a "bad substance." There is a fine balance of using marijuana as a recreational substance and as a substance of potential "medical" use. This balance may continue to shift as the United States becomes more receptive to the idea of "medical marijuana" or as research uncovers new details about its complicated effects.

*Antoine Al-Achi*

*See also* Cancer; Drugs, Recreational; Smoking.

## References

Aggarwal, S.K., G.T. Carter, M.D. Sullivan, C. ZumBrunnen, R. Morrill, and J.D. Mayer. "Medicinal Use of Cannabis in the United States: Historical Perspectives, Current Trends, and Future Directions." *Journal of Opioid Management* 5, no. 3 (2009):153–68.

Aldington, S., M. Harwood, B. Cox, M. Weatherall, L. Beckert, A. Hansell, A. Pritchard, G. Robinson, and R. Beasley. Cannabis and Respiratory Disease Research Group. "Cannabis Use and Risk of Lung Cancer: A Case-Control Study." *European Respiratory Journal* 31, no. 2 (2008): 280–86.

Budney, A.J., R.G. Vandrey, and C. Stanger. "Pharmacological and Psychosocial Interventions for Cannabis Use Disorders." *Revista Brasileira de Psiquiatria* 32, Suppl. 1 (2010): S46–S55.

Charuvastra, A., P.D. Friedmann, and M.D. Stein. "Physician Attitudes Regarding the Prescription of Medical Marijuana." *Journal of Addictive Diseases* 24, no. 3 (2005): 87–93.

Cohen, P.J. "Medical Marijuana: The Conflict between Scientific Evidence and Political Ideology." Part 1 of 2. *Journal of Pain & Palliative Care Pharmacotherapy* 23, no. 1 (2009): 4–25.

Efird, J.T., G.D. Friedman, S. Sidney, A. Klatsky, L.A. Habel, N.V. Udaltsova, S. Van den Eeden, W. Hall, and L. Degenhardt. "Medical Marijuana Initiatives: Are They Justified? How Successful Are They Likely to Be?" *CNS Drugs* 17, no. 10 (2003): 689–97.

Hosking, R.D., and J.P. Zajicek. "Therapeutic Potential of Cannabis in Pain Medicine." *British Journal of Anaesthesia* 101, no. 1 (2008): 59–68.

Liang, C., M.D. McClean, C. Marsit, B. Christensen, E. Peters, H.H. Nelson, and K.T. Kelsey. "A Population-Based Case-Control Study of Marijuana Use and Head and Neck Squamous Cell Carcinoma." *Cancer Prevention Research (Philadelphia PA)* 2, no. 8 (2009): 759–68.

Mouslech, Z., and V. Valla. "Endocannabinoid System: An Overview of Its Potential in Current Medical Practice." *Neuro Endocrinology Letters* 30, no. 2 (2009): 153–79.

Preet, A., R.K. Ganju, and J.E. Groopman. "Delta9-Tetrahydrocannabinol Inhibits Epithelial Growth Factor-Induced Lung Cancer Cell Migration in Vitro as Well as Its Growth and Metastasis in Vivo." *Oncogene* 27, no. 3 (2008): 339–46.

## MEDICAL POWER OF ATTORNEY

After involvement in an automobile accident in 1983, Nancy Cruzan lingered in a permanent vegetative state for seven years until the U.S. Supreme Court ruled her parents could have doctors take out her feeding tube. Nancy died in December 1990, the same month the feeding tube was removed. The court's Cruzan decision, one of several well-known right-to-die cases, represents the constitutional right to end life-sustaining treatment when it is clear such action is what the patient would have wanted.

Injury, illness, or death are difficult subjects to contemplate yet Americans need to consider the story of Nancy Cruzan and take steps to determine their own fate should something tragic happen in their lives. The medical power of attorney or proxy and living will are the two basic types of directives most frequently used for advance health care planning.

Following Nancy Cruzan's death, Congress passed the Patient Self-Determination Act (PSDA) to ensure individuals are informed of the right to participate in their own health care decisions, even when unable to speak for themselves. The act's intent is threefold: public education regarding state laws governing the refusal, withholding, and withdrawal of treatment at the end of life; encouragement of widespread use of advanced health care directives such as a medical power of attorney or living will to minimize the uncertainty among doctors and family members that can lead to protracted legal fights and prolonged treatment of the dying; and decreasing the cost of end-of-life treatment by reducing unnecessary or unwanted medical intervention. Under the act health care institutions are required to explain to patients that they have options to accept or refuse medical treatment. It also requires patients be made aware of their right to choose advance directives such as proxies and living wills.

The most common situations where people require someone to make medical decisions for them involve patients who have lost their capacity to understand their treatment options due to conditions such as dementia, Alzheimer's, brain injury, or some type of catastrophic accident.

A medical power of attorney, also known as a durable power of attorney for health care, enables patients to appoint a health care proxy or medical agent. This designated individual serves as a patient surrogate in situations when that person does not have the ability to make his own choices. The selected individual or "agent" may only make those decisions on behalf of the patient if the patient's physician certified in writing that he is incompetent. The medical power of attorney can be guided by an existing living will but the person acting for the patient also has the authority to interpret the patient's wishes in situations that are not described in that living will.

Anyone may hold a medical power of attorney except the patient's physician or health care provider or an employee of the health care provider unless that person is also a relative of the patient. Whoever is selected should be knowledgeable about the wishes, values, and religious beliefs of the patient, someone whom the patient trusts with what may become very difficult decisions.

A medical power of attorney differs from a living will, also referred to as a health care directive or declaration. The living will is a document that is limited in scope and addresses the withholding or withdrawing of medical treatment for patients who are terminal or have an irreversible condition. While a living will can help avoid disagreements over treatment options, it will not be enough in every circumstance, especially when treatment may be justified to increase the patient's comfort or has the potential to improve the patient's ability to communicate with others. In comparison, the medical power of attorney is broader in scope and includes all health care decisions with only a few exceptions.

Each state has specific laws governing the medical power of attorney. In some states it is possible to grant what is known as a springing power of attorney, which only takes effect after the patient is incapacitated. However, legal experts recommend those considering this option should specify exactly how and when the power would spring into effect. With the increase in health privacy laws in the United States physicians are not legally allowed to reveal information about the capacity of a patient unless the power of attorney specifically authorizes them to do so.

The necessary documentation for the medical power of attorney and living will may vary state by state, but the forms are usually available online at no or low cost. A person may prepare a directive on his own or consult with an attorney. In order for a medical power of attorney to be a legal document it must be signed and dated by the principal or patient, the agent, and other witnesses. Having the document reviewed and signed by a notary public increases the likelihood of it withstanding a legal challenge and is required by some states. Health care professionals and organizations can provide information and education. These legal directives can be canceled by the person it relates to at any time.

Decisions that need to be considered in this type of planning process include discussion of types of available life-sustaining treatments, what treatments a person would or would not accept if diagnosed with a terminal illness, along with an understanding of that individual's personal values and beliefs. All of these considerations should be formally documented in writing in the proper form, kept in an accessible place, and shared with appropriate individuals. Any type of advance health care directive should be reviewed and updated as a person's medical status changes over time.

While the content of any health care directive depends on an individual's personal scope, important questions to ask include: Will I use nonlife-sustaining measures to relieve pain and suffering? Will I accept resuscitation, mechanical ventilation, nutritional and hydration assistance? Do I have religious objections to any medical therapies? Do I want to be an organ donor?

Advance health care planning through the use of a medical power of attorney is not just for the very ill or very old. Anyone over the age of 18 would benefit from thinking ahead about their future health care preferences and medical treatments. Specifying someone as a medical proxy and providing instructions for medical care ahead of time ensures an individual's desires are met in the event of unexpected illness or injury that renders a person unable to make self-decisions, and minimizes the unknown for family, friends, and health care providers.

Research based on real and hypothetical patterns of patient preferences held by a majority of persons in like circumstances has been conducted by the Agency for Healthcare Research and Quality. The objective is to aid physicians and other health care professionals in their efforts to assist people with advance health care planning and the assessment and selection of end-of-life treatment options. Outcomes show that a person's doctor or primary care provider can help guide a patient's future treatment decisions and advance planning preparation. Caring conversations should lead to well-thought-out advance health care choices. The use of a medical power of attorney along with a living will provides emotional peace of mind when done prior to a person becoming incapacitated.

*Dianne L. Needham*

*See also* Alzheimer's Disease; Living Wills and Advance Directives; Primary Care Physicians.

## References

Advance Care Planning, Research in Action (Issue 12), Agency for Healthcare Research and Quality. www.ahrq.gov/research/endliferia/endria.htm.

"Advance Directives for Medical Decisions." Mayoclinic.com. www.mayoclinic.com/health/living-wills/HA00014.

Ashar, Linda C. *The Complete Power of Attorney Guide for Consumers and Small Businesses: Everything You Need to Know Explained Simply.* Ocala, FL: Atlantic, 2010.

"Caring Connections." National Hospice and Palliative Care Organization. www.caringinfo.org/i4a/pages/index.cfm?pageid=3277.

*Cruzan v. Director,* Missouri Department of Health, 497 U.S. 261 (1990).

Doukas, David John, and William Reichel. *Planning for Uncertainty: Living Wills and Other Advance Directives for You and Your Family.* Baltimore, MD: Johns Hopkins University Press, 2007.

Federal Patient Self-Determination Act (1991), 42 Code of Federal Regulations (CFR) 489.12.

"Preparing Your Advance Directives." National Hospice and Palliative Care Organization. www.caringinfo.org/i4a/pages/index.cfm?pageid=3287.

Shenkman, Martin M. *Estate Planning: For People with a Chronic Condition or Disability.* New York: Demos Medical, 2009.

"What Are Advance Directives?" National Hospice and Palliative Care Organization. www.caringinfo.org/i4a/pages/index.cfm?pageid=3285.

## MEDICARE

If you are over 65 years old or younger with permanent disabilities, you are among the more than 45 million Americans who have access to health insurance from Medicare. President Lyndon B. Johnson established this social insurance program in 1965 when many of today's newest recipients were just beginning their careers. Now, thanks to the 45-year-old program, the cost of health care services including doctor visits, hospital stays, and prescription drugs is less overwhelming for many Americans.

Medicare has been called socialized medicine by critics but at the time it was instituted roughly half of all U.S. senior citizens did not have medical insurance at an age when many needed it most. Still, Medicare takes a sizeable chunk out of the federal budget. In 2009, it made up 13 percent of the more than $3 trillion federal budget and equaled 17 percent of the total national health care spending of $2.5 trillion. And if figures from the Centers for Medicare and Medicaid Services (CMS) are correct, that number will almost double to $4.6 trillion by 2019 ("Get Health Reform," 2010).

Medicare is the elephant in the room during discussions about how to moderate the growth of both federal spending and health care spending. It was at the heart of the fierce debate over the Obama administration's health care reform efforts. Unfortunately, at the same time lawmakers were debating health care the number of uninsured Americans continued to grow at a rapid rate. Nationally, about 19 percent of people below the age of Medicare eligibility were uninsured in 2009, compared to 17 percent the previous year. This is the first year since 1987 that the number of people with health insurance has declined.

Plus, Americans who are eligible for government health insurance have now been enrolling in growing numbers, between 2008 and 2009 another 6 million additional people enrolled even as those covered by private employer-provided insurance dropped. This means the number of Americans receiving government insurance from Medicaid and Medicare was the highest ever in 2009, while the number of U.S. citizens privately insured was at its lowest (Benson, 2010).

American retirees turn to Medicare when they reach the age of 65. However, for some retirees Medicare becomes even more important when their employer-provided coverage plans increase premiums, raise rates, stop subsidizing costs, or are eliminated altogether. Following passage of the Patient Protection and Affordable Care Act in March 2010, analysts predict those numbers could grow even faster. Although under the new law, major provisions to expand insurance coverage do not go into effect until 2014, federal economists calculate an additional 32 million people will eventually be covered by government insurance as the changes unfold.

With those numbers in mind the debate has turned from criticizing the program to controlling its sharply risings costs, especially as the baby boom generation becomes eligible for coverage in larger and larger numbers.

**Basic Components**   What exactly will Medicare offer an aging American population? The program consists of four parts, each covering different benefits. Part A, also known as the Hospital Insurance (HI) program, covers hospital stays, costs for skilled nursing facilities, home health and hospice care. Part A is funded by tax dollars that are paid by employers and workers and it adds up to some 40 percent of Medicare spending ("Medicare: A Primer," 2009). Americans age 65 and older are almost all automatically entitled to Part A if they or their spouse are also eligible for Social Security payments and if they have made a payroll tax contribution for 10 or more years.

Anyone who is entitled to Part A does not pay premiums for covered services. They must be U.S. citizens or permanent legal residents. They can choose to enroll in a Medicare Advantage plan (see Part C), which is a specialized plan from a private insurer. For those individuals age 65 and over who did not pay enough Medicare taxes during their working years, they can pay a monthly premium to enroll in Part A.

Part B, called the Supplementary Medical Insurance (SMI) program, pays costs related to doctor visits, outpatient, home health and preventive services. Part B is funded by a combination of premiums paid by Medicare beneficiaries and general revenues. Medicare members who have higher annual incomes pay a higher monthly premium. Part B accounts for some 27 percent of Medicare spending and this section is voluntary, meaning enrollees who are still working and receive employer-sponsored health care can delay their Part B enrollment until they officially stop working.

Not surprisingly, although Part B is voluntary, about 95 percent of beneficiaries with Part A are also enrolled in Part B. Additionally, individuals who are not entitled to Part A may enroll in Part B, but those who are eligible must sign up when they are first eligible or face paying a penalty for late enrollment unless they are receiving employment-sponsored coverage.

Part C is called the Medicare Advantage program. It is unique because it allows beneficiaries to enroll in a private plan such as a health maintenance organization (HMO), a preferred provider organization (PPO), or a private fee-for-service plan (PFFS). Many people find the Advantage plans offer more flexibility. These plans receive payments from Medicare for their members when those members receive Medicare-covered benefits including hospital stays, doctor's visits, and in some cases, prescription drug benefits. Part C is financed with the same funds that cover Part A and it accounted for 21 percent of Medicare benefit spending in 2008. Individuals are eligible for Part C if they are entitled to Part A and enrolled in Part B.

Part D is the outpatient prescription drug benefit and is available to beneficiaries through private plans that contract with Medicare, including stand-alone prescription drug plans (PDP) or Medicare Advantage prescription drug plans (MAPD). The Medicare Modernization Act of 2003, which was retooled again in 2006 under President George W. Bush, called for Part D plans to provide a standard prescription benefit. Part D is funded through general revenues and premiums from Medicare beneficiaries. Those individuals eligible for Part A, and who are enrolled in Part B, are eligible for prescription drug coverage under a Part D plan as well. Just like Part B, there is a penalty for late enrollment for anyone who chooses to go without drug coverage from some type of provider. That coverage must be at least comparable to the Part D standard benefit.

**Annual Enrollment Choices** While basic Medicare options sound as easy as A, B, C, each year recipients face an overwhelming number of choices during their annual reenrollment period, which runs from November 15 through December 31. Of course, those whose coverage does not change and who are also satisfied with their plans can stand pat. But some recipients will have to make a change whether they want to or not. For many, their former Advantage plans no longer exist or their prescription drug coverage has gone away. In 2009, the Centers for Medicare and Medicaid Services (CMS) eliminated close to 18 percent of the Advantage plans, saying they had too few members or were too similar to other plans in terms of benefits provided (Konrad, 2009). That meant an additional 600,000 Medicare recipients had to change plans that year.

For those who were members of a private Advantage plan that was eliminated, they could do nothing and be automatically enrolled in the traditional Medicare A and B plans. But, if they were not enrolled in a prescription drug plan because drug coverage came with their previous Advantage plan, they would have to enroll separately through a private insurer for drug coverage during the end-of-the-year enrollment dates.

What if your plan did not change but your health or financial situation did? Then it might be important to reexamine coverage. The traditional Medicare coverage has monthly premiums and a deductible for hospitalizations and co-payments for many doctor visits. Some of the thousands of remaining Medicare Advantage plans can lower those costs. Or in some cases people choose to buy a Medigap or supplemental policy to cover costs Medicare will not. On the other hand, the Advantage plans work like the HMO or PPO systems and going to a doctor out of network can be expensive.

Don't forget to compare Medicare D drug plans as well. It is especially important to look at prices and at the drugs you use to see if they are covered by the plan you have selected and how those costs compare to other drug plan prices. Be careful, Medicare D plans change the list of covered drugs frequently, so a phone call to your prescription provider to check on your specific medications may be an important extra piece of "insurance."

**Donut Hole**   Of course, there is also the infamous "donut hole" to worry about as well. The "donut hole" is a coverage gap that people with Medicare hit after they spend a certain amount of money on their prescription drugs. This hole presents serious financial problems to many people on fixed incomes who may have to choose between their rent and groceries or their medicines. There is good news and bad news for seniors concerning improved coverage for that gap.

The bad news: according to a report released by the Kaiser Family Foundation, the hole has grown from $2,700 in 2009 to $2,830 in 2010 (Wechsler, 2010). Once these beneficiaries reach that amount they must pay the full cost of prescriptions. After individual costs exceed $6,440 the government will cover 95 percent of any additional drug charges (Wechsler, 2010). In an effort to provide more relief, the Obama administration is working to close the gap and pushing the pharmaceutical companies to pick up much of the cost by 2020. The federal government also offered a $250 rebate to "donut hole" beneficiaries in 2010. By the fall of 2010 more than 1.2 million people with Medicare had received rebate checks ("New Help for Seniors," 2010).

The good news is that the number of prescription drug plans now voluntarily filling the donut hole has increased. In August 2010, Department of Health and Human Services Secretary Kathleen Sebelius reported one more piece of good news, seniors with Medicare who fall into the hole can receive a 50 percent discount on brand-name drugs and will start to pay less for generic drugs starting in 2011 ("New Help for Seniors," 2010).

What if you make a mistake or change your mind when deciding on Medicare options and plans each year? You cannot switch or join a Medicare D plan unless you already have some plan with prescription drug coverage. You can switch from one Advantage plan to another during the open enrollment period from January 1 through March 31. You can also switch from an Advantage plan to the traditional Medicare or switch from Medicare to an Advantage plan during the January through March enrollment dates. Of course, there are also changes brought by the government, including proposed legislation to further cut payments to Medicare Advantage plans over the next 10 years.

**Medicare Recipients**   Who are Medicare recipients? Many enjoy good health but at least a quarter have serious problems and have multiple chronic conditions including diabetes, heart disease, cancer, arthritis, and hypertension. Although the majority is age 65 and older, some 16 percent of the 45 million Americans covered are under age 65 and are permanently disabled. These individuals tend to have lower incomes than other recipients. In fact, almost half of all Medicare beneficiaries have an income below 200 percent of the poverty level ($20,800 for an individual and $28,000 for a couple in 2008), and 16 percent have an income below 100 percent of the poverty level ("Medicare: A Primer," 2009). Most of these people live on modest incomes and depend on Social Security as their primary retirement income. Poverty rates are also substantially higher among women on Medicare than men. More than half of all female Medicare beneficiaries live on incomes below twice the poverty level, substantially higher than the rate for men on Medicare ("Medicare: A Primer," 2009).

America has changed in many ways since 1965 but one of the most significant changes was the creation of Medicare. At that time less than half of the elderly citizens in the United States had any help to pay for hospital or other medical services. Some were locked out of health insurance based on the cost of premiums; others were denied coverage due to preexisting health conditions. Funding for Medicare may be cut as the federal government works to balance the budget and deal with other financial issues. Will policy makers reduce Medicare, Medicaid, and Social Security? There are no guarantees, especially with increases in health care costs and increasing enrollment in the programs. However, seniors will continue to remind lawmakers that access to affordable health care must remain a high priority for the future.

*Sharon Zoumbaris*

*See also* Health Insurance; Managed Care; Medicaid.

### References

Benson, Judy. "Census Finds Fewer Have Health Insurance." *The Day, McClatchy-Tribune Information Services,* September 17, 2010.

"Census Bureau: High Unemployment Results in Huge Increase of Uninsured in 2009." *States News Service,* September 16, 2010.

Edlin, Mari. "Donut Hole Coverage Gap Grows: Bills Aim to Help Seniors: Only 20% of PDPs Will Offer Gap Coverage." *Managed Healthcare Executive* 19, no. 12 (December 2009): 23.

Evans, Melanie. "The Costs of Change: Reform Expected to Increase Average Annual Spending through 2019." *Modern Healthcare* 40, no. 37 (September 13, 2010): 8.

"Get Health Reform Up and Running." *Roanoke Times,* September 16, 2010. www.roanoke.com/editorials/wb/260534.

Konrad, Walecia. "Now Is the Time to Weigh Medicare Options." *New York Times,* October 31, 2009. www.nytimes.com/2009/10/31patient.html.

Lankford, Kimberly. "Filling the Gap: How to Pay the Bills That Medicare Won't." *Kiplinger's Retirement Planning Guide.* Washington, DC: Kiplinger Washington Editors, 2004, 102.

"Medicare: A Primer." Henry J. Kaiser Family Foundation. 2009. www.kff.org/medicare/upload/7615–03.pdf.

"New Help for Seniors Who Fall into the Medicare Donut Hole: 50% Discount Starts in 2011." *State News Service,* September 23, 2010.

Wechsler, Jill. "Donut Hole Closes." *Managed Healthcare Executive* 20, no. 5 (May 2010): 6.

## MEDITATION

Meditation involves focusing the mind intently on a particular thing or activity, while becoming relatively oblivious to everything else. Some meditation techniques trace their roots back to Eastern religious or spiritual practices. Today, however, people often use meditation in a secular context for inducing relaxation, reducing stress, and enhancing health and well-being. In addition, meditation is sometimes used to help decrease symptoms of depression.

A growing body of research supports the health benefits of meditation. But because many of the studies were not well designed, it is impossible to draw firm conclusions from them. Keeping that caveat in mind, some research suggests that meditation may help alleviate not only depression, but also anxiety disorders, substance abuse, binge-eating disorder, allergies, asthma, chronic pain, high blood pressure, and a host of other medical conditions.

There are several different forms of meditation, all aimed at focusing attention on one thing while freeing the mind of other distractions. The focal point can be a special word, a particular object, a repetitive activity, or even the simple act of breathing. Rather than actively trying to suppress other thoughts, the meditator passively lets them come and go without judgment, gently bringing attention back to the focal point. Most meditation techniques also emphasize finding a quiet spot to practice, assuming a comfortable position, and taking deep, even breaths to promote relaxation.

Meditation works partly by decreasing activity in the sympathetic nervous system, which mobilizes the body during stress, and increasing activity in the parasympathetic nervous system, which counteracts the body's stress response. Research

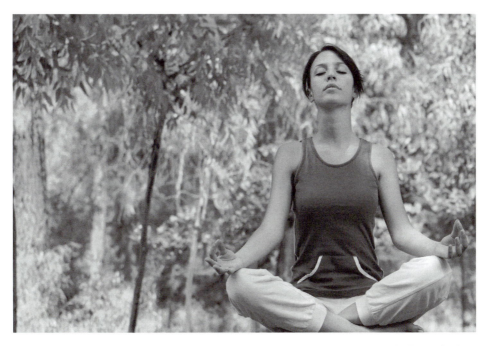

A young woman meditates in nature. Meditation can bring calmness and physical relaxation, and psychological balance. (Marco Lensi/Dreamstime.com)

has shown that sympathetic activity tends to be more pronounced in people who are depressed than in those who are not. Regular meditation also may improve the mind's ability to pay attention—an essential skill for regulating mood and getting along in everyday life.

**Breathe!**   Deep breathing exercises are meditation pared down to its most basic elements. The focal point is the breath going in and out. Because such mini-meditations can elicit the relaxation response, they may help control stress and depression. To practice a breathing exercise, find a quiet spot to sit or lie down. Rest a hand on your abdomen, just below the navel. Inhale through your nose as you slowly count to four, feeling your belly push out slightly against your hand as the air enters. Hold for a second. Then exhale through your mouth as you slowly count to four, feeling your belly fall back slightly toward your spine as the air exits. Repeat 5 to 10 times.

**Types of Meditation**   People do meditation to increase relaxation, enhance general well-being, or cope with mental or physical illness. Below are two types of meditation that are commonly used for health purposes.

*Mantra Meditation.* In mantra meditation, the focus is on a mantra—a special word, phrase, or sound that is repeated, either silently or aloud, to keep distracting thoughts from entering the mind. The goal is to achieve a state of pure, relaxed awareness. Transcendental Meditation, a modern variation derived from Hindu traditions, was introduced in 1958 by Indian guru Maharishi Mahesh Yogi (ca. 1918–2008).

*Mindfulness Meditation.* Mindfulness meditation, rooted in Buddhist practices, involves fully focusing on whatever is being experienced from moment to moment, without reacting to or judging that experience. This technique is a core feature of mindfulness-based cognitive therapy, a treatment approach specifically designed to help people who have recovered from depression avoid a recurrence in the future.

*Linda Wasmer Andrews*

*See also* Depression; Religion and Spirituality; Stress; Yoga.

### References

Andrews, Linda Wasmer. *Stress Control for Peace of Mind.* New York: Main Street, 2005.

Center for Mindfulness in Medicine, Health Care and Society, University of Massachusetts Medical School. 55 Lake Avenue North, Worcester, MA 01655. (508) 856–2656. www.umassmed.edu/cfm.

*Meditation: An Introduction.* National Center for Complementary and Alternative Medicine. February 2009. http://nccam.nih.gov/health/meditation/overview.htm.

*Meditation: Take a Stress-Reduction Break Wherever You Are.* Mayo Clinic. April 21, 2009. www.mayoclinic.com/health/meditation/HQ01070.

Ospina, Maria B., Kenneth Bond, Mohammad Karkhaneh, Lisa Tjosvold, Ben Vandermeer, Yuanyuan Liang, Yuanyuan Liang, Liza Bialy, Nicola Hooton, Nina Buscemi, Donna M. Dryden, and Terry Pl. Klassen. *Meditation Practices for Health: State of the Research.*

Evidence Report/Technology Assessment No. 155. Rockville, MD: Agency for Health-care Research and Quality, 2007.

*Relax in a Hurry.* Benson-Henry Institute for Mind Body Medicine. www.mbmi.org/basics/mstress_RIAH.asp.

Ruthven, Malise. "Maharishi Mahesh Yogi." Guardian.co.uk. February 6, 2008. www.guardian.co.uk/world/2008/feb/06/India.obituaries.

*Stress and Your Health.* National Women's Health Information Center. August 1, 2005. http://womenshealth.gov/faq/stress-your-health.cfm.

Transcendental Meditation Program. (888) 532–7686. www.tm.org.

## METABOLISM. *See* BASAL METABOLISM

## METHICILLIN-RESISTANT STAPHYLOCOCCUS AUREUS (MRSA)

Methicillin-Resistant Staphylococcus Aureus (MRSA) is a serious staph bacteria that has developed a resistance to many antibiotics. Historically, the most serious MRSA infections occurred in hospitals or other health institutions such as nursing homes and dialysis centers. However, in the past several decades these deadly infections have become more common in the community, where they also continue to develop resistance to treatment.

Where did MRSA come from and why is it now a major public health concern in the United States and in other countries around the world? The Staphylococcus aureus organism was first identified in the late 1800s by a Scottish surgeon named Alexander Ogston. Educated before the days of antisepsis, Ogston theorized that abscess formation was caused by a microorganism after he viewed pus under a microscope. What he saw were chains and bunches of cocci.

Ogston named them Staphylococci after the Greek word *staphyle,* meaning bunch of grapes. Based on their golden color he named the organism *Staphylococcus aureus.* Ogston was following in the footsteps of other pioneers such as Louis Pasteur and Joseph Lister, who early on had sought to connect the role of germs and antiseptic precautions in surgery. Scientists would later discover that it is not unusual for people to carry microscopic bacteria on their scalp, skin, and nasal passages. Statistics show some 80 percent of the general population carry around staph bacteria on an intermittent basis.

Penicillin was discovered by Sir Alexander Fleming in 1929, but it was not used against staph aureus until the 1940s. Prior to penicillin, bacterial infections could cause serious and many times fatal infections since there was no known treatment or cure. For nearly 50 years after penicillin became available, people gradually took antibiotics' effectiveness against bacterial infections for granted.

However, as penicillin was increasingly used for treatment, strains of the staph developed a resistance and by 1959 some 90 to 95 percent of all staph aureus strains were penicillin-resistant. Development of drug resistance in bacteria is an age-old battle between science and nature. When an antibiotic kills bacteria or slows their growth, natural selection helps the strongest bacteria then develop traits that aid in their survival against antibiotics. This also leads to the eventual reproduction of the surviving bacteria. Natural selection, an important component of evolution, is one of the main processes in creating genetically heritable traits, which then pass from one generation to the next.

In other words, when staph aureus is exposed to an antibiotic, some will survive while others will not. Those survivors will reproduce bacteria that have inherited that ability to survive. This is stored in the bacterium's genes and ultimately results in the development of complete resistance against a specific antibiotic. When a bacterium carries several resistant genes, it becomes known as a "superbug."

The longer a bacteria is exposed to an antibiotic, the bigger the risk of developing a resistance. Scientists believe the widespread use of antibiotics has played a key role in the evolution of the superbug, drug-resistant bacterium. This widespread use has included overuse of antibiotics by humans as well as the equally pervasive use of antibiotics in farm animal feed to promote growth and treat diseases caused by intensive agricultural practices. This means that people are unknowingly taking antibiotics in their food, milk, or meats. Antibiotics have even found their way into drinking water systems when the runoff from animal feedlots contaminates groundwater.

Also at issue are pharmaceutical companies and the incentives they have to develop new antibiotics as bacteria become resistant to current drugs. For years, there were new antimicrobials developed and released, but drug companies do not see much return on the money from these products or from antibiotics, which are prescribed for only 10 days. When one considers the newest antibiotics would be used very sparingly to prevent resistance, one sees that drug companies would rather put their research and development dollars into prescription drugs with more profit potential.

One new drug was approved by the FDA at the end of 2010 to treat MRSA. Called Teflaro, the drug is aimed at MRSA infections in the community rather than in health care settings ("FDA OKs Drug," 2010). The drug received approval for "acute bacterial skin and skin structure infections," which include but are not limited to MRSA. It was also approved for "community-acquired bacterial pneumonia," which develops in the lungs of patients exposed to bacteria outside of a hospital.

Over the years MRSA has developed resistance to penicillin, amoxicillin, oxacillin, and other antibiotics, making it impossible for all but the strongest or newest antibiotics to defeat the infection successfully. According to figures from the Centers for Disease Control and Prevention, MRSA strikes 32 out of every 100,000 Americans each year and causes more than 95,000 serious infections and some 19,000 deaths. The CDC figures suggest that MRSA now causes more deaths in the United States each year than AIDS (Klein, Smith, & Laxminarayan, 2007). No updated figures are available from the CDC on MRSA infections from 2005–2010, as hospitals in the United States must switch to the CDC's reporting system. Before the CDC reporting system was initiated, MRSA was reported to the Centers for Medicaid and Medicare. Still, according to the MRSA Survivors Network, other organizations estimate the true numbers to be more than

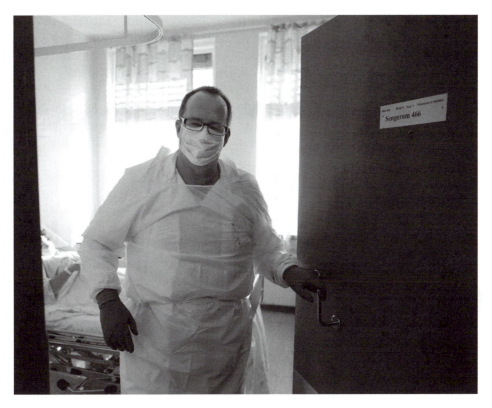

Doctor Jon Birger Haug leaves a quarantine room after visiting a patient at Aker Hospital in Oslo on October 8, 2009. The patient was quarantined after suspicion of H1N1. In Norway, the decreased use of antibiotics and strict routines have led to less cases of methicillin-resistant Staphylococcus aureus (MRSA), a virulent drug-resistant infection that kills more people in the United States each year than AIDS. (AP/Wide World Photos)

1 million Americans infected with MRSA and more than 100,000 deaths (MRSA Survivors Network, 2011).

There are some key differences in MRSA infections that occur in hospitals or nursing homes and those that occur in the community. Historically, those MRSA infections in hospitalized patients or those in medical institutions are often transmitted by health care workers into the body of patients via catheters, dialysis equipment, or on artificial joints or heart valves. When patients get MRSA in health care situations, those infections tend to be more severe when they enter the bloodstream. Although MRSA transmission in the community is growing, most people in this setting get infections of the skin, especially in dormitories, military barracks, correctional facilities, or day care centers.

MRSA infections, as with all staph infections, can be spread by having contact with someone's skin infection, personal items that person used such as towels or bandages. In close quarters, like a locker room, it is easy for the bacteria to spread. However, even if surfaces have MRSA on them, this does not guarantee transmission. The best defense is good hygiene, keeping hands clean, and showering immediately after activities that involve direct skin contact with others. Keeping clothes clean, especially athletic clothes, is also essential.

Symptoms of MRSA infection vary but include swollen, painful pimples or boils that may drain pus. They can quickly turn into deep, painful abscesses with the potential to infect bones, joints, surgical wounds, the bloodstream, heart valves, and lungs. MRSA is diagnosed by testing a tissue sample or nasal secretions for staph bacteria. The sample is examined in a lab where the specific type of staph can be identified.

Treatment of MRSA may include draining the infection and taking a prescription antibiotic. Health care workers caution that when individuals attempt to treat an MRSA skin infection, it could worsen the infection or spread it to others. Anyone suspecting an infection should cover the affected skin, wash their hands, and immediately contact their health care provider or primary care physician. According to researchers at Johns Hopkins Children's Center in Baltimore, a thorough and quick cleaning of the wound makes a significant difference in rapid healing versus persistent infection ("Timely Care," 2011).

It is also extremely important to take all doses of a prescribed antibiotic even if the symptoms improve unless instructed to stop taking the prescription by a doctor. Antibiotics are prescribed based on the specific bacterial profile of each individual infection. Not all skin sores are caused by MRSA but those that turn red, warm, or form pus should be tested so that they do not develop into more serious infections.

In January 2008 the U.S. Food and Drug Administration (FDA) approved the first rapid blood test that allows health care providers to identify the source of a staph infection in just two hours instead of the two days required by the old tests. This is a significant improvement in diagnosis and is important since an MRSA infection can quickly become serious. And those who have had an MRSA infection are not immune to future infections, making prevention extremely important.

Researchers consider preventative measures an important tool in the fight against infections. Women have been drinking cranberry juice to help treat urinary tract infections for generations. Researchers from Worcester Polytechnic Institute in Massachusetts found that cranberry juice blocks a strain of staphylococcus aureus from initiating infection. The results were presented at the American Chemical Society's national meeting in Boston in August 2010 by Terri Camesano, professor of chemical engineering at WPI (Worcester Polytechnic Institute, 2010). Although the study's main focus was with E. coli and urinary tract infections, the Staphylococcus aureus was included because it can cause a range of staph infections from minor rashes to MRSA. According to the study's author, the S. aureus showed the most significant results in the study and may help researchers in their fight against a number of serious bacterial infections.

In another pioneering study, researchers at the University of Strathclyde, Glasgow, have developed a lighting system based on a narrow spectrum of visible-light wavelengths to decontaminate and prevent the transmission of hospital superbugs including MRSA ("Superbugs Could Be Destroyed," 2010). The lighting system was discovered and developed by a team of experts that included an electrical engineer, an optical physicist, a microbiologist, and others. According to clinical trial results the technology kills pathogens but is harmless to patients and health care workers and has provided a greater reduction of bacterial pathogens than can be obtained from cleaning and disinfecting alone.

Others are calling attention to the seriousness of MRSA by pushing international health organizations, the CDC, and state health departments to declare MRSA an epidemic and pandemic. The Chicago-based MRSA Survivors Network launched World MRSA Day on October 2, 2009, after it lobbied the U.S. Senate to name October MRSA Awareness Month and designate October 2 as World MRSA Day. Jeanine Thomas, a woman who nearly died from an MRSA infection following surgery, started the U.S. organization. Thomas has combined forces with MRSA Action UK members to raise global awareness about antimicrobial resistance. The groups advocate changes in health care procedures, such as early screening and isolation for MRSA.

*Sharon Zoumbaris*

*See also* Bacteria; Food and Drug Administration (FDA); Staphylococcus.

## References

"FDA Clears First Quick Test for Drug-Resistant Staph Infections." *FDA News.* January 2, 2008. www.fda.gov/bbs/topics/NEWS/2007/NEW01768.html.

"FDA OKs Drug to Treat Resistant Infections." *CQ Healthbeat (Congressional Quarterly).* November 1, 2010. General Reference Center Gold.

Jones, Peter F. "Two Nineteenth Century Surgeons." *British Medical Journal* 305, no. 6868 (December 19, 1992): 1546.

Klein, E., D. L. Smith, and R. Laxminarayan. "Hospitalizations and Deaths Caused by Methicillin-Resistant Staphylococcus aureus, United States 1999–2005." *Emerging Infectious Diseases* 13 (December 2007): 1840–46.

"MRSA Activists Call for Action during World MRSA Awareness Month." *USNewswire,* October 13, 2009.

"MRSA Infection." Mayo Clinic. December 21, 2010. www.mayoclinic.com/health/mrsa/DS00735.

MRSA Infection Webpage, Medline Plus (December 21, 2010) www.nlm.nih.gov/medlineplus.mrsa.html.

"MRSA Infections." Centers for Disease Control and Prevention (CDC). www.cdc.gov.

MRSA Survivors Network. "Statistics: United States." www.mrsasurvivors.org/statistics.

"MRSA Update." *Saturday Evening Post* 282, no. 2 (March–April 2010): 66.

National Institute of Allergy and Infectious Diseases (NIAID). "Methicillin-Resistant *Staphylococcus aureus* (MRSA)." www3.niaid.nih.gov.

Spurgeon, D. "Prevalence of MRSA in U.S. Hospitals Hits New High." *British Medical Journal* 335, no. 7627 (November 2007): 961.

"Superbugs Could Be Destroyed Using Beams of Light That Decontaminate the Air." *Daily Mail Reporter,* November 15, 2010. www.dailymail.co.uk/sciencetech/article-13297778/Superbugs.

"Timely Care May Be Key to Treating Infected Cuts: Type of Antibiotic Mattered Less Than Good First-Aid Even for Resistant Staph, Study in Kids Suggests." *Consumer Health News.* February 23, 2011. General Reference Center Gold.

Worcester Polytechnic Institute. "Cranberry Juice Shows Promise Blocking Staph Infections." *ScienceDaily.* September 3, 2010. www.sciencedaily.com/released/2010/09/100901 132233.htm.

## MIND-BODY HEALTH. *See* PSYCHOSOMATIC HEALTH CARE

## MINERALS (FOOD)

Minerals are inorganic elements that cannot be made by the human body. They are stored in varying amounts and along with vitamins are essential for good health. Most minerals, categorized as either major or trace minerals, come directly from plants and water or indirectly from animal foods. One of the most important tasks minerals perform is their ability to maintain the proper balance of water in the human body. The most important water-regulating minerals are sodium, chloride, and potassium. The major minerals include these three as well as calcium, magnesium, phosphorus, and sulfur. Trace minerals include chromium, copper, fluoride, iodine, iron, manganese, molybdenum, selenium, and zinc.

Major minerals are required in amounts of 100 milligrams or more while trace minerals are required in amounts less than 100 milligrams per day. The amount of a mineral or trace mineral that is absorbed and available to any individual is called its bioavailability, which is determined by several factors. Different elements in the diet can decrease the availability of different minerals and excess intake can negatively affect the absorption of other minerals. Minerals can, of course, be obtained from supplements but research suggests that for optimum health, eating a balanced diet is superior to depending on supplements.

Some minerals travel through the body by being absorbed into the bloodstream like water-soluble vitamins. Others, like calcium, act like fat-soluble vitamins and require a carrier for absorption and transport. However, vitamins and minerals differ in one key aspect: vitamins are organic and can be broken down by heat, air, or acid while minerals are inorganic and hold on to their chemical structure. That makes it easier to ingest minerals because they are found in soil and water, through the plants, animals, or fluids consumed each day. Vitamins are more fragile and can be weakened by cooking, storage, and even exposure to air.

Of all the minerals in the human body calcium is the best known because it is most abundant. Approximately 98 percent of calcium is found in bones and teeth as is widely known. Osteoporosis, a disorder linked to inadequate calcium intake and fragile bones, has become a serious public health problem for many U.S. women. However, many Americans may not be aware that calcium also plays a role in the proper functioning of the heart, muscles, and nerves that maintain blood flow.

While requirements for calcium change depending on age, gender, and other factors, a healthy adult should take in between 1,000 and 1,300 milligrams per day.

Good dietary sources of calcium include kale, broccoli, dried peas and beans, collard greens, and calcium-fortified foods such as orange juice and cereals. Having too much calcium can create a problem when combined with excess sodium. The calcium binds with the sodium and is excreted when the body attempts to lower sodium levels. Too much sodium in the diet, whether through table salt or processed foods, can mean too much calcium is lost. On the other hand, excess calcium also interferes with the absorption of iron, zinc, and manganese.

Chloride is a component of hydrochloric acid, an important part of gastric juice, which is secreted by glands in the stomach lining and works to digest food. Chloride or sodium toxicity can be caused by dehydration or excess loss of water. Suggested daily intake of chloride is 3,400 milligrams according to government guidelines.

Magnesium is necessary in a number of essential metabolic reactions from energy production to the synthesis of DNA. In some cases it has been shown to protect the heart, improve vision in glaucoma patients, and even reduce hyperactivity in children with low magnesium levels. Whole grains were once an excellent source of magnesium. Today, the beneficial qualities have been refined out of many processed foods, making it harder for some adults to get the recommended 400 milligrams of magnesium. Still, a healthy diet full of fruits and vegetables should provide an adequate amount of magnesium.

Phosphorus is the second most abundant mineral in the human body, just behind calcium. While calcium is largely found in bones and teeth, phosphorus appears in every cell in the body and plays a role in most of the body's chemical reactions. Researchers are now looking at whether calcium and phosphorus need to be kept in balance for optimum bone health but studies are still inconclusive. Phosphorus is found in many foods but there is some concern that Americans may be getting much more than the 1,000 milligrams required each day thanks to the growing consumption of soft drinks and food additives, which contain high levels of phosphorus.

Potassium is essential to every cell in the human body and works in tandem with sodium. Together they regulate water balance and stimulate nerve impulses for the heart and other muscle contractions. Unfortunately, the typical American diet of processed, convenience, and fast foods may contain insufficient potassium along with excess sodium. That imbalance can create high blood pressure, kidney or heart disease. Good sources of potassium include bananas, avocados, potatoes, and whole grains. Daily recommended intake of potassium is 3,500 milligrams.

Sodium has different effects on different people. Some individuals can eat large quantities of salt and processed foods and have no problems while others who eat lots of sodium develop high blood pressure or other adverse effects. Many Americans consume from 2,300 to 4,700 milligrams a day of salt. Nutrition experts recommend limiting sodium intake to no more than 2,300 milligrams per day.

Sulfur is essential for good health and is found in two amino acids: cysteine and methioninein. In its native form, it is a bright yellow crystalline solid. In nature, it can be found as the pure element and as sulfide and sulfate minerals. Adults require relatively large quantities of sulfur. Many people may not be aware that there are no government recommended guidelines for sulfur. Since the sulfur comes from and is used by amino acids, any diet with an adequate protein intake should have sufficient amounts of sulfur.

The trace minerals found in the human body are just as important as their major mineral counterparts and they too carry out a diverse set of tasks. Trace minerals can interact with one another, and these interactions can trigger imbalances. Too much of one can cause or contribute to a deficiency of another. For instance, excess manganese can cause iron deficiency. Also, when the body has too little of a trace mineral problems can develop as in the case with iodine. Too little iodine causes thyroid hormone production to slow down, too much can create a different problem.

Iron is best known for carrying oxygen throughout the body. It also aids in energy metabolism and DNA synthesis. Almost two-thirds of iron in the body is found in hemoglobin, the protein in red blood cells that carries oxygen to tissues. Smaller amounts of iron are found in myoglobin, a protein that helps supply oxygen to muscle. Iron stores are regulated by intestinal absorption.

Although iron is largely associated with animal foods such as red meat, liver, and fish, nonmeat iron sources include spinach and chard, molasses, dried fruits, and whole grains. Quinoa and amaranth contain about four to six times more iron than other grains. Low iron levels can cause anemia, so teens and young women of child-bearing age often need iron supplements. A healthy adult should get at least 18 milligrams daily. However, excess iron can accumulate in the body to toxic levels, so iron supplements should only be prescribed by a doctor.

Chromium is a trace mineral important for the production of a substance called glucose tolerance factor (GTF), a compound that works with insulin to move glucose into cells where it can be used to produce energy. A diet that includes mostly processed foods can deplete chromium because so much chromium is taken up when it is used to metabolize sugary foods. Dietary guidelines call for 120 micrograms (mcg) each day.

Copper plays an essential role in the body's ability to produce energy as well as in iron metabolism, brain and nervous system function, and the formation of connective tissue. Zinc is important in reproduction and, like copper, in neurological function. Additionally, nearly 100 enzymes are dependent on zinc for their function. Zinc comes from the soil where plants are grown, making grains a good food source for zinc, especially quinoa and amaranth. Copper and zinc have similar properties and provide a balancing effect on each other.

Selenium is a natural antioxidant that assists the immune system, protects against cancer, and may play a role in fertility. Research continues to look at selenium's role in preventing or lowering the rates of lung, colorectal, prostate, and skin cancers. Research is continuing as scientists also work to clarify its overall importance in maintaining good health. The richest plant source for selenium is the Brazil nut; a single nut contains double the daily requirement of 50 micrograms (mcg). Other good sources include nuts, seeds, and grains. However, high doses of selenium are toxic and recommendations call for no more than 400 mcg a day.

Selenium deficiency due to low levels of the mineral in the soil is still found in parts of China and has been linked to Keshan disease, a heart disorder prevalent in that country.

Fluoride acts to stabilize bone mineral and harden tooth enamel, increasing resistance to tooth decay. Fluoride deficiency leads to problems with dental caries and is common in areas of the world where water has low fluoride concentrations. The discovery of fluoride's effects on dental health led to the use of fluoridated water in the United States and other parts of the world. Iodine is essential for normal thyroid function, which is important for growth and development, particularly brain development. Iodization of salt, especially in the United States, has all but eliminated goiter and other iodine-related physical and mental development issues in this country.

Manganese is found as a free element in nature (often in combination with iron), and in many minerals. It activates several enzymes, which then contribute to the metabolism of carbohydrates, amino acids, and cholesterol. Manganese is found in leafy green vegetables, fruits, nuts, and whole grains. The nutritious kernel, called wheat germ, contains the most minerals and vitamins of the grain. Processed foods like white bread have the germ removed. Many common vitamin and mineral supplements fail to include manganese. Relatively high dietary intake of other minerals such as iron, magnesium, and calcium can also inhibit the proper intake of manganese and a deficiency can slow the production of collagen in wound healing.

Molybdenum can be found in very small quantities in the human body, and like the other trace minerals, is essential for healthy nutrition. It assists in processes such as the development of the nervous system, removal of kidney waste, and energy production in cells. Proponents claim molybdenum may also act as an antioxidant by protecting cells from free radicals. Researchers are continuing their efforts to understand how it interacts with other chemicals. Molybdenum is used as a treatment in rare cases of inherited metabolic diseases like Wilson's disease, in which the body cannot process copper.

Molybdenum comes from foods including legumes, grains, leafy vegetables, liver, and nuts. The actual amount of molybdenum in plants varies according to the amount in the soil. Healthy individuals require a very small amount of this trace mineral. Because so little is needed, just 2.3 milligrams daily, deficiency is rare and occurs only in situations such as when an individual requires long-term intravenous feeding. While knowledge of molybdenum dates back to the Middle Ages, actual research into its importance in the human body began only within the past couple of decades. In 2001, the U.S. Food and Nutrition Board established the recommended dietary allowance, or RDA, of molybdenum for most adults at 45 micrograms, with an RDA of 50 micrograms for women who are pregnant or breast-feeding.

*Sharon Zoumbaris*

*See also* Dental Health; Vitamins.

### References

"Dietary Guidelines for Americans." www.cnpp.usda.gov/dietaryguidelines.htm.

"Dietary Reference Intakes (DRI) and Recommended Dietary Allowances (RDA)." www. nal.usda.gov/fnic.

"Getting Your Vitamins and Minerals through Diet." *Harvard Women's Health Watch,* July 1, 2009.

"Position of the American Dietetic Association: Food Fortification and Dietary Supplements." American Dietetic Association. www.eatright.org.

"Research on Cancer Discussed by Scientists at Harvard University, Department of Nutrition." *Biotech Week,* October 6, 2010, 1360.

"Research on Minerals Detailed by Scientists at Hebei University, College of Life Sciences." *Science Letter,* October 5, 2010, 2689.

Stampfer, Meir J. "The Benefits and Risks of Vitamins and Minerals." *Harvard Special Health Report,* March 2006, 16.

## MYPLATE

Move over MyPyramid and say hello to MyPlate, the latest government effort to battle America's obesity epidemic and to get families eating healthier meals. MyPlate replaces the U.S. Department of Agriculture's MyPyramid, introduced in 2005 to spice up the original Food Guide Pyramid unveiled in 1992.

According to nutritionists the pyramid had grown too complicated for average Americans to understand. The plate is a basic concept and was introduced by First Lady Michelle Obama during a press briefing where she was joined by U.S. Agriculture Secretary Tom Vilsack and Surgeon General Dr. Reginal Benjamin. Obama called it "a quick, simple reminder for all of us to be more mindful of the foods that we're eating" ("First Lady, Agriculture Secretary," 2011).

The USDA MyPlate logo uses the image of a round dinner plate to provide consumers with a visual representation of a balanced meal consisting of servings of fruits, vegetables, grains, protein, and a small amount of dairy. At the same time the USDA introduced an updated link on its website called ChooseMy Plate.gov.

The ChooseMyPlate.gov site offers consumers everything from informative articles on the food groups to a personalized eating plan, weight loss information, even assistance with planning healthy menus. The site offers the opportunity to ask questions and to analyze individual food choices. There is also a tip of the day, recommendations on foods to reduce such as those high in sodium, and specific nutrition information for special groups including pregnant and breast-feeding women.

The MyPlate program recommends Americans pay attention to portion size or serving size when eating and switch to low-fat or fat-free dairy products, especially milk. The USDA deputy director of the Center for Nutrition Policy and Promotion, Robert C. Post, in discussing the MyPlate program cited federal estimates that show some two-thirds of U.S. adults and as many as one-third of children are now overweight or obese (Reinberg, 2011).

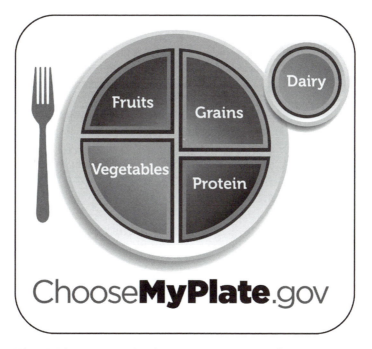

The MyPlate program by the USDA encourages all Americans to make healthy food choices. (U.S. Department of Agriculture)

The First Lady added that as a mom this new logo makes it easier for her when she looks at her kids' plates to remember each plate should be half full of fruits and vegetables, leaving room on the rest of the plate for a lean protein, low-fat dairy, and whole grains choices ("First Lady, Agriculture Secretary," 2011). Nutritionists and supporters of the new logo call the plate a universally used utensil and a recognized part of nutrition education.

The USDA has a history of creating food guides to motivate American consumers to make healthy food choices. Early guidelines were established in 1916 with a focus on protective foods. Later, in the 1940s the government released a guide that included the Basic Seven, which it later updated to the Basic Four in the 1950s. The USDA also created Dietary Guidelines for Americans, with the first goals released in 1977. The Dietary Guidelines continue to be evaluated every five years, with the latest update released in 2010 to support the introduction of MyPlate.

*Sharon Zoumbaris*

*See also* Basic Four (Foods); Nutrition; U.S. Department of Agriculture (USDA).

### References

"ChooseMyPlate.gov." U.S. Department of Agriculture. www.choosemyplate.gov.

"First Lady, Agriculture Secretary Launch *MyPlate* Icon as a New Reminder to Help Consumers to Make Healthier Food Choices." U.S. Department of Agriculture (USDA) Office of Communications. June 2, 2011. www.usda.gov.

Haven, J., A. Burns, P. Britten, and C. Davis. "Developing the Consumer Interface for the MyPyramid Food Guidance System." *Journal of Nutrition Education and Behavior* 38 (2006): S124–S135.

Reinberg, Steven. "U.S. Serves up New Nutrition Guidelines on 'MyPlate'; The Logo, Which Replaces the Food Pyramid, Is Designed to Encourage Healthful Eating." *Consumer Health News,* June 2, 2011.

Welsh, S., C. Davis, and A. Shaw. "A Brief History of Food Guides in the United States." *Nutrition Today* (November/December 1992): 6–11.

# N

## NATIONAL CANCER INSTITUTE

In 1937, the U.S. government passed the National Cancer Institute Act, and by doing so, made a commitment to its citizens to support and coordinate cancer research through its own laboratories and by others and, it is hoped, to one day find a cure for cancer. Over seven decades later this primary tool of the government in the fight against cancer, the National Cancer Institute (NCI), is still a vital part of the National Institutes of Health (NIH) and also one of the 11 agencies that compose the Department of Health and Human Services (HHS). Most important, the NCI is still working to improve the lives and futures of American cancer patients.

In its early days, additional legislation, including the 1944 Public Health Service Act (PHSA), expanded the NCI's role in getting information out to patients and the public. The PHSA has been broadened and expanded many times since then. The National Cancer Act of 1971 added even more responsibilities to the NCI.

It was the 1971 legislation that expanded the scope of the NCI activities to include support of international cancer research and added information dissemination and education programs for patients and the public to the NCI list of duties. To help individuals deal with cancer, the NCI provides programs to doctors and the public about the treatment of individual types of cancer. It also identifies clinical trials that might benefit patients and it provides information to improve long-term survival while educating the public on early detection techniques.

The National Cancer Amendment of 1974 went on to establish the President's Biomedical Research Panel, which keeps the president and Congress informed on policies and issues as well as research with respect to the programs of the National Institutes of Health. Other legislation that increased the NCI's mission include the Biomedical Research Training Amendments of 1978; the Health Research Extension Act of 1985, which consolidated cancer communication activities and highlighted the International Cancer Research Data Bank; and the

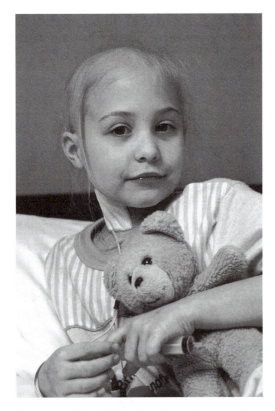

A young girl with leukemia undergoes chemotherapy. The National Cancer Institute is responsible for conducting and supporting cancer-related research; sharing state-of-the-art information about cancer detection, diagnosis, treatment, prevention, control and survivorship; and training physicians and scientists. (Bill Branson/National Cancer Institute)

Health Omnibus Program Extension of 1988,which added rehabilitation research to NCI's duties.

The NCI now has a budget of more than $5 million ("NCI Annual Fact Book"). Those dollars support the NCI's main responsibilities, which include coordinating the National Cancer Program; conducting and supporting cancer-related research; sharing state-of-the-art information about cancer detection, diagnosis, treatment, prevention, control, and survivorship; and training physicians and scientists. According to the National Institutes of Health, most of the NCI budget goes to fund grants and contracts awarded to laboratories, universities, medical schools, and private companies in the United States and around the world to fund their efforts to treat and understand cancer in all its manifestations.

According to the NCI, real progress is being made in the fight against cancer. The U.S. government statistics show the rate of new cancer cases overall has gone down since 1999 and the rate of overall cancer deaths has also been declining for more than a decade ("Fact Sheets about NCI"). In other words, cancer is no longer an automatic death sentence, a fact illustrated by the more than 11 million cancer survivors in the United States. The NCI joined with the World Health Organization (WHO) in 2006 as part of its global cancer prevention and control resolution. Resolution WHA58.22 aims to improve cancer prevention, early detection and treatment, as well as provide better care for cancer patients in all WHO member state countries.

*Sharon Zoumbaris*

*See also* Cancer; U.S. Department of Health and Human Services (HHS); World Health Organization (WHO).

### References

"Fact Sheets about NCI." National Cancer Institute. www.cancer.gov.cancertopics.fact-sheets.NCI.

"National Cancer Act of 1937." National Cancer Institute. http://legislative.cancer.gov/history/1937.

"NCI Annual Fact Book." National Cancer Institute. http://obf.cancer.gov/financial/factbook.htm.

"NCI International Portfolio." National Cancer Institute. www.cancer.gov/nci-international-portfolio.

"NCI Professional Judgment Budget: 2012." National Cancer Institute. www.cancer.gov/PublishedContent/Files/aboutnci/budget_planning_leg/plan-archives/nci_plan.pdf.

## NATIONAL CENTER FOR COMPLEMENTARY AND ALTERNATIVE MEDICINE (NCCAM)

The National Center for Complementary and Alternative Medicine (NCCAM) is the U.S. government agency dedicated to using scientific analysis and research to explore complementary and alternative healing practices for American consumers.

The NCCAM is one of 27 entities that make up the National Institutes of Health (NIH), which is within the Department of Health and Human Services (HHS). The NIH is one of eight agencies that compose the Public Health Service (PHS) branch of HHS.

The NCCAM was first established in the fall of 1991 as the Office of Alternative Medicine (OAM) and was then renamed the NCCAM in October 1998. The four primary areas of focus for the NCCAM include research; research training and career development; outreach; and integration. As part of its research efforts the center supports clinical and scientific research projects that focus on complementary and alternative medicine. It provides national and international grants. The office also analyzes clinical and laboratory-based studies at its Bethesda, Maryland, offices on the NIH campus.

The NCCAM offers training and career development opportunities for predoctoral, postdoctoral, and other researchers through its grant awards. The NCCAM also sponsors educational programs, exhibits and conferences, and operates an information clearinghouse for consumers to answer questions and update information through written publications and via a government website.

Its fourth area of focus includes efforts to integrate scientifically proven complementary and alternative medicine practices into conventional medicine via publication of studies; by supporting its inclusion into the curriculum of medical, dental, and nursing schools; and by supporting others who incorporate those changes. The NCCAM received some $122 million for 2009, which is just a small piece of the total NIH budget of $29 billion for that same year ("NIH Announces Five," 2010).

Research funded by NCCAM includes a $6 million grant to the University of Chicago to study antitumor effects of ginseng on cancer. The 2008 award was made to the university's Center for Herbal Research on Colorectal Cancer. In

2009, the NCCAM also announced a $2.5 million grant for research of asthma disparities among Latino children, awarded to the College of Nursing and Health Innovation at Arizona State University. Statistics show a steadily growing rate of asthma among Latino children, and the grant will seek to determine the causes of different health outcomes among children of different ethnic origins. The study results are expected in late 2013.

International awards included a grant of more than $200,000 for the Chinese University of Hong Kong (CUHK) for a research project dealing with Chinese medicine. The project plans to develop an International Center for Research on Complementary and Alternative Medicine to examine the uses of promising herbal medicines for untreatable diseases like cancer. At that same time a grant was also given to CUHK in partnership with the University of Maryland and University of Illinois at Chicago to set up a Center for Functional Bowel Disorders and Traditional Chinese Medicine, which will study the potential uses of Traditional Chinese Medicine in the treatment of irritable bowel syndrome.

**Critics**   Over the years since its inception NCCAM has more than doubled its budget from $49 million its first year to more than $122 million in 2009, and has grown its research division to more than 25 researchers and support staff. While many support its mission, there are critics of the department who suggest that since its creation in 1991 the NCCAM has not been effective in confirming the success or failure of any alternative medical method. Other critics have questioned whether NCCAM grants are decided based on politics or science. In a 2008 interview, NCCAM director Josephine P. Briggs, MD, a kidney expert specializing in translational research, outlined the center's goals. She stated she would like to have more support and outreach materials available to increase the education of American consumers and to provide them with information about treatments that could improve their health. She also called for continued efforts by NCCAM to enable the integration of complementary and alternative medicine practices that can be shown to be helpful into modern medical practices ("Exploring the Alternatives"). Briggs recommended that people share information with their primary physician about any supplements they may be taking to prevent any adverse interactions.

*Sharon Zoumbaris*

*See also* Dietary Supplements; National Institutes of Health; Traditional Chinese Medicine.

## References

"Exploring the Alternatives: How the National Center for Complementary and Alternative Medicine Looks for Treatments on the Cutting Edge." *Tufts University Health and Nutrition Letter* 26, no. 7 (September 2008): 4.

"HK Receives Grants for Traditional Chinese Medicine Projects." *Xinhua News Agency.* February 4, 2004. General Reference Center Gold.

Hurley, Dan. *Natural Causes.* New York: Broadway Books, 2006.

"Lack of Lab Space and Need for More Trials Slow NCCAM Progress." *Science and Government* 34, no. 1 (January 15, 2004): 6.

Marcus, Donald M., and Arthur P. Grollman. "Review for NCCAM Is Overdue." *Science* 313, no. 5785 (July 2006): 301–2.
"NIH Announces Five Botanical Research Centers." *National Institutes of Health: News and Events.* August 31, 2010. www.nih.gov.
"NIH Center Awards $2.5 Million Grant to ASU College of Nursing and Health." *States News Service,* September 14, 2009.

## NATIONAL INSTITUTES OF HEALTH (NIH)

The National Institutes of Health (NIH) is a collection of 27 different institutes and centers, headquartered in Bethesda, Maryland, whose mission is to enhance health and reduce the burdens of illness and disability for all Americans. The NIH actually dates back to 1887 to the Marine Hospital Service (MHS) and its laboratory on Staten Island in New York City. The MHS was set up by the government to offer medical care for merchant seamen and later took on the task in the 1880s of examining immigrant passengers for infectious diseases when they arrived in America. The examinations were used to try and stop the spread of diseases such as cholera and yellow fever. The MHS was the predecessor of the U.S. Public Health Service (PHS), renamed with its current name in 1948. The NIH is one of the eight health agencies included in the Department of Health and Human Services.

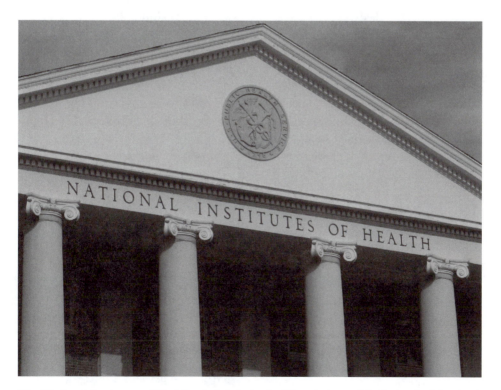

The National Institutes of Health administrative building is located in Bethesda, Maryland. (AP/Wide World Photos)

The NIH is funded by Congress, which approved an almost $32-billion budget for 2012. The NIH functions as the nation's largest advocate of biomedical research and now supports more than 40,000 competitive research grants and 325,000 research staff at more than 3,000 research facilities across America according to its director, Dr. Francis S. Collins (2011).

The goal of that research is to find new ways to prevent, detect, diagnose, and treat diseases with the ultimate goal of better health for all Americans. While the majority of NIH research activities are conducted by scientists working in laboratories around the country and the world, the central office or NIH headquarters in Maryland is located on a 300-acre campus that includes some 75 buildings. The various institutes and centers that make up the NIH specialize in specific areas including cancer; heart, lung, and blood diseases; allergy and infectious diseases; human genome research; mental health; dental health; and aging.

Examples of specific research supported by the NIH include a study that developed a screening test to aid in the early detection of autism spectrum disorders and other developmental delays in young children. The study results, covered in the *Journal of Pediatrics* online edition, described the screening program that correctly spotted a problem 75 percent of the time ("Simple Checklist").

Other research conducted by the National Cancer Institute of the NIH came from a study of the effects of a high-fiber diet on longevity. The NIH-AARP Diet and Health Study reported that participants in the nine-year study who consumed the highest amount of fiber were less likely to die from heart disease or other chronic diseases compared to those who consumed little fiber ("High-Fiber Diet").

Infectious diseases, chronic medical conditions, maternal and child health, even dental research are all research priorities under the NIH umbrella of agencies and institutes along with the National Library of Medicine (NLM). The NLM is the world's largest medical library, and it works to support other medical libraries as well as the training of medical librarians and health specialists. In an increasingly technological society, the NLM can provide up-to-date research and information around the globe as it works to support the mission of the NIH and the health of the American public.

*Sharon Zoumbaris*

*See also* Autism; U.S. Department of Health and Human Services (HHS).

### References

Collins, Francis S. "Fiscal Year 2012 Budget Request." National Institutes of Health, Department of Health and Human Services. May 11, 2011. www.nih.gov/about/director/budgetrequest/fy2012budgetrequest.pdf.

"High-Fiber Diet Linked with Longevity." *Environmental Nutrition* 34, no. 5 (May 2011): 8.

"Simple Checklist Can Catch Early Signs of Autism." *States News Service,* May 9, 2011.

U.S. Department of Health and Human Services (HHS). "NIH History." National Institutes of Health. March 4, 2011. www.nih.gov/about/history.htm.

U.S. Department of Health and Human Services (HHS). "NIH Mission." National Institutes of Health. March 4, 2011. www.nih.gov/about/mission.htm.

## NATIONAL ORGANIC PROGRAM (NOP)

The National Organic Program (NOP) is part of the U.S. Department of Agriculture's Agricultural Marketing Service (AMS) agency and does not deal directly with nutrition or food safety. Instead, it is a marketing program, started in 2002, that focuses on organic products. The NOP was set up to establish regulations to assure U.S. consumers that any organic products would meet consistent and uniform standards. The importance of the NOP regulations to individual Americans varies and ultimately depends on that individual's food concerns. For example, if a consumer wants to avoid genetically modified foods, or GMOs, she might look for the USDA Organic Seal as a guarantee that GMO ingredients are not included in a particular product since NOP regulations do not allow them in organic products.

The history of the NOP in the United States actually goes back to the 1950s and 1960s when a handful of American consumers started buying products grown without chemicals. Farmers experimenting with organic systems would market directly to those consumers or to small health food stores. By the late 1960s, a new generation of environmentally friendly consumers demanded more and more products grown or created without chemicals, which in turn increased the need for more organic items. As the sales of those foods rose so did interest from mainstream agriculture in this new niche market.

However, the issue of what it meant for something to be organic was different for different producers. The first organization to offer organic certification was the California Certified Organic Farmers, a group formed in 1973. Still, different states passed different legislation, some allowed voluntary certification while others demanded that all organic products be certified by their standards. There were no national guidelines.

The first attempt on the national level to develop a common language and uniform standards for organic food came via the Organic Foods Production Act (OFPA). It was included in the 1990 farm bill. At that point organic farming was becoming one of the fastest-growing segments of American agriculture. The United States had under a million acres of organic farmland when Congress passed the OFPA. By 2002 it had doubled and then doubled again between 2002 and 2005. Unfortunately, as the business of organics grew, so did the friction between small organic farmers and large factory farms. Following passage of the OFPA, a National Organic Standards Board (NOSB) was formed to act as an advisory panel and help both sides reach a consensus and decide what the term *organic* really meant.

The board of 15 members appointed by the secretary of agriculture included a diverse group of farmers, retailers, scientists, certifiers, and consumers. Even though the regulations for organic farming seemed fairly clear-cut, the rules needed for processing organic food proved a more difficult issue. Both sides had strong opinions and neither wanted to compromise. The board finished its first draft of recommendations and submitted them to the USDA in 1995.

For two years the USDA reviewed the standards and then released a document in 1997 that surprised the small organic farmers and producers. The USDA standards had allowed genetically modified organisms (GMOs), irradiated foods, and sewage sludge into "organic" products. The organic community was furious and bombarded the USDA with the largest recorded response to a proposed rule; some 275,000 negative comments poured into the agency (Greene, 2001). There was speculation that the USDA had been under political pressure from the Clinton administration to improve U.S. exports of genetically modified foods in Europe. Still, it would be another three years before the USDA reissued the standards. When those new standards were unveiled, they no longer allowed GMOs, irradiation, and sewage sludge in organic production.

At the same time another debate had developed between big organics and the small organic growers and producers. The big corporations wanted relief from the 1990 legislation that prohibited synthetic food additives and manufacturing agents, which they claimed were vital to large-scale production of organic processed foods. They pressed for the standards to include a list of synthetic substitutions that could be used if the organic versions were not commercially available. The USDA did not help the situation; it left the decision of what it meant for a product to be "unavailable" in organic form to each certifying agency and organization.

Another 12 years passed before the NOP was finally launched in 2002. Then it was immediately challenged. A Georgia chicken producer had persuaded his congressional representative to loosen the rules requiring organic feed for organic livestock. The congressman had responded by adding a rider to a congressional spending bill that would allow livestock producers to use cheaper, nonorganic feed and still call themselves organic if the price of the organic feed was more than double the cost of regular feed. The bill passed but consumers and organic producers again protested in overwhelming numbers and it was repealed a few months later.

This constant assault on the intent of the 1990 Organic Foods Production Act (OFPA) frustrated many organic growers, including a blueberry farmer from Maine who filed a lawsuit against the USDA and then secretary of agriculture Ann Veneman. Arthur Harvey charged that the 2002 rule did not conform to the OFPA. During the course of his lawsuit he gained the support of organizations including the Center for Food Safety, Beyond Pesticides, the Organic Consumers Association, Greenpeace, and the Sierra Club.

Harvey's biggest complaint was over the NOSB approved list of 38 synthetic ingredients that were allowed in processed organic food. Harvey and his supporters argued that synthetics would damage the integrity of organic foods and if any prohibited substances were ever added to the list the organic industry's credibility with U.S. consumers would be destroyed. At the same time the large organic operations were calling on the board to protect the list of ingredients; otherwise, they argued, it would be impossible to successfully produce organic foods for national distribution.

The 2005 court decision ruled in favor of Harvey on three of his seven points and gave the USDA one year to write new rules to match the law. The changes included a limitation on the prohibition of synthetic ingredients. While this left the national list in place and gave industrial organics a set list of synthetic materials for use in organic production, it also provided a tool for eventually adding more ingredients to that list. The Organic Trade Association (OTA), which represents organic producers such as Kraft Foods and Archer Daniels Midland Company, supported those changes while small, independent organic growers and producers called it one more example of how agribusiness was gaining control in the organic market.

NOP regulations describe organic crops as those raised without using conventional pesticides, petroleum-based fertilizers, or sewage sludge–based fertilizers. Animals raised on an organic operation must be fed organic feed and given access to the outdoors or pasture. They cannot be given any antibiotics or growth hormones. To become USDA certified organic, applicants must submit a plan that describes practices and substances used in their production, recordkeeping procedures, and practices to prevent comingling of organic and nonorganic products. The growers and producers must be accredited by USDA-approved agents who conduct on-site inspections. However, any operation that sells less than $5,000 a year in organic agricultural products is exempt from the certification process. While they can label their products organic if they follow the NOP standards, they cannot attach or display the official USDA Organic seal. Also, retail operations, such as grocery stores or restaurants, do not have to be certified organic.

The percentage of organic ingredients in a product determines its label. Products labeled "100 percent organic" by law must contain only organically produced ingredients. Anything labeled "organic" must have at least 95 percent of its ingredients organically produced, and both the "100 percent organic" and the "organic" products are allowed to display the official USDA Organic seal.

Any product that is made up of at least 70 percent organic ingredients but less than 95 percent can use the phrase "made with organic ingredients" on its label and is allowed to list up to three of the organic ingredients or food groups on its principal display panel. For example, soup made with at least 70 percent organic ingredients and all organic vegetables may state on the label "made with organic peas, potatoes and carrots," or "made with organic vegetables." However, at 70 percent or less of organic ingredients, the USDA Organic seal may not be added to the packaging. Finally, products that contain less than 70 percent organic ingredients cannot use the word *organic* on their packaging. They can identify the specific ingredient that is organically produced in their ingredient list but cannot add the word *organic* anywhere else on the label or packaging.

USDA figures show that close to 5 million acres of land in the United States are now dedicated to organic production. In order to increase that number the U.S. government has set up programs to help farmers convert to organic methods.

The USDA initiative called "Know Your Farmer, Know Your Food" benefits organic farmers according to Bob Scowcroft, executive director of the Organic Farming Research Foundation in Santa Cruz, California. Programs being supported by the initiative include the Environmental Quality Incentives Program, which had a budget of $50 million in both 2009 and 2010 to provide technical support for organic farmers or those planning to convert to organic farming. The program offers individual farmers up to $20,000 a year and also provides funds for local farmer's markets and a hoop house program to extend the growing season for organic family farmers. While researchers are still evaluating possible nutritional benefits to eating organic foods, studies also continue to raise questions about the association between pesticides from foods and an increased risk for diseases such as Parkinson's or other cancers.

The USDA's Agricultural Marketing Service announced in 2010 a move to increase its enforcement of national organic standards. The increase came in response to reviews that found major gaps in federal oversight of organic foods, in particular, frequent failure to perform spot testing for pesticides required in the 1990 law. The USDA also released its first edition of its program handbook in 2010. The manual is designed for anyone who owns, manages, or certifies organic operations. Prepared by the NOP, the handbook offers guidance about the national organic standards and also includes instructions that outline best practices in such areas as the use of green waste in organic production systems, the approval of liquid fertilizers as well as recordkeeping, steps to certification, accreditation procedures, and how to apply to become an accredited certifying agent.

*Sharon Zoumbaris*

*See also* Genetically Modified Organisms (GMOs); Organic Food.

### References

Clapp, Stephen. "USDA Issues New Procedures for Enforcing Organic Standards." *Food Traceability Report* 10, no. 10 (October 2010): 12.

Clute, Mitchell. "The New USDA: Look for Big Changes in Agency Priorities and Funding under Obama." *Natural Foods Merchandiser* 31, no. 10 (October 2010): 70.

Fromartz, Samuel. *Organic Inc.: Natural Foods and How They Grew.* Orlando, FL: Harcourt, 2006.

Grandjean, Phillippe, David Bellinger, Ake Bergman, Sylvaine Cordier, George Davey-Smith, Brenda Eskenazi, Devid Gee, Kimberly Gray, Mark Hanson, Peter Van Den Hazel, Jerrold J. Heindel, Birger Heinzow, Irva Hertz-Picciotto, Howard Hu, Terry T-K Huang, Tina Kold Jensen, Phillip J. Landrigan, I. Caroline McMillen, Katsuyuki Murata, Beate Ritz, Greet Schoeters, Niels Erik Skakkebaek, Staffan Skerfving, and Pal Weihe. "The Faroes Statement: Human Health Effects of Developmental Exposure to Chemicals in Our Environment." *Basic and Clinical Pharmacology and Toxicology* 102, no. 2 (February 2008): 74.

Greene, Cathy. "Organic Labeling." In *Economics of Food Labeling,* edited by Elise Golan, Fred Kuchler, and Lorraine Mitchell. Agricultural Economic Report No. 793. USDA

Economic Research Service. January 2001. www.ers.usda.gov/publication/aer793/aer793g.pdf.

"National Organic Program." USDA Agricultural Marketing Service. www.ams.usda.gov/NOPProgramHandbook.

"USDA Publishes Organic Program Handbook." *Food Traceability Report* 10, no. 10 (October 2010):12.

## NATIONAL SCHOOL LUNCH PROGRAM (NSLP)

Everyday more than 32 million U.S. schoolchildren buy their lunch as part of the National School Lunch Program (NSLP) thanks to a law passed by President Harry S. Truman more than 50 years ago. However, the program may need a serious overhaul to combat the nation's growing obesity rates among American schoolchildren. Today students are being fed French fries, pizza, and chicken nuggets as school food service managers wrestle with the problem of creating meals that are appealing, low cost, but still follow Dietary Guidelines for Americans for nutrition.

Good news for NSLP arrived late in 2010 thanks to the Healthy, Hunger-Free Kids Act, which was signed into law and will provide an additional $4.5 billion for children's nutrition, including money for school lunches for the next decade. The law will also open up school lunch enrollment for more children and will provide funds to improve food choices, which could translate into less pizza and more salads. The bill is part of President Barack Obama's efforts to end childhood hunger by 2015.

First Lady Michelle Obama voiced additional support for the bill as a way to bolster her "Let's Move" campaign against childhood obesity. By increasing the number of students eligible to enroll in school meal programs and by improving the quality of the food served, Obama and U.S. Secretary of Health and Human Services Kathleen Sebelius supported the bill as a way to meet goals of ending hunger and cutting obesity levels at the same time. Sebelius was among government officials who publicly praised its passage.

Nowhere is poor nutrition more noticeable than among America's youngest citizens. Statistics from the White House Task Force on Childhood Obesity Report, released in May 2010, show that more than 30 percent of American children ages 2 to 19 are overweight or obese. Data from the National Health and Nutrition Examination Survey (NHNES) found the percentage of overweight and obese children has tripled since those figures were first collected in the early 1970s.

Future improvement in lunch food choices may come just in time as research now reveals that children who eat lunch as part of the National School Lunch Program have an increased likelihood of becoming overweight as adults (Millimet, 2010). This is bad news for a generation of young Americans since studies show that children who are obese or have high cholesterol are more likely to develop heart disease as they age. Doctors are already seeing an increase in Type 2 diabetes in children, believed to be a direct consequence of their increased obesity (Belluck, 2008).

Part of the problem comes from the food currently being served in school lunches. By law no more than 30 percent of each meal's calories may come from fat, and less than 10 percent from saturated fat. Regulations also established a standard for school lunches to provide one-third of the RDA of protein, vitamin A, vitamin C, iron, calcium, and calories. However, schools can serve individual food items à la carte, those items can fall outside the scope of the nutrition guidelines and are where schools often try to balance their budgets. These foods include choices children will like and purchase such as pizza, French fries, and fried chicken nuggets.

This budgetary balancing act has been in effect since the late 1960s and early 1970s when President Richard Nixon dramatically increased funding for the NSLP. The problem arose when Congress only increased federal dollars for food costs, not for operating expenses, equipment, or labor, making it necessary for school food service programs to try to walk the line between cost and nutrition. School lunch programs are nonprofit but given the tight budgets faced by many school districts, sales of à la carte lunch items are an important part of their overall operating funds.

Later, to help school lunchrooms improve their budgets, the USDA eased restrictions banning commercial operations from school cafeterias. This was ultimately a poor nutritional choice because it opened the door for fast-food corporations and giant food service companies to introduce burgers, fries, pizza, and chicken nuggets, which were inexpensive and pushed sales up. Children were happy to buy the same high-fat, sugary, salty foods they were often eating at night with their families in fast-food restaurants. Today, high schools across the country sell everything from Subway sandwiches to Taco Bell products, Pizza Hut, Domino's, and McDonald's. The American School Food Service Association estimates that about 30 percent of public high schools in the United States offer branded fast food.

The U.S. Department of Agriculture (USDA) oversees both the federal lunch and breakfast programs. In its initial days, the National School Lunch Program was born out of New Deal politics. Signed into law in 1946, right from the start the program linked nutrition to the priorities of agricultural and commercial food interests; they have always donated surplus agricultural food items to be used as part of the program. During its early years, the number of free lunches served was small. Still, that ability to give farmers an outlet for their surplus commodities was significant and helped the government stabilize prices for a number of products.

In 1994, the USDA launched the School Meals Initiative for Healthy Children (SMI) to improve nutritional quality of school meals. Until the SMI, federal nutritional requirements had not changed since the program's beginning in 1946. As part of the initiative the USDA published regulations to help schools bring their meals up to date with the Dietary Guidelines even as the schools were still required to use federally approved commodity foods, many of which are high in fat.

In addition, a report released in 2008 by the Robert Wood Johnson Foundation's Healthy Eating Research showed more than 50 percent of the commodity foods were sent to processors before they were sent to schools (Muzaurieta, 2008). The processing adds fat, sugar, and sodium. For example, cheese becomes the topping on pizza rather than being served as just cheese, poultry becomes chicken nuggets, and fruit shows up in dessert items rather than used as simple fruit. The commodity foods that schools must use include frozen ground beef, canned or frozen fruits and vegetables, cheese and cheese products, and rice, pasta, and other grains. The schools are allowed to use other bonus foods over and above entitlement foods that come to schools as agricultural surpluses. Those bonus foods might include things such as canned sweet potatoes, canned pineapples, or dehydrated potatoes.

The surplus USDA food, the growth of the fast food industry, and a changing American diet have all contributed to the growing school lunch dilemma. Findings from the second School Nutrition Dietary Assessment Study (SNDA II) showed that schools are falling far short of meeting USDA health requirements. According to the SNDA report the meals are too high in fat, with on average 33 percent of calories in elementary school lunches coming from fat; only 20 percent of all schools met the guidelines for total fat in the average lunch and only 14 percent of schools met the guidelines for saturated fat.

The White House Task Force on Childhood Obesity was established as part of the "Let's Move" campaign, and the 124-page report of recommendations released in May 2010 detailed a total of 70 recommendations including improved food choices and increased lunch program enrollment. The report also suggested better federal nutrition standards for the NSLP and supported additional funding for school meals. The task force called on private companies to lower the fat content and calories from their foods. Mrs. Obama announced that members of her Healthy Weight Commitment Foundation, food firms including Kellogg's, Mars, and PepsiCo, have pledged to cut 1.5 trillion calories from their products by the end of 2015 ("Fighting the Flab").

While any child at a participating school may purchase a meal through the NSLP, children from families with incomes at or below 130 percent of the poverty level are eligible for free meals ("National School Lunch Program"). About 7 million children were enrolled in the program its first year in 1946. By 1970, 22 million children were participating, and in fiscal year 2009, more than 31 million children got their lunches through the NSLP ("National School Lunch Program"). The program cost the federal government $70 million in 1947 and cost $9.8 billion in 2009 ("National School Lunch Program"). The program is administered through the Food and Nutrition Service at the federal level and by state education agencies on the local level.

Students are being encouraged to change their food choices through efforts like the movie *Lunch Line,* presented by Applegate Farms. The documentary follows six high school students from Chicago who enter a cooking contest to create a healthier school lunch and end up serving their winning meal to congressional leaders and touring the White House with its chefs. The students had been asked to create a meal that would exceed the USDA standards and use only $1 per meal for ingredients as part of the "Cooking Up Change" contest, sponsored by the nonprofit organization Healthy Schools Campaign. The film has been shown in Detroit, Chicago, Denver, and Washington, DC, along with screenings in Atlanta, Houston, and Los Angeles.

*Sharon Zoumbaris*

*See also* Dietary Guidelines for Americans; Obesity; U.S. Department of Agriculture (USDA).

### References

Belluck, Pam. "Obese Kids Show Early Signs of Heart Disease." *Virginian Pilot,* November 12, 2008, 4.

"Fighting the Flab; Nutrition in Schools." *The Economist* (June 5, 2010): 38.

"Healthy School Lunches: National School Lunch Program Background." Physicians Committee for Responsible Medicine. www.healthyschoollunches.rg/background/nutrition.html.

"Lunch Line." www.facebook.com/lunchlinefilm or www.applegatefarms.com.

Millimet, Daniel L., Rusty Tchernis, and Muna Husain. "School Nutrition Programs and the Incidence of Childhood Obesity." *Journal of Human Resources* 45, no. 3 (2010).

Muzaurieta, Annie Bell. "Are School Lunches Causing Childhood Obesity?" DailyGreen.com. November 3, 2008.

"National School Lunch Program." U.S. Department of Agriculture. September 2010. www.fns.usda.gov.

"President Obama Signs Healthy, Hunger-Free Kids Act of 2010 into Law." The White House Press Office. December 13, 2010. www.whitehouse.gov/the-press-office/2010.

## NATUROPATHIC MEDICINE

The underlying philosophy of naturopathic medicine dates back to 400 BCE, with a focus on helping the body heal itself by increasing vitality through natural means or the healing power of nature. In some ways, this is an approach of many medical healing traditions. In the United States naturopathic medicine is considered part of the complementary and alternative medicine (CAM) approach to healing. The basic philosophy of healing that underlies the field is different from regular medicine, which includes allopathic medicine, or physicians with an MD degree, along with a DO, doctor of osteopathic medicine degree.

The essence of the naturopathic philosophy is vitalism. At its core, vitalism argues that life is too complex to be explained as just an assemblage of chemical and physical reactions. Living organisms are more than just the sum of their parts; they include a vital spark or energy that bears some relationship to the concept of a soul. This is in contrast to the allopathic approach, a mechanistic philosophy that sometimes views living organisms as machines, composed of material parts and biochemical processes that interact according to the laws of nature.

Allopathic medicine focuses on identification of the signs and symptoms of diseases linked to malfunctions in the body. In some ways, older theories such as the Hippocratic four humors and Chinese chi are similar approaches to vitalism as they all argue that disease is a result of an imbalance in the vital force. The goal of naturopathic medicine is to maintain or restore the homeostatic balance of the organism, up until the point of death.

Naturopathic practitioners use an eclectic array of treatment modalities. Some practitioners believe in a strict nature-cure foundation and use only hydrotherapy, diet, detoxification, and lifestyle modification; others include homeopathic medications, acupuncture, botanicals, or physical manipulation. Both mechanistic and vitalistic healing philosophies believe in the healing power of nature, but mechanistic healing works at the symptom level to eradicate the pathogenic agent that is causing harm, while the vitalistic approach focuses on restoring the body's homeostatic balance and keeping that balance through prevention.

Naturopathy was one of many competing ideologies that increased during the unregulated free market period of many different healers in 19th-century America. The naturopathic philosophy of natural healing appealed to sick people who were disenchanted with the aggressive therapies of "regular" allopathic physicians, like purging, bleeding, and treating with addictive patent medicines.

The beginning of naturopathy in North America can be traced to Benedict Lust, who believed he was cured of tuberculosis by Father Sebastian Kneipp's water treatments in Germany in the late 19th century. Lust then immigrated to the United States where he worked on developing naturopathy. In 1901, Lust opened the first school to award the degree of Naturopathic Doctor (ND) in New York. During this same time period, Henry Lindlahr, another follower of Kneipp, began his own practice in Illinois. Rather than using the term *naturopathy,* Lindlahr called it "natural therapeutics" to emphasize that the practice was about "nature—cure" rather than "nature—disease."

At this period in the United States, licensure of physicians, where it existed, was optional. Anyone in the United States could state they were a doctor whether they had attended a college or not. Admission to proprietary schools offering medical "degrees" was relatively easy, with no clear requirements for formal education. Many of the 160 medical schools in the United States in 1900 were for-profit businesses with minimal entrance requirements. Competing theories of disease flourished, and naturopathy was only one area of medicine along with such fields as chiropractic medicine.

Naturopaths established formal training and achieved state licensure in the United States at the turn of the 20th century. Although they eventually won licensure in 25 states, this was not a steady progression in licensure or in recognition. Rather, at different points and in different states, the legal right of naturopaths to practice has been won, lost, and won again. For example, these professional privileges were in jeopardy in the 1910s and 1920s when the leading allopathic medical organization, the American Medical Association (AMA), increased the scientific rigor of medical education.

By the early 20th century, allopathic physicians had abandoned the most dangerous and ineffective heroic therapies and had embraced science as an underpinning for treatment including the new science of "germ theory." Germ theory provided a highly successful model for preventing and eventually treating infectious diseases, the major cause of death at the time, and for improving surgical outcomes with antiseptic protocols.

Allopathic physicians began to campaign against competing "irregular practitioners" such as naturopaths, who continued to espouse alternative philosophies about disease. The allopathic model of medicine, with its assumption of specific etiology, reductionism, and separation of mind and body, dominated 20th-century health care. It became the conventional model of health care, adopted by allopathic doctors and eventually by osteopathic doctors (DOs). Both of these groups of physicians use a more reductionistic, mechanical, and intervention-oriented approach to illness in contrast to naturopathic physicians.

The ideology of natural healing lost much of its intuitive appeal when the "wonder drug" of penicillin and other antibiotics proved effective in curing many common, communicable diseases. The increased use of antibiotics, coupled with declining public interest in naturopathic medicine and the infighting within the naturopathic profession itself, pushed the field toward extinction. In 1968, in a report released by the U.S. Department of Health, Education, and Welfare on "Independent Practitioners under Medicare," the U.S. House of Representatives recommended Medicare not be expanded to cover naturopathic services because naturopathy was not grounded in medical science and practitioners were inadequately prepared to offer appropriate diagnoses and treatments (Baer, 1994). This report reflected the prevailing view of naturopathy by the U.S. scientific community in the 1960s.

However, by the end of the 20th century, interest in CAM once again increased thanks to public disenchantment with conventional medicine and a desire for a more holistic, preventive approach to health care. Since that time, the naturopathic medical profession has enjoyed significant growth, with an increase in the number of schools in North America, the number of students, and consequently the ranks of practitioners. The number of states currently regulating and licensing naturopathic physicians has enlarged with naturopaths currently authorized to diagnose and treat diseases in 15 U.S. states, the District of Columbia, Puerto Rico, and the U.S. Virgin Islands.

Since naturopathy remains a form of CAM and is considered outside of mainstream medicine and since practitioners cannot prove scientifically that naturopathic medicine benefits its patients, any evidence of demonstrated effectiveness would need to follow a rigorous, scientific, standard of empirical, controlled, double-blind studies. Still, naturopaths argue their approach goes further than what can be seen in clinical trials due to the fact that their healing focus is on the whole body, rather than the impact of a single drug or treatment.

There are three recognized categories of practitioners who utilize naturopathic medicine (National Center for Complementary and Alternative Medicine, 2011).

Those include naturopathic physicians, lay naturopaths, and regular physicians who also incorporate naturopathic approaches.

**Naturopathic Physicians**   Naturopathic physicians practicing in North America utilize naturopathic medicine as their primary health care modality. They are mostly primary care physicians who focus on preventive care by employing the body's natural healing processes. They may also incorporate some allopathic treatments and will refer cases to other medical doctors when they determine those patients are beyond their scope of practice. Naturopathic physicians are graduates of one of seven four-year, accredited, naturopathic medical schools in North America and have passed licensing exams in one of the 15 U.S. states, 2 U.S. territories, and 4 Canadian provinces that currently offer licensure.

**Lay Naturopaths**   Practitioners who adhere to a natural health care ideology but lack licensure are known as lay naturopaths, sometimes also called traditional naturopaths, true naturopaths, or nature—cure doctors. They are an eclectic group and include people trained in informal apprenticeships as well as people who have attended unaccredited schools. Unaccredited schools might include correspondence schools such as Clayton College of Natural Health or Trinity School of Natural Health. These lay practitioners oppose state licensing of naturopathic physicians and instead argue for certification, a voluntary form of accreditation that lacks the force of regulatory law over the occupation's work.

**Physicians Incorporating Naturopathy**   Finally, more allopathic and osteopathic physicians have begun to utilize modalities in CAM, including naturopathic modalities. Andrew Weil and Deepak Chopra are examples of two well-known, media-savvy allopathic physicians who have brought attention to and integrated some forms of CAM into what is considered mainstream medicine. As naturopathic medicine gains media recognition, the ranks of allopathic physicians incorporating it into their treatment programs may continue to grow.

*Jennie Jacobs Kronenfeld*

*See also* Acupuncture; Antibiotics; Homeopathy; Primary Care Physicians.

### References

Baer, Hans. *Towards an Integrated Medicine: Merging Alternative Theories with Biomedicine.* Walnut Creek, CA: Altamira Press, 1994. chirobase.org. 2011.

Kirchfeld, Friedham, and Wale Boyle. *Nature Doctors: Pioneers in Naturopathic Medicine.* Portland, OR: Medicina Biologica, 1994.

National Center for Complementary and Alternative Medicine. 2011. http://nccam.nih.gov/health/naturopathy/.

Starr, Paul. *The Social Transformation of American Medicine: The Rise of a Sovereign Profession and the Making of a Vast Industry.* New York: Basic Books, 1982.

## NESTLE, MARION

Marion Nestle, influential and award-winning nutritionist, author, scholar, and teacher, is a leading independent voice in the food politics arena. Since the 2002 publication of her seminal book *Food Politics: How the Food Industry Influences Nutrition and Health,* Nestle has been at the forefront of the food social movement, raising awareness, and shaping the debate around the often insidious interplay of food, nutrition, and politics in the United States.

Through her research, writing, and lectures, Nestle has profoundly impacted Americans' understanding of the relationship between their food choices and consumption patterns on the one hand and the food industry's marketing and lobbying efforts that drive those choices on the other.

Her own recognition of that intrinsic relationship between consumer choice and food industry lobbying was forged in 1986 to 1988 during her brief stint in government as senior nutrition policy advisor in the Department of Health and Human Services (HHS) and managing editor of the 1988 *Surgeon General's Report on Nutrition and Health.* Nestle observed firsthand "that everything is political, especially when it comes to dietary advice."

Her real "lightning bolt moment," as Nestle describes it, came in the early 1990s during a National Cancer Institute meeting on behavioral approaches to cancer prevention, when a fellow presenter pulled back the curtain on the cigarette industry's strategy of marketing to youngsters. Immediately making the connection to child-directed marketing by food companies, Nestle began compiling research and writing articles on the subject, out of which the highly influential and controversial *Food Politics* was born, inciting a new food-focused dialogue across the country.

Nestle originally tackled food industry marketing toward children, but gradually her policy reform target expanded to include aspects of both production and consumption while she explored the raging obesity epidemic debilitating Americans. In part, Nestle attributes rising obesity rates to the Reagan administration's deregulating industry and lessening agricultural controls, which indirectly encouraged American farmers to produce more food. As the daily available per capita caloric supply increased to 3,900, Americans consumed more food, making obesity commonplace.

On Wall Street, far from the agricultural production venues, the "shareholder value movement" had stockholders demanding that food manufacturing companies create higher yields by increasing revenues in already excessive caloric foods and food categories. The American three-meal-a-day norm, practiced for decades, quickly gave way to between-meal snacks, increased and excessive portion sizes, packaged convenience foods, and frequent meals consumed outside the home. Americans grew accustomed to and expected lower food prices, ease of access, and "super-sized" portions. Nestle exposed and argued that the food industry and its lobbying groups effectively created a new platform for U.S. food consumption and with that a platform for obesity and related health risks.

As the food industry grew and refocused its attention on high-caloric, high-fat, low-nutrient, and high-profit food, it attempted publicity spins by aligning itself with nonprofit organizations, health-related publications, sponsored journals, and research—all attempting to promote positive health images to products. The result is increasingly tainted scientific claims and a more confused public, unsure of whom to believe. Nestle argues that suspect nutrition labeling, such as "low-fat," "heart healthy," "anti-oxidant," and "organic," functional foods, and supplements promulgated by the food industry further confuse the general public. Nestle has become a vocal watchdog and inquisitor of the food industry.

Following the success of *Food Politics,* Nestle's scope broadened to include food safety (*Safe Food: The Politics of Food Safety,* 2003, updated edition 2010); public guidance on healthy food choices in the face of often intentionally misleading dietary messages and advertising claims (*What to Eat,* 2006); practices and perils of the pet food industry (*Pet Food Politics: The Chihuahua in the Coal Mine,* 2008, and *Feed Your Pet Right,* 2010, with co-author Malden Nesheim); front-of-package food labeling; and, in a forthcoming book, the myths and science surrounding calories. Throughout all of Nestle's publications and international speaking engagements runs the common thread of the role of politics—both governmental and big business—in shaping policy and behavior, often in spite of the science and to the detriment of the consumer.

In addition to writing books and articles, Nestle influences and directs nutrition and food policy dialogues through ongoing public health nutrition research and advisory work. She has served on a wide array of government, professional, and community advisory committees and boards, among them the Food and Drug Administration Food Advisory Committee and Science Board; the U.S. Department of Agriculture/DHHS Dietary Guidelines Advisory Committee; the Commission on Federal Leadership in U.S. Health and Medicine at the Center for the Study of the Presidency and Congress; the Harvard Business School and John F. Kennedy School of Government's Private and Public, Scientific, Academic and Consumer Food Policy Committee; and the *Journal of Public Health Policy.* Her research interests have continued to evolve throughout her eclectic academic career, centering on the development and analysis of food policy and dietary guidelines; social and political drivers of food choice; the politics of food safety; and the impact of corporate food advertising on children's eating habits and health.

Nestle has a PhD in molecular biology and an MPH in public health nutrition from the University of California, Berkeley. She has taught at Brandeis University and the University of California–San Francisco School of Medicine. From 1988 until 2003, Nestle chaired New York University's Department of Nutrition, Food Studies, and Public Health, in 1996 launched the pioneering graduate program in Food Studies, and laid the groundwork for a food movement and today's food revolution sweeping the nation.

She teaches courses in food policy, the ethics of nutrition and nutrition in the public health arena. She is Paulette Goddard Professor in the Department of Nutrition, Food Studies, and Public Health at New York University; professor of sociology at New York University; and visiting professor of nutritional sciences at Cornell University.

Although sometimes derided in a sexist manner by pro-industry groups as "hysterical," Nestle's style tends on the contrary to be characterized by reasonableness and common sense, her outrage generally tempered by amusement and grounded in scientific fact. Her impact on policy and regulations, while largely indirect, has been substantial.

*Meryl Rosofsky and Jennifer Berg*

*See also* Nutrition; U.S. Department of Agriculture (USDA); U.S. Department of Health and Human Services (HHS).

### References

Nestle, Marion. *Food Politics: How the Food Industry Influences Nutrition and Health.* Rev. ed. Berkeley: University of California Press, 2007.

Nestle, Marion. *Food Politics* blog. www.foodpolitics.com/.

Nestle, Marion. *Safe Food: The Politics of Food Safety.* 2nd ed. Berkeley: University of California Press, 2010.

## NURSE PRACTITIONERS

The United States is facing a shortage of primary care providers and one key solution may be the more than 125,000 trained nurse practitioners. A nurse practitioner (NP) is a registered nurse who has completed an advanced educational program with the minimum of a master's degree and has also received a national certification in an area of specialty such as family health, pediatrics, acute care. or others.

The role of the NP developed in 1965 in response to a nationwide shortage of physicians. That predicted shortage brought an increase in funding for NP programs, and the availability of programs caused enrollment to grow as well. During the 1970s the NP requirements shifted to include continuing education programs, which helped accommodate the demand for NPs. After completing an education program, the NP candidate must be licensed by the state in which he or she plans to practice. The state boards of nursing regulate nurse practitioners, and each state has its own licensing and certification criteria.

The NP often works closely with doctors and consults with them as needed, and in most cases, provides much of the same care as provided by doctors. In fact, an NP can serve as a patient's regular health care provider. Their training emphasizes disease prevention, reduction of health risks, thorough patient education, research, and patient advocacy, allowing a medical practice or medical care facility to see more patients without the doctor having to spend more time in the office.

On the job an NP will collaborate with doctors and other health professionals as needed; counsel and educate patients on treatment options; diagnose and treat acute illness, infections, and injuries; diagnose and treat chronic diseases; perform physical examinations; order and interpret diagnostic studies such as lab tests, x-rays, or EKGs; prescribe medications; prescribe physical therapy; provide prenatal care; and provide health maintenance care for adult patients.

There are a variety of institutions where NPs work. Those include community clinics, health departments, HMOs, hospitals, hospice centers, doctor's offices, school or college clinics, Veterans Administration facilities, and nursing homes. Since nursing is the largest of the health care occupations, nurse practitioners are in high demand. According to the American Nurses Association, approximately 60 to 80 percent of primary and preventive care in the United States can be performed by an NP, and with the changes in health care law the need for qualified nurse practitioners will continue to grow. Statistics show that the nursing field, especially NPs, is one of the 10 occupations projected to have the largest numbers of new jobs in the near future ("Nurse Practitioner").

Information about programs for nurse practitioners is available from the American Academy of Nurse Practitioners (AANP). Other organizations that oversee NP certification include the American Association of Critical-Care Nurses, the Board of Certification for Emergency Nursing, the National Certification Board of Pediatric Nurse Practitioners and Nurses, the National Certification Corporation for the Obstetric, Gynecologic and Neonatal Nursing Specialties, and the Oncology Nursing Certification Corporation.

*Sharon Zoumbaris*

*See also* Primary Care Physicians.

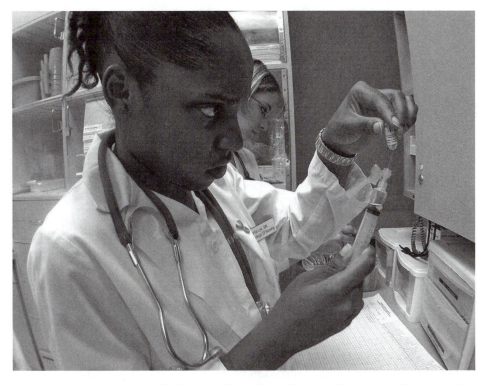

A nursing student from the University of Southern Mississippi draws medication at Forrest General Hospital in Hattiesburg on October 15, 2003. Nursing students at the university spend two days a week at the hospital, taking care of patients under the supervision of registered nurses as part of their training. (AP/Wide World Photos)

## References

Carryer, J., G. Gardner, S. Dunn, and A. Gardner. "The Core Role of the Nurse Practitioner: Practice, Professionalism and Clinical Leadership." *Journal of Clinical Nursing* 16 (2007): 1818–25.

"Nurse Practitioner." Mayo Foundation for Medical Education and Research. www.mayo.edu/mshs/np-career.html.

"125,000 Solutions to the Primary Care Shortage—Nurse Practitioners (NPs)." *Obesity, Fitness and Wellness Week,* August 8, 2009, 2252.

"Specially Trained Nurse Practitioner Detected Same Breast Abnormalities as Surgeon." *Women's Health Weekly,* July 1, 2010, 110.

## NUTRIENTS

At its most basic level, nutrition is the process by which we take in food, food provides energy, and energy powers the body and keeps us alive. There are six groups of essential dietary elements, called nutrients, required for a body to remain healthy. These nutrients provide energy, help us grow, and allow us to repair damaged tissues. They include proteins, carbohydrates, fats, vitamins, minerals, and water.

**Proteins**   Proteins are made up of chemicals called amino acids. There are 22 different amino acids; the body can make 13, but the other 9 must come from the food we eat. All amino acids contain carbon, oxygen, nitrogen, and hydrogen. The main work of proteins is to grow and repair body tissue such as bones, skin, and organs. Proteins make up much of the body's muscles and organs, and even some hormones. Proteins also make up hemoglobin, the part of the red blood cells that carries oxygen around the body. Finally, proteins provide a small source of energy. Humans get the protein they need from animal or plant foods, including meat, chicken, fish, eggs, nuts, dairy products, and legumes.

**Carbohydrates**   Carbohydrates provide energy needed for the brain, central nervous system, and muscle cells. Carbohydrates are an often misunderstood nutrient, but they are the biggest source of energy for the human body. They come in two forms, simple and complex. The simple carbohydrates, including sugars such as glucose and fructose, are quickly digested and used for immediate energy. Simple carbohydrates can be found in white potatoes, white rice, and foods made with white, refined flour. Complex carbohydrates—starches and glycogen—take longer to digest, and provide a slow but steady supply of energy. Complex carbohydrates are found in whole grain breads, cereals, and pasta, as well as grains such as bulgur and brown rice.

**Fats**   The various types of fats continue to confuse American consumers. Fats come in three varieties—saturated, monounsaturated, and polyunsaturated fats—and, like carbohydrates, they contain carbon, oxygen, and hydrogen. Basically, different fats get their names from their patterns of hydrogen atoms. All fatty acids, which make up fats, contain chains of carbon atoms, with hydrogen atoms attached to some or all of the carbon atoms. These fatty acids differ in the amount of hydrogen they contain.

In carbon chains in which the carbon atoms are bonded to the maximum number of hydrogen atoms—that is, "saturated" with hydrogens—the carbon atoms are linked to each other only by single bonds. Conversely, in an "unsaturated" carbon chain, with carbon atoms bonded to fewer hydrogens, some carbon atoms are linked to each other by double bonds. The more double bonds, the fewer hydrogen molecules. Fats with one double bond are called monounsaturated; those with two or more double bonds are called polyunsaturated. Both monounsaturated and polyunsaturated fats are considered good fats by nutritionists. The monounsaturated and polyunsaturated fats found in olive oil, other vegetable oils, nuts, and fish are considered part of a healthy diet. These fats provide the high-density lipoprotein (HDL) cholesterol that protects artery walls by carrying away low-density lipoprotein (LDL), or "bad," cholesterol.

Saturated fats are found in whole milk, red meats, and other animal products, as well as in palm oil and processed foods such as margarine and pastries. These fats lack double bonds between their carbon atoms, and encourage the body to make more LDL cholesterol. LDL cholesterol, considered the harmful type of cholesterol, damages artery linings and forms deposits on artery walls. Nutritional studies clearly link saturated fats and cholesterol in the diet to increased blood cholesterol levels and a greater risk of heart attack, heart disease, stroke, and other health problems. However, nutritionists caution that it is important to have some fat in a healthy diet. Healthy, unsaturated fats build cell membranes and store the fat-soluble vitamins A, D, E, and K. Most important, fats are the body's most concentrated sources of energy, and take longer than proteins or carbohydrates to digest.

*Trans Fats*   Trans fats or trans fatty acids are just about everywhere in the typical American diet. Created through a process called hydrogenation that turns liquid oils into stick margarines or shortening, they are used to increase the shelf life and stability of processed foods. Trans fats are found in many crackers, cookies, and doughnuts, to name just a few snack foods. There is a growing concern among scientists and nutritionists that, gram for gram, trans fats are more damaging than saturated fat. In other words, French fries cooked in partially hydrogenated vegetable shortening have as much artery-clogging potential as potatoes fried in lard or beef fat. In 2006, the U.S. Food and Drug Administration (FDA) added trans fat to the nutrition label requirements established by the National Labeling and Education Act (NLEA) of 1990. Now, food manufacturers must list trans fatty acids or trans fat if a food includes at least 0.5 grams of trans fat.

**Vitamins**   There are 13 vitamins needed by the body for normal growth, digestion, and resistance to infection. They also assist the body in utilizing carbohydrates, fats, and proteins more efficiently. Vitamins are found naturally in many foods, and come in two forms, fat-soluble and water-soluble. The fat-soluble vitamins, A, D, E, and K, are dissolved and stored in fats, meaning that they remain in the body longer than the water-soluble vitamins. The water-soluble vitamins, C and the eight B-complex vitamins, are dissolved and stored in water. This means they pass quickly through our bodies and must be replenished on a regular basis.

Overall, our bodies need varying amounts of vitamins to prevent vitamin deficiency diseases such as scurvy and rickets. Fifty-two percent of Americans take dietary supplements and vitamins in an attempt to compensate for their poor eating habits or other perceived nutritional deficiencies, according to an October 2007 survey by the Council for Responsible Nutrition (Solorio, 2007). Others rely on foods that are enriched with vitamins. For example, milk and milk products are enriched with vitamin A and often with vitamin D. Vitamins are also found naturally in a variety of foods.

Vitamin A is found in fruits, and in dark green or deep yellow and orange vegetables such as carrots, pumpkins, and spinach. It is linked to improved vision and healthy skin. "Vitamin B" refers to a group of vitamins, comprising B1, B2, B6, and B12 as well as niacin, folic acid, biotin, and pantothenic acid. The B vitamins are involved in making the red blood cells that carry oxygen throughout the body. Folic acid, one of the B vitamins, is thought to lower the risk of neural-tube birth defects such as spina bifida. In 1996, the FDA introduced a requirement that folic acid be added to white "enriched" flour to raise the average intake for consumers. A decade later, scientists are looking at the impact of high folic acid intake on cancer. Sources of vitamin B include fish, beef, pork, chicken, whole wheat grains, green leafy vegetables, enriched breads and cereals, and dried beans.

Vitamin C helps build bones and muscles and improves some infection-fighting capabilities, but large quantities can result in kidney problems. Good sources of vitamin C include citrus fruits, strawberries, melons, sweet potatoes, cabbage, tomatoes, and broccoli.

Vitamin D plays an important role in building strong healthy bones and teeth, and also assists the body in absorbing calcium. Along with its addition to foods such as milk and orange juice, vitamin D can be found in egg yolks and fish, and is also synthesized in the body after exposure to sunshine.

Vitamin E is found in vegetable oils, dark green vegetables, nuts, poultry, seafood, and wheat germ. It helps form red blood cells, muscles, and other tissues. Vitamin K is essential for effective blood clotting. It is found in dark green vegetables, whole grains, potatoes, cabbage, and cheese.

**Minerals** Minerals come from the foods we eat, both plants and plant-eating animals. Our bodies need 21 minerals; 7 of these are considered major minerals, and 14 are called trace minerals. They all contribute to a healthy body in many ways, from regulating chemical reactions, to building bones and teeth, to making hemoglobin in red blood cells. The major minerals comprise sodium, calcium, potassium, magnesium, phosphorus, chloride, and sulfur. Well-known trace minerals include iron, iodine, zinc, manganese, selenium, chromium, and fluorine.

**Water** Finally, water is the most important nutrient of all. We need more than 2 quarts of water per day to function. The exact amount needed depends on many factors, including activity levels, temperature, and humidity. A person can live for several weeks without food and other nutrients, but cannot survive for more than one week without water. Even though water does not supply any energy, it does other important work. It makes up part of our blood, cools our bodies, and carries waste away as urine. We drink water, but we also get up to 20 percent of our water from the foods we eat.

It is important to remember that all foods are not created equal; some have more nutrients than others. In fact, *nutrient density* is the term used when measuring the nutrients a food provides when compared to the calories it also provides. Nutritionists recommend eating lots of foods that are nutrient dense, meaning they are high in nutrients and low in calories. The opposite would be nutrient poor foods, those are the foods high in calories and low in nutrient content. These should be eaten sparingly. Nutrient poor diets over time can lead to malnutrition. Malnutrition can be caused by a lack of the proper nutrients over time, or it can also be caused by health problems.

*Sharon Zoumbaris*

*See also* Carbohydrates; Fats; Malnutrition; Minerals (Food); Trans Fats; Vitamins; Water.

### References

Nestle, Marion. *What to Eat.* New York: North Point Press, 2006.

Reinhard, Tonia. *Superfoods: The Healthiest Foods on the Planet.* Buffalo, NY: Firefly Books, 2010.

Shulman, Martha Rose. *The Very Best of Recipes for Health: 250 Recipes and More from the Popular Feature on NYTimes.com.* Emmaus, PA: Rodale, 2010.

Solorio, Season. "More Consumers Consider Themselves Regular Supplement Users, Annual Survey Results Show." *Council for Responsible Nutrition.* October 4, 2007. www.crnusa.org/CRN_PR_100407_ConsumerConfidence.html.

## NUTRIGENOMICS

If you are what you eat as the saying goes, it may be possible in the future to select foods that will make a better you. Molecular biologists and other researchers are working to combine discoveries in human genetics with a broader knowledge of the compounds in food and the complex interactions between you and your diet.

In nutrigenomics they have embraced the idea of individual nutrition, giving a futuristic twist to the concept of personal nutrition. Nutrigenomics is the study of how foods affect our genes and how individual genetic differences affect the way our bodies process nutrients. *Nutrigenomics* is also referred to as *nutritional genomics* and both terms have been used interchangeably.

The European Nutrigenomics Organization (NuGO) is among the leaders in this field. The NuGO is made up of a network of scientists funded by the European Union with 23 partners including research organizations, universities, and small businesses from 10 European countries with the common goal of improving nutrigenomics research. The second nutritional genomics symposium was held in the summer of 2010 in Adelaide, Australia, to provide its members with an up-to-date overview of the field with a special focus on identifying gaps in the research that might help prevent or better manage early childhood diseases such as autism and cancer.

Those involved with nutrigenomics believe that the information they uncover will ultimately prevent nutritional deficiencies. For example, consider the question of how many cups of coffee you should drink per day. Genetic tests can determine whether you have a specific genetic variation that makes it hard to absorb calcium in the presence of caffeine. Or consider the question, is a high-fat diet damaging to your health? Scientists now know that about 15 percent of people are born with a form of liver enzyme that causes their good cholesterol to go down in response to dietary fat. This is opposite of what should happen when dietary fat is eaten: in most people the HDL or good cholesterol level goes up.

Scientists suggest that by understanding the role of specific nutrients in foods and how they might cause disease, scientists could one day recommend specific diets for treatment rather than medication. Imagine a time when you could go to a genetic counselor or a physician who would determine your genetic makeup, and then customize your diet to improve your health or heal your disease.

This area of research is new, but the field is growing rapidly. There are companies already offering testing for a limited number of gene-nutrient interactions. Testing kits, available in some supermarket pharmacies and online, have users swab the inside of the cheek then send the sample and a questionnaire about diet and lifestyle back to the company's laboratories. Within weeks, a computerized analysis arrives offering highlights of the genetic test results.

Yet, there is still work to be done to figure out how all the genetic variables in humans relate to health and disease. Add the fact that food is full of hundreds of bioactive compounds, each influenced by where plants are grown or how and where animals are raised, and it is clear that nutrigenomics is in its infancy. But the fantasy of a personalized set of dietary guidelines is tantalizing to those with a family history of chronic disease or weight management issues.

The International Food Information Council surveyed consumer attitudes and determined that 71 percent of Americans favor the idea of using genetic information to improve their nutrition. Another 70 percent of those surveyed were interested in learning more about how genetic information can help improve their diets and overall health. That's impressive given that only 11 percent of American adults consume the USDA recommended daily portions of fruits and vegetables.

However, public health officials worry that without proper consumer education the benefits of nutrigenomics may be lost. European consumers are very skeptical of genetically modified foods, for example, a process where scientists modify the DNA of a food and add genes to improve its qualities. While this is different from nutrigenomics, which pays attention to the natural components in each food, it is easy to see how there could be confusion over the two terms.

There are already certain obvious rules of healthy nutrition that can improve individual health, like reducing the amount of sodium in your diet to improve hypertension or reducing the amount of saturated fat you eat to improve heart health, but scientists are anxious for the day when they will be able to provide comprehensive genetic examinations that can easily pinpoint specific nutritional needs to improve health and eliminate disease.

Researchers already have a good reference guide for the 25,000 or so genes of the human genome and the some 3 million common variants that reside within those genes. All they need to do now is to figure out how all those genetic variables interact with each individual. In fact, the day will come when you will find out exactly why you still need to eat your broccoli. Maybe Hippocrates was right when he wrote, "Leave your drugs in the chemist's pot if you can heal the patient with food."

*Sharon Zoumbaris*

*See also* Genetically Modified Organisms (GMOs); Nutrition.

### References

Colby, Brandon. *Outsmart Your Genes: How Understanding Your DNA Will Empower You to Protect Yourself against Cancer, Alzheimer's, Heart Disease, Obesity and Many Other Conditions.* New York: Penguin, 2010.

Collins, Francis S. *The Language of Life: DNA and the Revolution in Personalized Medicine.* New York: Harper, 2010.

El-Sohemy, Ahmed. "The Science of Nutrigenomics." *Health Law Review* 16, no. 3 (Summer 2008): 5 (4).

Gorman, Christine. "Does My Diet Fit My Genes?" *Time* 167, no. 24 (June 12, 2006): 69.

"Kansas State University Researchers Say Nutrigenomics Likely to Change the Future of Public Health." *Ascribe Higher Education News Service,* March 5, 2010, www.highbeam.com/doc/1G1-221355723.html.

Milunsky, Aubrey. *Your Genetic Destiny: Know Your Genes, Secure Your Health and Save Your Life.* Cambridge, MA: Perseus, 2001.

Ottewell, Sean. "Future Foods: The Latest Research Reveals Tantalizing Links between Gene Function and Nutrition." *International Food Ingredients* 4 (August–September 2007): 30 (3).

Schwartz, James. *In Pursuit of the Gene: From Darwin to DNA.* Cambridge, MA: Harvard University Press, 2008.

Stephenson, Frank Harold. *DNA: How the Biotech Revolution Is Changing the Way We Fight Disease.* Amherst, NY: Prometheus Books, 2007.

## NUTRITION

At its most basic level, nutrition is the process by which we take in food, food provides energy, and energy powers the body and keeps us alive. There are six groups of essential dietary elements, called nutrients, required for a body to remain healthy. These nutrients provide energy, help us grow, and allow us to repair damaged tissues. They include proteins, carbohydrates, fats, vitamins, minerals, and water.

**Proteins** Proteins are made up of chemicals called amino acids. There are 22 different amino acids; the body can make 13, but the other 9 must come from the food we eat. All amino acids contain carbon, oxygen, nitrogen, and hydrogen.

The main work of proteins is to grow and repair body tissue such as bones, skin, and organs. Proteins make up much of the body's muscles and organs, and even some hormones. Proteins also make up hemoglobin, the part of the red blood cells that carries oxygen around the body. Finally, proteins provide a small source of energy. Humans get the protein they need from animal or plant foods, including meat, chicken, fish, eggs, nuts, dairy products, and legumes.

**Carbohydrates**   Carbohydrates provide energy needed for the brain, central nervous system, and muscle cells. Carbohydrates are an often misunderstood nutrient, but they are the biggest source of energy for the human body. They come in two forms, simple and complex. The simple carbohydrates, including sugars such as glucose and fructose, are quickly digested and used for immediate energy. Simple carbohydrates can be found in white potatoes, white rice, and foods made with white, refined flour. Complex carbohydrates—starches and glycogen—take longer to digest, and provide a slow but steady supply of energy. Complex carbohydrates are found in whole grain breads, cereals, and pasta, as well as grains such as bulgur and brown rice.

**Fats**   The various types of fats continue to confuse American consumers. Fats come in three varieties—saturated, monounsaturated, and polyunsaturated fats—and, like carbohydrates, they contain carbon, oxygen, and hydrogen. Basically, different fats get their names from their patterns of hydrogen atoms. All fatty acids, which make up fats, contain chains of carbon atoms, with hydrogen atoms attached to some or all of the carbon atoms. These fatty acids differ in the amount of hydrogen they contain.

In carbon chains in which the carbon atoms are bonded to the maximum number of hydrogen atoms—that is, "saturated" with hydrogens—the carbon atoms are linked to each other only by single bonds. Conversely, in an "unsaturated" carbon chain, with carbon atoms bonded to fewer hydrogens, some carbon atoms are linked to each other by double bonds.

Fats with one double bond are called monounsaturated; those with two or more double bonds are called polyunsaturated. Both monounsaturated and polyunsaturated fats are considered good fats by nutritionists. The monounsaturated and polyunsaturated fats found in olive oil, other vegetable oils, nuts, and fish are considered part of a healthy diet. These fats provide the high-density lipoprotein (HDL) cholesterol that protects artery walls by carrying away low-density lipoprotein (LDL), or "bad," cholesterol.

Saturated fats are found in whole milk, red meats, and other animal products, as well as in palm oil and processed foods such as margarine and pastries. These fats lack double bonds between their carbon atoms, and encourage the body to make more LDL cholesterol. LDL cholesterol, considered the harmful type of cholesterol, damages artery linings and forms deposits on artery walls. Nutritional studies clearly link saturated fats and cholesterol in the diet to increased blood cholesterol levels and a greater risk of heart attack, heart disease, stroke, and other health problems. However, nutritionists caution that it is important to have some fat in a healthy diet. Healthy, unsaturated fats build cell membranes and store the fat-soluble vitamins A, D, E, and K. Most important, fats are the body's most concentrated sources of energy, and take longer than proteins or carbohydrates to digest.

*Trans Fats* Trans fats or trans fatty acids are just about everywhere in the typical American diet. Created through a process called hydrogenation that turns liquid oils into stick margarines or shortening, they are used to increase the shelf life and stability of processed foods. Trans fats are found in many crackers, cookies, and doughnuts, to name just a few snack foods. There is a growing concern among scientists and nutritionists that, gram for gram, trans fats are more damaging than saturated fat. In other words, French fries cooked in partially hydrogenated vegetable shortening have as much artery-clogging potential as potatoes fried in lard or beef fat. In 2006, the U.S. Food and Drug Administration (FDA) added trans fat to the nutrition label requirements established by the National Labeling and Education Act (NLEA) of 1990. Now, food manufacturers must list trans fatty acids or trans fat if a food includes at least 0.5 grams of trans fat.

**Vitamins** There are 13 vitamins needed by the body for normal growth, digestion, and resistance to infection. They also assist the body in utilizing carbohydrates, fats, and proteins more efficiently. Vitamins are found naturally in many foods, and come in two forms, fat-soluble and water-soluble. The fat-soluble vitamins, A, D, E, and K, are dissolved and stored in fats, meaning that they remain in the body longer than the water-soluble vitamins. The water-soluble vitamins, C and the eight B-complex vitamins, are dissolved and stored in water. This means they pass quickly through our bodies and must be replenished on a regular basis.

Overall, our bodies need varying amounts of vitamins to prevent vitamin deficiency diseases such as scurvy and rickets. Vitamin A is found in fruits, and in dark green or deep yellow and orange vegetables such as carrots, pumpkins, and spinach. It is linked to improved vision and healthy skin. "Vitamin B" refers to a group of vitamins, comprising B1, B2, B6, and B12 as well as niacin, folic acid, biotin, and pantothenic acid. The B vitamins are involved in making the red blood cells that carry oxygen throughout the body. Folic acid, one of the B vitamins, is thought to lower the risk of neural-tube birth defects such as spina bifida.

In 1996, the FDA introduced a requirement that folic acid be added to white "enriched" flour to raise the average intake for consumers. A decade later, scientists are looking at the impact of high folic acid intake on cancer. Sources of vitamin B include fish, beef, pork, chicken, whole wheat grains, green leafy vegetables, enriched breads and cereals, and dried beans.

Vitamin C helps build bones and muscles and improves some infection-fighting capabilities, but large quantities can result in kidney problems. Good sources of vitamin C include citrus fruits, strawberries, melons, sweet potatoes, cabbage, tomatoes, and broccoli.

Vitamin D plays an important role in building strong healthy bones and teeth, and also assists the body in absorbing calcium. Along with its addition to foods such as milk and orange juice, vitamin D can be found in egg yolks and fish, and is also synthesized in the body after exposure to sunshine.

Vitamin E is found in vegetable oils, dark green vegetables, nuts, poultry, seafood, and wheat germ. It helps form red blood cells, muscles, and other tissues.

Vitamin K is essential for effective blood clotting. It is found in dark green vegetables, whole grains, potatoes, cabbage, and cheese.

**Minerals**    Minerals come from the foods we eat, both plants and plant-eating animals. Our bodies need 21 minerals; 7 of these are considered major minerals, and 14 are called trace minerals. They all contribute to a healthy body in many ways, from regulating chemical reactions, to building bones and teeth, to making hemoglobin in red blood cells. The major minerals comprise sodium, calcium, potassium, magnesium, phosphorus, chloride, and sulfur. Well-known trace minerals include iron, iodine, zinc, manganese, selenium, chromium, and fluorine.

**Water**    Finally, water is the most important nutrient of all. We need more than 2 quarts of water per day to function. The exact amount needed depends on many factors, including activity levels, temperature, and humidity. A person can live for several weeks without food and other nutrients, but cannot survive for more than one week without water. Even though water does not supply any energy, it does other important work. It makes up part of our blood, cools our bodies, and carries waste away as urine. We drink water, but we also get up to 20 percent of our water from the foods we eat.

*Sharon Zoumbaris*

*See also* Carbohydrates; Fats; Nutrients; Vitamins; Water.

**References**

Kingsolver, Barbara, Steven L. Hopp, and Camille Kingsolver. *Animal, Vegetable, Miracle: A Year of Food Life.* New York: HarperCollins, 2007.

Knight, Judson, and Neil Schlager. "Nutrients and Nutrition." *Science of Everyday Things.* Vol. 3. Detroit: Gale, 2002.

Nestle, Marion. *What to Eat.* New York: North Point Press, 2006.

Reinhard, Tonia. *Superfoods: The Healthiest Foods on the Planet.* Buffalo, NY: Firefly Books, 2010.

U.S. Department of Health and Human Services, Centers for Disease Control and Prevention. "Physical Activity and Good Nutrition: Essential Elements to Prevent Chronic Diseases and Obesity 2008." February 2008. www.cdc.gov/nccdphp/publications/aag/pdf/dnpa.pdf.

## NUTRITION FACTS LABEL

To reassure American consumers about the content of the foods they buy and eat, the federal government passed the National Label Education Act in 1990 requiring all packaged foods in the United States to have a Nutrition Facts label on them. These labels provide information on certain nutrients and are one of the best sources of understanding the quality of an overall diet. The labels must contain information about calories, fat, carbohydrates, fiber, sodium, cholesterol, and vitamin and mineral content of the food. In 2006 trans fats were added as a requirement. Now the labels break down the fat counts into total fat, saturated fat, trans fat, and in many cases, polyunsaturated fat and monounsaturated fat. They may also list essential vitamins and minerals beyond the required ones. Here's what can be learned from a Nutrition Facts label.

**Calories** A calorie is a measurement of heat needed to raise 1 kilogram of water 1 degree Centigrade. Since food "stokes the furnace" of the human body, foods have assigned calorie values. Fat and alcohol are high in calories. Foods high in both sugars and fat contain many calories but often are low in vitamins, minerals, or fiber. There are numerous calorie counters readily available—online

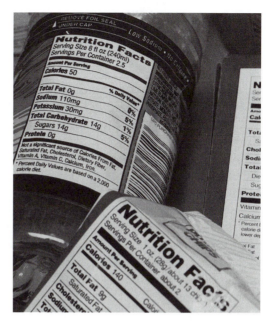

Nutrition facts labels give consumers important information about processed foods. (Photo Disc, Inc.)

and often in cookbooks. If you reduce your caloric intake, you'll lose weight. If you increase the amount of calories you consume, you'll gain weight. But that doesn't mean that a low-calorie diet is the best way to lose weight. That's how those awful grapefruit and black-coffee diets originated. Sure, severe reductions in calories for a week will cause weight loss. However, once old eating habits return, so will the lost weight. A pound equals 3,500 calories. So to lose a pound in, say a week, an individual would have to eat 3,500 calories less or burn off 3,500 calories in exercise or some combination of the two.

Exercise burns calories. For example, walking briskly can burn off about 100 calories per mile. Bicycling for a half hour at nearly 10 mph will burn about 195 calories. The specific number depends on the person's weight and the intensity of the activity. A variety of interactive exercise counters, available on the Internet, allow individuals to plug in their weight, age, and change variables such as the length of time and intensity of the activity.

The following formula will help determine the approximate number of calories needed per day to maintain body weight. Moderately active males should multiply their weight in pounds by 15. For example, if a man weighs 170 pounds, he needs to eat about 2,500 calories per day to maintain his current weight. Moderately active females should multiply their weight by 12. A 130-pound female needs about 1,560 calories per day. However, the number of calories needed per day decreases as the level of activity goes down. Relatively inactive men should multiply their weight by 13 pounds and women in that category should multiply their weigh by 10. So that 170-pound man who is relatively inactive needs only 2,210 calories and the 130-pound inactive woman needs only 1,300 calories to maintain body weight.

The information on nutrition labels is based on a 2,000-calorie-per-day diet, an important fact to remember for those working to maintain their weight.

**Calories from Fat** Numerous health and government authorities, including the U.S. Surgeon General, the National Academy of Sciences, the American Heart Association, and the American Dietetic Association, recommend reducing dietary fat to 30 percent or less of total calories. However, that doesn't mean an individual has to pass by all high-fat food products. For example, peanut butter with sugar added has 190 calories in a 2-tablespoon serving. Of those, 130 calories are from fat—68 percent. Add that peanut butter to two slices of whole wheat bread, which have 120 calories and 20 calories from fat, and the equation is different: now the fat is down to about 48 percent. It's still higher than the recommendation, but by adding a glass of skim milk and an apple, it is possible to reduce the fat content to a healthy level.

*Trans Fat* This is measured in grams and food manufacturers are required to list trans fats, or trans fatty acids, if a food contains at least 0.5 grams. The FDA did not establish a Daily Value or % DV for trans fats, but scientists have reported links between trans fat and saturated fat and increased levels of LDL cholesterol, which can increase coronary heart disease. Trans fat is commonly found in margarine, commercial baked goods, and in fried foods. Scientists suspect that gram for gram, trans fats are twice as damaging to the heart as saturated fat. Trans fat is made by adding hydrogen to vegetable oil during hydrogenation to keep the fat from turning rancid and to increase the shelf life of processed foods.

*Total Fat* This is also measured in grams. For someone eating a 2,000-calorie-per-day diet, daily fat intake should not exceed 65 grams. Fatty foods are always high in calories. Despite its bad image, though, fat isn't all bad. Some fat is needed because fats supply energy and help the body absorb fat-soluble vitamins A, D, E, and K. Fats contain both saturated and unsaturated fatty acids. Saturated fat raises blood cholesterol more than other forms of fat. Limiting saturated fats to less than 10 percent of calories will help lower blood cholesterol levels. High levels of saturated fats and cholesterol in the diet are linked to increased blood cholesterol levels and a greater risk for heart disease.

While polyunsaturated and monounsaturated fats could help lower blood cholesterol levels, the recommendation still holds that total fat account for no more than 30 percent of daily calorie intake.

**Cholesterol** The human body makes cholesterol, but it is also obtained from food. Animal products, such as egg yolks, higher-fat milk products, poultry, fish, and meat are high in cholesterol—and usually also in saturated fats. The daily value for cholesterol should be 300 milligrams. There are two kinds of cholesterol: LDL, the "bad cholesterol," and HDL, or "good cholesterol." LDL stands for low-density lipoproteins. If there's too much LDL cholesterol in the bloodstream, it can build up within the walls of the arteries and contribute to the formation of plaque, which can ultimately clog the arteries. That blockage could affect the flow of blood to the heart, and cause a heart attack, or to the brain, and result in a stroke. Doctors can measure the level of LDL in the blood—ideally it should be below 130.

High-density lipoproteins (HDL) is the "good" cholesterol because experts believe HDLs can carry cholesterol away from the arteries and to the liver, where it's passed from the body. HDL levels typically range from 40 to 50 milligrams/dL for men and 50 to 60 milligrams/dL for women. Levels below 35 milligrams/dL are abnormally low and a risk factor for cardiac problems. Low HDL levels can be caused by cigarette smoking, obesity, and physical inactivity.

**Sodium** Sodium is a trace mineral that helps maintain body fluid balance. Salt is an excellent source of sodium. One-quarter teaspoon, the typical serving, provides 540 milligrams of sodium, or 25 percent of the daily recommended allowance. Milk and processed foods are other sources. Sodium intake should stay below 2,400 milligrams. That might sound like a lot, but realize how quickly these sources add up. A frozen turkey pot pie, single serving, contains about 29 percent of the recommended daily sodium intake. Hot dogs typically have at least 21 percent of the daily total of sodium per hot dog. Even a tablespoon of ketchup has 190 milligrams of sodium or 8 percent of the daily value. Lower sodium intake could help people avoid or control high blood pressure—a risk factor in heart disease and strokes. For anyone eating many processed, packaged foods and exceeding daily sodium intakes, doctors recommend looking for ways to duplicate those foods while cooking using fresh ingredients. Many herbs and spices have no sodium and can add tremendous flavor to foods. These include garlic, basil, pepper, parsley, chives, vinegar, sage, cinnamon, nutmeg, and cloves.

**Total Carbohydrates** Carbohydrates provide energy for the brain, central nervous system, and muscle cells. They are found largely in sugars, fruits, vegetables, and cereals and grains. Meats generally have no carbohydrates. There are simple carbohydrates, such as sugars, and complex carbohydrates, such as breads and pastas, that the body breaks down into sugars. Someone with a 2,000-calorie-per-day diet should limit carbohydrates to 300 grams. Someone with a 2,500-calorie-per-day diet can consume up to 375 grams of carbohydrates. A medium baked potato with skin has 51 grams of carbohydrates. An apple has about 21 grams of carbohydrates, a tablespoon of sugar has 12 grams, and a slice of pie can pack 60 or more grams of carbohydrates.

Carbohydrates are divided into three kinds: monosaccharides or simple sugars, such as glucose and fructose; disaccharides—composed of two monosaccharides—such as maltose, sucrose, and lactose; and polysaccharides, which are starches and glycogen. On the Nutrition Facts label, total carbohydrates are broken down into two categories: fiber and sugar.

**Dietary Fiber** Fiber helps the body digest food. Soluble fiber, combined with a low-fat diet, may reduce levels of bad cholesterol. The RDA for fiber is 25 grams. Generally, grains, such as oat, wheat, and rice products, are good sources of fiber, as are some vegetables. Some foods that might seem as though they would be high in fiber, such as cereals, in fact have very little. High-sugar cereals often have just 1 gram of fiber; a high-fiber hot wheat cereal could have 5 and a 100 percent bran cereal could have up to 8 grams or more. Some fruits, such as an apple (3.5 grams), a banana (2.4 grams), three prunes (3 grams), and a half grapefruit (3.1 grams), also have high fiber content.

**Sugar**  Sugars in foods are the monosaccharides and disaccharides described above. In some foods, carbohydrate makeup is almost entirely sugar. For example, a tablespoon of fruit preserves, sweetened only with fruit juices, derives 9 of its 10 grams of carbohydrates from sugar. Breads and pastas, on the other hand, have much higher polysaccharide contents. One pita bread pocket, for example, has 2 grams of sugar out of its 24 grams of total carbohydrates. Looking at the Nutrition Facts label becomes especially important for anyone seeking to cut down on the simple sugars.

**Protein**  Protein is actually a combination of 22 amino acids. The human body makes 13 of these amino acids on its own. These are called nonessential amino acids. But 9 of the amino acids—essential amino acids—must come from food. Protein builds up and maintains the tissues in the body. Protein comprises much of the muscles, organs, even some hormones. Protein also makes hemoglobin, the part of the red blood cells that carries oxygen around the body. Protein makes antibodies to help fight off infections and disease. Protein is found in meat, chicken, fish, eggs, nuts, dairy products, and legumes.

**Vitamins and Minerals**  These are expressed on Nutrition Facts labels as a percentage of the Recommended Dietary Allowance (RDA). Anyone eating a varied diet most days, and not severely limiting calories, should not need additional vitamin or mineral supplements.

Some foods are enriched with additional nutrients. For example, enriched flour and bread contain added thiamine, riboflavin, niacin, and iron; skim milk, low-fat milk, and margarine are usually enriched with vitamin A; and milk is usually enriched with vitamins A and D. The ingredient list on packaging will provide information on which nutrients are in the food. In a nutshell, vitamin A is found in fruits and dark green and deep yellow vegetables, such as carrots, pumpkins, and spinach. Vitamin A is important to your vision and healthy skin.

Vitamin B actually refers to a group of vitamins—B1, B2, B6, B12, niacin, folic acid, biotin, and pantothenic acid. These vitamins play a role in making red blood cells, which carry oxygen to all the parts of the body. In other words, the B vitamins help with energy. Fish, beef, pork, chicken, whole wheat grains, green leafy vegetables, dried beans, and enriched breads and cereals are sources of vitamin B. Vitamin C strengthens bones and muscles and also has some infection-fighting capabilities. However, large doses can result in kidney problems. Good natural sources of vitamin C are citrus fruits, strawberries, melons, sweet potatoes, cabbage, broccoli, tomatoes, and peppers. Vitamin D contributes to strong healthy bones and teeth and it also helps the body absorb calcium. Vitamin D can be obtained through fortified milk products, egg yolks, and fish. Another great source for vitamin D is sunshine. Vitamin E helps form red blood cells, muscles, and other tissues throughout the body. Vitamin E also helps the body store vitamin A. It's found in vegetable oils and dark green leafy vegetables, nuts, poultry and seafood, and wheat germ and fortified cereals. Vitamin K is essential for blood clotting. It's also found in dark green vegetables, whole grains, potatoes and cabbage, and cheese.

**Calcium**   Calcium warrants special attention because new research is pointing to an even more crucial role than previously thought and because calcium requirements are highest for young people whose bones are developing. Calcium is used in building bone mass and also plays a role in the proper functioning of the heart, muscles, and nerves maintaining blood flow. Adequate calcium can also reduce the risk of osteoporosis, a weakening of the bones that can occur late in adulthood. Calcium is found naturally in dairy products and in dark green leafy vegetables.

**Iron**   Iron is a trace mineral found in red meat, liver, fish, green leafy vegetables, enriched bread, and some dried fruits such as prunes, apricots, and raisins. Recommended iron intake for young women is 15 milligrams per day; for boys aged 15 to 18, it's 12 milligrams per day, decreasing to 10 milligrams per day after age 19. The level of iron required for women stays the same until menopause. Blood loss, such as menstrual cycles, is a major cause of iron deficiency. Low iron levels can result in iron-deficiency anemia. Iron supplements can be taken, and individuals can eat more foods that are higher in iron content. Vitamin C can help iron absorption, while coffee, tea, wheat bran, eggs, and soy inhibit iron absorption. Medications such as antacids, for example, can also interfere with iron absorption.

Iron demands are typically highest for pregnant women. The requirement for iron doubles in the second trimester and triples in the third as blood volume increases and the fetus grows dramatically.

*Marjolijn Bijlefeld and Sharon Zoumbaris*

*See also* Calcium; Calories; Cholesterol; Fats; Fiber; Trans Fats; Vitamins.

## References

"FDA Trans Fat Nutrition Label Claim Unnecessary; GMA Opposes Misleading Footnote Statement." *PR Newswire,* December 17, 2002. DCTU05617122002.

"Food Advertising: Separating Fact from Fiction." *Mayo Clinic Health Letter,* March 2006, 6.

"Good News/Bad News." *Current Health 2. A Weekly Reader Publication* 32, no. 3 (November 2005): 4.

Kessler, David A. "Building a Better Food Label." *FDA Consumer* 25, no. 7 (September 1991): 10–14.

Lee, Elizabeth. "Report Urges Food Label Revamp." *Atlanta Journal-Constitution,* December 12, 2003, F1.

Lofshult, Diane. "New User-Friendly Food Database (Food for Thought)." *IDEA Fitness Journal* 5, no. 1 (January 2008): 72. www.NutritionPedia.com.

Nestle, Marion. *What to Eat.* New York: North Point Press, 2006.

"Rebuilding the Pyramids (Governments Hope to Reduce Consumption of Trans Fatty Acids)." *Better Nutrition* 65, no. 9 (September 2003): 28.

Taub-Dix, Bonnie. *Read It before You Eat It: How to Decode Food Labels and Make the Healthiest Choice Every Time.* New York: Penguin, 2010.

Ursell, Amanda. *What Are You Really Eating? How to Become Label Savvy.* Carlsbad, CA: Hay House, 2005.

Waxman, Henry A. *The Waxman Report: How Congress Really Works.* New York: Twelve, 2009.

## NUTRITIONAL DISEASES

To many Americans, nutritional diseases are considered a thing of the past, relegated to history thanks to modern medicine, vitamins, and the industrial agriculture that fills our stores and our cupboards. Unfortunately, nutritional diseases still exist in the world thanks to food shortages, poverty, and malnutrition. There are also new, modern twists on nutritional diseases, like obesity. According to the most recent figures, some 33 percent of adult Americans are overweight or obese (Flegal et al., 2010).

Nutritional disorders exist in other cases because eating too much of one thing can create a deficiency in another, as in the case of sodium and calcium. Excess sodium intake often brings calcium deficiency due to the fact that sodium and calcium metabolism are linked and higher sodium intake may increase calcium excretion.

This lack of vitamins, minerals, and other essential nutrients can result in osteoporosis from too little calcium; anemia from an iron deficiency; osteomalacia and rickets from too little vitamin D; beriberi and Korsakoff's syndrome due to a lack of vitamin B1, also known as thiamine; and scurvy from a lack of vitamin C.

Scurvy, among the first of the nutritional diseases to find a cure, is caused by a lack of vitamin C and was common among sailors centuries ago. Those sailors were eventually known as "limeys" when it was discovered that eating limes or lemons during a voyage cured the condition.

Rickets, another disease of deficiency, develops when there is a lack of vitamin D in the diet. Although some vitamin D is produced by the body when it is exposed to sunlight, some must be supplied through food. Simply eating foods high in vitamin D such as milk, fish, or liver and an increase in exposure to sunlight can correct the condition. In many cases the bone deformities from the rickets will improve over time.

Beriberi is another disease that improved when thiamine, or vitamin B1, was added to the diet. Symptoms of beriberi, a nervous system disease, include lethargy and fatigue as well as pain, an irregular heart rate, and swelling. Beriberi is rarely diagnosed in developed countries thanks to the amount of vitamin-enriched foods now available. However, today the disease is seen in alcoholics since excess alcohol makes it hard for the body to absorb thiamine but also increases the body's need for B vitamins. Korsakoff's syndrome, a memory disorder, also comes from a lack of vitamin B1.

Osteomalacia and osteoporosis are both diseases caused by a lack of vitamin D. Osteomalacia should not be confused with osteoporosis, which is caused by a lack of calcium and leads to decreased amounts of bone. Instead, osteomalacia produces a softening of bones that can then bend or become misshapen. The prognosis for curing most of these diseases is excellent if they are diagnosed and treated with supplements or food choices that provide the needed nutrients. Individuals should not attempt to diagnose perceived nutritional imbalances without consulting their primary care physician or a registered dietitian or qualified nutritionist.

*Sharon Zoumbaris*

*See also* Nutrition; Osteoporosis; Primary Care Physicians; Vitamins.

## References

Flegal, Katherine M., Margaret D. Carroll, Cynthia L. Ogden, and Lester R. Curtin. "Prevalence and Trends in Obesity among US Adults, 1999–2008." *Journal of the American Medical Association* 303, no. 17 (2010): 1695–96. doi:10.1001/jama.2010.518.

Larson Duyff, R. *ADA Complete Food and Nutrition Guide.* 3rd ed. Chicago: American Dietetic Association, 2006.

Spence, Jean T., and Janet R. Serwint. "Secondary Prevention of Vitamin D–Deficiency Rickets." *Pediatrics* 113, no. 5 (January 2004): 129.

Wharton, Brian, and Nick Bishop. "Rickets." *The Lancet* 362, no. 9393 (October 2003): 1389.

# *O*

## OBESITY

When a person's caloric intake (food consumption) exceeds his or her energy expenditure (exercise and daily activity), the net calories are stored in fat cells in the body. (Fat cells are built during childhood and are never lost, though they can shrink by dieting.) If this imbalance continues, the individual will gain significant weight. We call this extreme weight *obesity*. The most common definition of *obesity* is a body mass index (BMI) over 30. An index between approximately 19 and 24 is considered healthy. *Overweight* is defined as a BMI of 25 to 29.9. A BMI of 40 or higher, *morbid obesity,* is an immediate health threat. The Belgian anthropometrist Adolphe Quetelet developed the BMI equation. It uses a formula to compare an individual's weight-to-height ratio. BMI does not, however, indicate what percent of an individual's weight is fat. Some extremely muscular individuals, for instance, have a BMI that indicates they are overweight, despite the fact that they are in peak physical shape.

This equation, however, tells us little about the full story of obesity. The inability to keep calorie intake and energy output balanced predisposes the fat man, woman, and child to medical, social, emotional, and even financial hardships. Despite the fact that many American adults are now either overweight (61%) or obese (20%), fat prejudice, ironically, is still pervasive. In fact, the International Size Acceptance Association claims that a bias against fat is the last legally allowed—and even encouraged—form of discrimination.

Most doctors would not dispute the health dangers of obesity (though fat activists might). However, the social implications of obesity have fluctuated wildly throughout history. Figurines of earth goddesses are common archeological finds from across many eras and cultures. Used in rituals, these naked images of small, plump women suggest that, prehistorically, obesity was desirable. No doubt the images symbolized fertility and sexuality (some are very explicit). Even as late as the 16th century, the most erotic female form was the rubenesque, named for Peter Paul Rubens, who immortalized the obese female nude in his paintings.

During much of European history, a fat body type advertised wealth (necessary to purchase large quantities of food) and social standing (hard physical labor prevents weight gain). Many societies in Africa, Asia, and the Pacific still value the large body.

Science has uncovered some strong evidence for the causes of obesity in our culture: increasingly sedentary lifestyle; high consumption of simple carbohydrates and fats (especially the refined sugars and greasy preparations common in junk and fast foods); and stress. To a lesser degree illnesses such as hypothyroidism (underactive thyroid), genetic predisposition, and psychotropic (mind-altering) medications may lead to excessive weight gain. The cause of American obesity is a combination of bodily predispositions or abnormalities and environmental factors.

Evolution and modernization may have collided to produce an environment where obesity is not only likely but unavoidable for many people. Evolution of our bodies, brains, hormonal and neurobiological systems, and our metabolisms is imperceptibly slow, taking thousands of years to complete even a simple biological change. However, cultural changes are often revolutionary—occurring rapidly, even in a matter of years—rather than evolutionary. The development of our species was marked by struggle. Scarcities of food could last several months. The human, like many other mammals, adjusted to a "feast or famine" environment created by seasonal changes. In periods of abundance, our primitive ancestors probably gorged themselves, acquiring layers of fat tissue. In seasons of scarcity, their bodies burned their own fat to survive. Modern science has nearly eliminated the seasonal fluctuation of food availability. Unfortunately, no one told our metabolisms.

The results of this phenomenon can be very troubling, but also interesting. Dieting to lose weight, in fact, might tell our brain that the body is starving. When the brain receives this message, it slows the metabolism down to conserve fat. When the dieter stops dieting and food is once again plentiful, our body tells us to feast and gain weight for the next period of starvation (dieting). Obesity, from the body's point of view, is desirable.

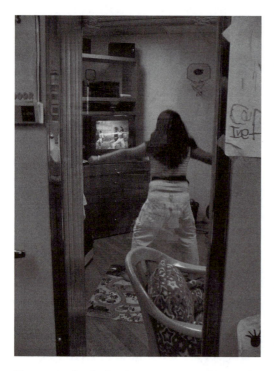

Room-sized calorimeters are one tool to assist in the fight against obesity. (U.S. Department of Agriculture)

We can see why obesity has become a modern-day problem, a problem of affluence. Unfortunately, even poor countries are experiencing sharp rises in obesity as they become more Westernized. Consequently, obesity has become a focus for both national and international organizations, particularly health organizations. The World Health Organization (WHO) now considers obesity to be a global epidemic with more than 250 million adults obese, and many more who are overweight. The United Nations Educational, Scientific, and Cultural Organization (UNESCO) has organized a fact-finding committee to assess the obesity problem in third world countries. In 2004, the U.S. Department of Health and Human Services (HHS), for the first time, classified obesity as a disease. In 2005, the U.S. Department of Agriculture (USDA) and HHS jointly published the Dietary Guidelines for Americans, the culmination of a five-year cooperative project to assist overweight Americans in their search for a healthier lifestyle.

Unfortunately, obesity will continue to be a problem until the world—particularly the West—deemphasizes junk and fast foods, the sedentary lifestyle (both at work and at play), and, ironically, its obsession with dieting. Scientists are beginning to voice the belief that dieting does not work for at least 90 percent of the people who diet. Obesity can best be managed by the adoption of a healthy lifestyle that emphasizes exercise, conscious and careful eating habits, and acceptance of one's body, no matter what shape it is in.

**Outlook**   According to journalist Mike Adams (2004), "There's a war brewing over obesity. [T]he leaders and promoters of western medicine, who are saying that obesity is now a disease, [are on one side]. . . . [A] growing group of people who are fighting against this idea [are on the other]." Overweight Americans question the cultural fiat that stigmatizes obesity. Even the word *obesity* itself has come under attack by large-size Americans who find *fat* honest and descriptive of a certain body type. *Obesity,* they insist, is identified with an obsessive food consumer, a glutton. In as much as gluttony is one of the seven deadly sins, overweight people are judged as moral misfits. Many fat activist groups contest this assumption; the most vigilant is the National Association to Advance Fat Acceptance (NAAFA), founded in 1969. NAAFA feels that discrimination against fat Americans is nowhere more true than in the scientific professions, which have consistently failed fat people. According to many fat Americans, *obesity* is not only a clinical diagnosis, it is also a moral indictment.

The scientific community bases its opinions on the grounds that obesity is unhealthy. Many health issues are either unique to or exacerbated by obesity: cardiovascular, endocrinal, metabolic, gastrointestinal, renal and genitourinary, integument (skin and appendages), musculoskeletal, neurological, respiratory, and psychological disorders. Organizations such as NAAFA point to the dismal statistics of weight loss programs: 95 to 98 percent of diets fail over three years; furthermore, science can't decide whether excess weight or excessive dieting is the real culprit. As a result, NAAFA wants the research agenda to change from a focus on finding ways to make fat people thin to ways to make fat people healthy. NAAFA also accuses the diet industry of setting dieters up to fail in order to keep the market for their products.

**Healthy or Unhealthy: What the Health Professional Sees**    According to the World Health Organization (WHO), obesity is spreading throughout the world as more and more nations adopt Western diets. Obesity burdens the most vulnerable people in society: children and adolescents, the poor and working poor. Experts believe that 300,000 people a year die because of obesity. Furthermore, obesity is one of the most preventable causes of death, second only to smoking. Obesity, according to these experts, causes or exacerbates almost every major health problem including cancer and hearth disease. The National Institutes of Health (NIH), the Office of the Surgeon General, and the WHO also point to the double-bind of fat people: they suffer physically, and they are then punished socially. A study that followed obese adolescents found that "compared to thinner peers, overweight girls completed fewer years of school, were twenty percent less likely to be married, and had ten percent higher rates of household poverty." Although health professionals agree that fat people face discrimination, they criticize any movement that would casually accept obesity. This concern is voiced by Susan S. Bartell, a psychologist who specializes in women's weight issues: "it is a part of a greater tendency in this country toward not working hard to do what we should be doing. We want to take the easy way out. Fat acceptance is about taking the easy way out" (Skomal, 2005).

**Healthy or Unhealthy: What the Fat Person Sees**    Fat activists vehemently challenge these assertions, particularly that obesity causes death. Representing the estimated 38 million Americans whose weight is above average, NAAFA responds to the health issue this way: "Just being fat does not signify poor health. In fact, research shows that the health risks once associated with weight may instead be attributable to yo-yo dieting. Because fatness is most often caused by heredity and dieting history [and because most diets fail], it is becoming apparent that remaining at a high, but stable weight and concentrating on personal fitness rather than thinness may be the healthiest way to deal with the propensity to be fat."

Furthermore, fat activists point out that because fat people must deal with insensitivity in the medical profession, many do not seek treatment for illnesses clearly unrelated to their weight. Doctors often insist that fat patients, regardless of their complaint, must lose weight. As one fat activist suggested, if you go to your doctor because your feet hurt, and she says you need to lose weight, ask her, "And what do you do for thin people whose feet hurt?" This sarcastic response raises a serious point. If prejudicial doctors assume weight is always related to their fat patient's illness, they might overlook a real cause. Some professionals may see obesity as an exaggerated threat, especially in cases of prescribed treatment. Fat activists are shocked by the use of bariatric surgery to "cure" obesity; having a part of one's stomach removed, they insist, is an amputation that should only be considered for immediate life-and-death situations, such as unresponsive infections and cancers.

According to activist Marilyn Wann, fat Americans are not supporting overeating or unhealthy relationships with food. The goal of fat activism for a healthy lifestyle is not far from mainstream medical advice: emphasizing general health over any specific focus on one problem. People of all sizes should be encouraged to eat sensible, well-balanced meals. All people should avoid refined sugars and fatty foods as much as possible. Most important—and the issue about which both sides find common ground—is the need for regular exercise. Dieting alone is not a panacea for good health and a happy life. The issues surrounding obesity are not likely to go away any time soon.

*Mary Jo Thomas*

*See also* Atkins, Robert C.; Bariatric Surgery; Body Mass Index (BMI); Diabetes: Nutrition; Ornish, Dean; Pritikin, Nathan; Weight Watchers.

### References

Adams, Mike. "Anti-Obesity Activists Fight for Fat Acceptance: Here's Where They're Right and Wrong on Issues of Obesity." *News Target,* August 6, 2004.

Fairburn, Christopher G., and Kelly D. Brownell. *Eating Disorders and Obesity: A Comprehensive Handbook.* 2nd ed. New York: Guilford Press, 2005.

Gard, Michael. *The Obesity Epidemic.* New York: Routledge, 2005.

Rothblum, Esther, Sondra Solovay, and Marilyn Wann. *Fat Studies Reader.* New York: New York University Press, 2009.

Skomal, Lenore. "Love the Shape You're In: A National Movement Is Afoot to Redefine Way We See Ourselves." *Her Times,* September 16, 2005.

## OBSESSIVE-COMPULSIVE DISORDER (OCD)

The defining features of obsessive-compulsive disorder (OCD) are recurrent, uncontrollable thoughts (obsessions) and actions (compulsions). The most common mental disorder coexisting with OCD is depression. Prevalence estimates vary widely, but researchers have reported that up to two-thirds of people with OCD may develop depression at some point in their lives.

Obsessions are intrusive, upsetting thoughts that keep coming back despite efforts to push them away. Because the thoughts cause so much anxiety, people try to counteract them with some physical or mental act, which is where compulsions come into play. Compulsions are ritualistic actions that people feel driven to perform in an effort to reduce the anxiety produced by an obsession.

Typical obsessions involve frequent, exaggerated thoughts about being diseased, dirty, or sinful, or doing abhorrent things. Examples of common compulsions include repetitively washing one's hands, cleaning, checking the locks, putting objects in order, counting, or silently saying a phrase. Such obsessions and rituals control people with OCD rather than the other way around, preoccupying their thoughts and consuming time that could otherwise have been spent doing more productive things.

OCD affects about 2.2 million U.S. adults, striking men and women in roughly equal numbers. It usually starts in childhood, adolescence, or early adulthood. Compared to those with OCD alone, people whose OCD is combined with major depression tend to have more severe and longer-lasting OCD symptoms as well as a greater number of hospitalizations and suicide attempts.

Although adding depression to the mix makes treatment a bit more complicated, both disorders usually respond well to medication and/or psychotherapy. With appropriate treatment, most people are able to feel better, reduce their obsessions and compulsions, and regain control of their lives.

**Criteria for Diagnosis** The symptoms of OCD are defined by the *Diagnostic and Statistical Manual of Mental Disorders,* 4th edition, text revision (*DSM–IV–TR*), a diagnostic guidebook published by the American Psychiatric Association (2000) and widely used by mental health professionals from many disciplines. People with OCD have obsessions and compulsions that cause serious distress, take up more than an hour a day, or interfere with daily activities. Most adults with the disorder recognize that their obsessive thoughts and compulsive behaviors are excessive or unreasonable, but they feel powerless to stop. Children may not realize that their behavior is out of the ordinary, however.

Obsessions are recurring, unwanted thoughts, impulses, or mental images that intrude into people's minds and cause great distress or anxiety. These thoughts are more than just excessive worries about real-life problems. Typical themes include being very fearful of dirt or disease, having repeated doubts, and keeping things orderly or symmetrical. Some people experience disturbing aggressive impulses or mental images of distressing sexual scenes. Despite efforts to ignore or suppress such thoughts, the obsessions keep coming back time and again.

**Treatment** When people have OCD and depression simultaneously, both conditions need to be addressed during treatment. Below are some of the main treatment options for OCD. For psychotherapy treatment, cognitive-behavioral therapy (CBT) helps people identify maladaptive thought and behavior patterns and replace them with more adaptive ones. One offshoot of CBT developed specifically for treating OCD is called exposure and response prevention. The exposure part of the treatment involves confronting thoughts and situations that provoke obsession-related distress. The response-prevention part involves voluntarily refraining from using compulsions to reduce distress during these encounters. For medication treatment, selective serotonin reuptake inhibitors (SSRIs), a widely prescribed class of antidepressants, can help relieve symptoms of anxiety as well as depression. SSRIs are considered a first-choice treatment for OCD. If these medications do not provide enough relief, a tricyclic antidepressant called clomipramine may be used instead.

**Compulsions** Compulsions are ritualistic behaviors (e.g., washing and cleaning, arranging objects in order, checking something repeatedly) or mental acts (e.g., counting, repeating words silently) that people feel driven to do over and over in response to an obsession or according to rigid rules. The rituals are aimed at reducing distress or preventing some calamity from occurring. However, they are either clearly excessive or not connected in a realistic way to what they are intended to prevent. At best, the rituals provide only temporary relief from the anxiety caused by obsessions.

Shared genetic factors may help explain why OCD and major depression occur together so often. Major depression is more common in the close family members of people with OCD than in the family members of those without the disorder. Biological and environmental factors may play central roles as well. When people have both OCD and major depression, the OCD usually comes first.

Obsessions and compulsions can be very demoralizing and disruptive to everyday life, and the stress created by them may trigger depression in some people. It is also possible that abnormalities in brain function and chemistry associated with OCD could render the brain itself more vulnerable to the development of other disorders, including depression.

There is some evidence that depression in people with OCD may differ somewhat from garden-variety depression. Both people with OCD plus depression and those with major depression alone are prone to experiencing a low mood, loss of interest in most activities, lack of energy, trouble concentrating, and suicidal thoughts. But those with OCD plus depression are less likely to have difficulty sleeping and changes in appetite, and they are more likely to experience inner tension and pessimism.

These differences in symptoms may derive from differences in brain physiology. For instance, researchers have found that people with major depression alone tend to have increased metabolic activity in the thalamus, a structure inside the brain that acts as a relay station for sensory input, filtering out important information from the mass of incoming signals. In contrast, people with both major depression and OCD tend to have decreased activity in the thalamus.

The response to antidepressants also differs, suggesting that there may be underlying differences in brain chemistry as well. SSRIs, which increase the available supply of a chemical called serotonin in the brain, can help relieve symptoms of both OCD and depression. But higher doses may be needed when OCD is present, compared to the doses needed to treat major depression by itself. Other types of antidepressants that work well for people with major depression alone do not seem to be as effective for those with OCD.

*Linda Wasmer Andrews*

*See also* Depression; Stress; Suicide.

## References

American Psychiatric Association. *Diagnostic and Statistical Manual of Mental Disorders.* 4th ed., text rev. Washington, DC: American Psychiatric Association, 2000.

*Anxiety Disorders.* National Institute of Mental Health. 2007. www.nimh.nih.gov/health/publications/anxiety-disorders/summary.shtml.

Fineberg, Naomi A., Hannelie Fourie, Tim M. Gale, and Thanusha Sivakumaran. "Comorbid Depression in Obsessive Compulsive Disorder (OCD): Symptomatic Differences to Major Depressive Disorder." *Journal of Affective Disorders* 87 (2005): 327–30.

Fineberg, Naomi A., Sanjaya Saxena, Joseph Zohar, and Kevin J. Craig. "Obsessive-Compulsive Disorder: Boundary Issues." *CNS Spectrums* 12 (2007): 359–64, 367–75.

Foa, Edna B., and Linda Wasmer Andrews. *If Your Adolescent Has an Anxiety Disorder: An Essential Resource for Parents.* New York: Oxford University Press, 2006.

Hong, Jin Pyo, Jack Samuels, O. Joseph Bienvenu III, Paul Cannistraro, Marco Grados, Mark A. Riddle, et al. "Clinical Correlates of Recurrent Major Depression in Obsessive-Compulsive Disorder." *Depression and Anxiety* 20 (2004): 86–91.

*Obsessive-Compulsive Disorder (OCD).* Mayo Clinic. December 21, 2006. www.mayoclinic.com/health/obsessive-compulsive-disorder/DS00189.

Obsessive-Compulsive Foundation, P.O. Box 961029, Boston, MA 02196. (617) 973–5801. www.ocfoundation.org.

*Practice Guideline for the Treatment of Patients with Obsessive-Compulsive Disorder.* American Psychiatric Association. July 2007. www.psychiatryonline.com/pracGuide/pracGuide Topic_10.aspx.

*When Unwanted Thoughts Take Over: Obsessive Compulsive Disorder.* National Institute of Mental Health. June 26, 2008. www.nimh.nih.gov/health/publications/when-unwanted-thoughts-take-over-obsessive-compulsive-disorder/summary.shtml.

## OMEGA 3/6 FATTY ACIDS. *See* FATS

## ONLINE HEALTH RESOURCES

The past two decades have seen the use of the Internet for everything, ranging from leisure to business. The reason for this growth is simple—the Internet provides an easy medium for the widespread dissemination of information to the public. In the area of health care, a plethora of Internet health resources have cropped up, ranging from information websites to direct online consultation with physicians or other health care professionals. The advent of these online health resources has allowed patients quick access to basic medical information. It is increasingly common for patients to search for tips on how to live healthfully or to search for possible explanations to their symptoms.

As of 2002, as many as 80 percent of individuals reported having looked up health information online at least once, with even more among select demographics, such as college graduates (Pew Research Center, 2005). This trend holds incredible potential. This means that patients can readily access basic health information without having to contact a health care professional. Furthermore, it enables patients to educate themselves and take on a greater role in managing their own health, helping patients ask the right questions of their physicians, and more.

Unfortunately, the flip side to this trend is the danger of misinformation present on the Internet. While there are accurate, credible sources available online, unfortunately many are not without factual problems. Whether intentionally erroneous, biased, or just incomplete—online health resources can give patients inappropriate expectations when they visit their physicians. This can have deleterious effects on the patient-physician relationship if the physician is unable to provide the treatment or course of action that a patient expects from reading online resources (Erdem and Harrison-Walker, 2006).

The Medical Library Association (MLA) maintains a guide to help patients navigate the maze of online health resources (Medical Library Association, n.d.).

First, the guide recommends that patients identify the sponsorship of the website. Government, educational institution, and professional organization websites are generally reliable sources (.gov, .edu, and .org addresses). While commercial and independent websites may still contain good information, it is important for patients to recognize that commercial information may be biased in order to promote a particular treatment or product. Furthermore, patients should attempt to identify whether information given is referenced from a professional or otherwise reliable source, as well as checking to see if the information is current or recently updated. The MLA guide keeps a brief list of useful, credible online health resources for consumers to go to for information, available at www.mlanet.org/resources/userguide.html.

However, even with credible sources such as these, it is important for patients to remember online health resources are not a substitute for the evaluation or diagnosis by their physician or primary care provider. Additionally, individuals should follow their physicians' instructions, even if those instructions do not agree with information they may have discovered online. With a little bit of care and effort, consumers can check the credibility of online health information. With the right attitude, online resources will be able to serve as a valuable tool for patients to use to educate themselves and enhance the quality of their care.

*David Chen*

*See also* Doctors in the Media; Primary Care Physicians; Virtual Hospital.

## References

Erdem, Altan S., and Harrison-Walker, Jean L. "The Role of the Internet in Physician-Patient Relationships: The Issue of Trust." *Business Horizons* 49 (2006): 387–93.

Medical Library Association. "A User's Guide to Finding and Evaluating Health Information on the Web." www.mlahq.org/resources/userguide.html.

Pew Research Center. Pew/Internet and American Life Project. *Health Information Online,* by Susanna Fox. 2005. www.pewinternet.org/reports/2005/Health-Information-Online.aspx.

## ORGANIC FOOD

Organics are the new darling of the food industry. More than a niche market, they have expanded during the past decade by a healthy 20 percent annually, while other industries struggle to stay afloat. Statistics from the Organic Trade Association's "2011 Organic Industry Survey" showed total sales of U.S. organic products at more than $28 billion for 2010, a 7 percent increase from the previous year (Roberts, 2011). The 2010 sales figures were well above organic food and beverage sales of $17 billion in 2006, according to U.S. Department of Agriculture (USDA) figures (Food and Drug Administration, 2008). Everyone from Trader Joe's and Whole Foods to Wal-Mart and the big-box supermarkets are rushing to fill their shelves, produce bins, and meat counters with anything and everything organic.

## Dirty Dozen of Foods with Most Pesticide

The "dirty dozen" of foods that are most likely to have pesticide and chemicals include apples, cherries, grapes, peaches, nectarines, pears, lettuce, strawberries, bell peppers, celery, potatoes, and spinach. The U.S. Food and Drug Administration (FDA) routinely tests produce for harmful chemicals like pesticides, fungicides, and herbicides. The FDA rates the foods on a scale of 1 to 100 based on how much measurable pesticide residue it contains after the produce is washed. A low rating means a food has small amounts of chemical residue; numbers closest to 100 represent the highest pesticide levels.

Strawberries have one of the highest levels of pesticide residue. Their score of 82 is influenced by their soft skin. Strawberries are among the most heavily chemically treated fruits in this country.

Apples top the list with a score of 89. U.S.-grown cherries rated a 75, although domestically grown cherries contained significantly higher pesticide levels than imported cherries. Grapes were the opposite; domestic grapes had a rating of 43, but imported grapes had a higher rating of 65.

Of all the fruits, peaches received the highest rating of 100, making them the fruit with the most harmful residue levels in the United States. Nectarines, a sister to the peach, were lower at 84. Pears also have a lower number of 65.

The vegetables on the list included lettuce with an FDA rating of 59. The other vegetables on the list ranged from bell peppers, celery, and potatoes to spinach. The peppers and celery rated between 85 and 86; both contained high pesticide residues.

More than 60 percent of nonorganic spinach tested by the FDA showed traces of pesticides, including DDT. It has an FDA rating of 60. Finally, potatoes had the lowest rating of the "dirty dozen," at 58.

*—Sharon Zoumbaris*

As the small and large organic producers jockey to get their products to consumers, the big corporations new to organics are working to change the stringent organic rules to avoid the higher costs that come from having to meet such exacting standards. This leaves small-scale organic farmers struggling to keep their customers in the face of rising food prices and fierce competition from the big players.

In this mad dash to give consumers unprecedented organic choices, the questions remain, are organics healthier or just more expensive? And are they better for the environment, farmers, or consumers? Another major issue looming over the organic food industry is the question of scale. Does the move toward industrial-sized organic farming undermine the benefits and identity of organic food itself? Or is it a logical way to introduce more consumers to organics? That red-hot debate between "little organics" and "big organics" is a factor in purchasing decisions for some Americans. From the earliest days, supporters of organic farming envisioned a way to feed people and build a food ecosystem using sustainable practices, working with rather than against nature. Another aim of organic agriculture was to nurture the earth and achieve a harmonious fit with the land and the local community. Organic food today remains a reaction to the use of synthetic fertilizers in industrial agriculture, which depletes the soil, pushes small farmers off the land, and replaces them with single-crop agribusiness operations.

**Labels**   In the food industry, labels are a tool consumers use to gauge the value of a product. *Organic* is one of the most recognized labels in today's supermarkets, but many consumers remain confused about the different organic designations. According to the USDA, all packaged or processed food using the term *100% Organic* must contain all organic ingredients. Production processes have to meet federal organic standards and be independently verified by accredited inspectors. A different label, *USDA Organic,* faces less strict standards: up to 5 percent of their total ingredients excluding salt and water may come from nonorganic or synthetic sources. Items labeled *Made with organic ingredients* must include at least 70 percent organic components; the remaining 30 percent must come from the USDA-approved list of additives and synthetic ingredients. Produce, fruits, and vegetables labeled organic have to be grown without synthetic pesticides and synthetic fertilizers, and cannot be genetically engineered or irradiated.

Organic beef or chicken may not be cloned animals; must be raised on 100 percent organic feed; may not be given growth hormones, antibiotics, or other drugs; and cannot be irradiated. The USDA has no laws concerning seafood standards. This means fish can be labeled organic even if it contains contaminants such as mercury or polychlorinated biphenyls (PCBs) as long as it doesn't use *certified organic* logos.

The use of *natural* or *all natural* on a label by the USDA for meat and poultry means the meat contains no artificial flavorings, colors, chemical preservatives, or synthetic ingredients. *Grass-fed* on a label suggests a diet of natural grass, but it also applies to cattle fed grass indoors in a pen or only allowed outside for the first few months of their lives. The label *pasture-raised* refers to animals that were allowed to roam freely outdoors where they ate grasses and other plants.

Any dairy product with an organic label comes from cows fed 100 percent organic feed but no bovine growth hormone (BGH) or antibiotics. Organic eggs come from hens fed 100 percent organic feed, raised without growth hormones or antibiotics. The term *cage-free* for poultry or eggs means little because the birds may still live in crowded, unhealthy conditions.

The label *free-range* or *free-roaming* on eggs or chicken suggests the animals spent time outdoors. However, U.S. government standards for these terms are vague and do not guarantee different conditions than those for animals raised in conventional factory farms. In other words, if a coop door is open for five minutes a day and the birds remain packed inside, the eggs or chicken can legally be labeled free-range.

**Is Organic Food Better or Just More Expensive?**   Organic food products routinely cost more than their conventional counterparts, which supporters say just means organic farmers get paid a fair price for their food and their labor. Ask supporters of organic food, and they will tell you the extra money spent on organic products is part of a daily contribution to their health and the health of the planet. These advocates say there are hidden costs in cheap conventional foods, including the price of environmental damage from pesticides and synthetic fertilizers; waste and overuse of energy resources needed for fertilizing, harvesting, and processing food and for transporting it thousands of miles; the effects on human health from toxic residues left by arsenic, added hormones, and antibiotics; worsening soil quality; and an increasing lack of biodiversity.

Supporters of organics say that if these elements were factored into conventional food prices, consumers would pay less in comparison for organics. Another reason organic food is more expensive, advocates say, is that the U.S. government pays subsidies to conventional growers. That money keeps prices low in the grocery stores even though consumers eventually pay for the subsidies through increased taxes. According to supporters of organics foods, this amounts to corporate welfare for big agribusiness from the USDA and the federal government.

Over time, the formula for subsidies based on crop type and volume has changed; now two commodities, corn and soybeans, receive more than 70 percent of the earmarked federal funds. USDA statistics for the period from 1995 to 2003 showed that three-quarters of the subsidies went to the top 10 percent of growers. In other words, the government subsidies supported big industrial operations rather than small family farms (Kingsolver, Hopp, & Kingsolver, 2007). In 2007, Indiana Senator Richard Lugar criticized those subsidies, still in place today, and said they hurt the family farmer. Ironically, the Federal Farm Bill that governs subsidies was originally introduced after the Great Depression as a way to alleviate poverty among small farmers and rural communities.

By providing subsidies for commodities the government creates a situation where fruits and vegetables, which do not receive the same price supports, are more expensive calorie for calorie. For example, a dollar can buy more than 1,000 calories of fast food but only 200 or so calories of fresh fruit. For families with a limited income, the choice comes down to having a larger quantity of food to eat instead of having a smaller amount of fresh fruits and vegetables. Another issue for low-income families is access to fresh fruits and vegetables due to what authorities are calling food deserts. The term *food desert* is defined as a geographic area that lacks access to affordable healthy foods due to distance from a supermarket or large grocery store combined with no easy access to transportation. According to the Centers for Disease Control and Prevention, food deserts exist in the United States, although estimates of how many Americans are affected varies greatly.

Add to this equation the fact that organic food continues to cost on average more than its conventional counterparts and it is easy to see that low-income Americans face significant hurdles in finding and purchasing organic food. Price remains a big obstacle even as the government supports projects such as farmer's markets, community gardens, and other types of programs aimed at increasing the availability of fresh food in urban and rural settings. The USDA's Community

Food Projects Competitive Grant program is an example of the government's support of these programs.

**Nutritional Values** For decades studies that compared the nutrition of conventional crops and their organic counterparts could find little difference. However, as the organic market grows, so does the body of research and scientists are now producing results that dispute earlier industry-sponsored studies. The "Fruit and Soil Quality of Organic and Conventional Strawberry Agroecosystems," a study led by a Washington State University professor, while limited to organic strawberries, is being called the most comprehensive, and persuasive, of the new studies showing clear nutritional benefits from organic farming. Scientists have applauded the design of the research as both comprehensive and meticulous. Those researchers concluded that the organically grown strawberries were superior in taste and nutritional quality as well as being better for the soil than conventional strawberries (Reganold, 2010).

A 2009 French study, which also concluded there were nutritional benefits to organically grown food, went on to dispute earlier data released by the United Kingdom's Food Standards Agency. That report found no difference between conventionally grown food and organically grown food. The French scientists criticized the British report, suggesting their conclusions were based on extremely limited data and at the same time ignored the potential chemical or pesticide exposure to consumers and also ignored environmental issues.

These results followed another study led by Charles Benbrook, former executive director of the Board of Agriculture of the National Academy of Sciences, which concluded that "the average serving of organic plant-based food contains about 25 percent more of the nutrients encompassed in the study than a comparable-sized serving of the same food produced by conventional farming methods" (Benbrook, 2008). Although the two-year project focused on plant foods, it also suggested that there was strong evidence that poultry and livestock raised on organic food produced meat, milk, and eggs with higher levels of protein, more vitamins and minerals, and improved levels of heart-healthy fats.

As new research results continue to be released organic supporters say the argument needs to shift from an examination of differences between organically and conventionally grown food and focus instead on the potential health benefits of eating organic foods rather than foods treated with chemicals, pesticides, drugs, or hormones.

**The Future of Organics** Americans are willing to pay for something they place a high value on, but they are extremely value-conscious consumers. What does that mean for organic food? Stores such as Whole Foods and Trader Joe's are thriving, thanks in part to their ability to sell at increasing volumes, while offering organic products at lower prices. The increase in organics in many more stores, including Wal-Mart, means that families of all economic levels will have increased access to organic choices. In fact, up to 57 percent of organic shoppers now buy their food at mainstream grocery stores and discounters rather than at smaller health food stores, according to statistics from the Food Marketing Institute

(Fromartz, 2006). Still, in tough economic times American consumers may not care where or how their chicken or beef was grown as long as the cost is low.

On the other hand, American consumers are turning in increasing numbers to farmer's markets and the growing number of community gardens, especially in urban areas to find low-cost organically grown food. A growing number of Americans interested in supporting small organic farms are buying directly from farmers through efforts called community-supported agriculture programs or CSAs. For a yearly or monthly fee, members receive fresh, organic produce throughout the growing season. For example, one week's order might include broccoli, peppers, zucchini, and melon but not out-of-season produce such as potatoes, grapes, or strawberries.

Will the power of this alternative food economy be able to shape Americans' opinions about the benefits of organic food? Although no one can be absolutely certain of the outcome, supporters of organics hope time will prove them right before too much damage is done to the environment or to our nation's health.

*Sharon Zoumbaris*

*See also* Antibiotics; Irradiation; Nutrition.

## References

Benbrook, Charles, Xin Zhao, Jaime Yanez, Neal Davies, and Preston Andrews. "New Evidence Confirms the Nutritional Superiority of Plant-Based Organic Foods." *Organic Center Critical Issue Report,* March 2008, 42. www.organic-center.org.

Center for Food Safety. "Organic and Beyond." www.centerforfoodsafety.org/organic_an.cfm.

Food and Drug Administration. "National Organic Program: Proposed Amendment to the National List of Allowed and Prohibited Substances." *Federal Register* 73, no. 135 (July 14, 2008): 40200.

Fromartz, Samuel. *Organic, Inc.: Natural Foods and How They Grew.* Orlando, FL: Harcourt, 2006.

Greene, Cathy. "Organic Labeling." In *Economics of Food Labeling,* edited by Elise Golan, Fred Kuchler, and Lorraine Mitchell, Agricultural Economic Report No. 793. USDA Economic Research Service. January 2001. www.ers.usda.gov/publications/aer793/aer 793g.pdf.

Kingsolver, Barbara, Steven L. Hopp, and Camille Kingsolver. *Animal, Vegetable, Miracle: A Year of Food Life.* New York: HarperCollins, 2007.

Lawrence, Felicity. "Organic Milk Higher in Nutrients." *Guardian,* January 7, 2005, 10.

Mosteller, Rachel. "Thinking Globally, Eating Locally in the USA." *USA Today,* May 4, 2007, sec. D, 6.

Parks, Louis B. "Getting to the Root of the Issue: New USDA Labels Cultivate Recognition of Organic Industry." *Houston Chronicle,* October 13, 2002, 1.

Reganold, J.P., P.K. Andrews, J.R. Reeve, L. Carpenter-Boggs, C.W. Schadt, et al. "Fruit and Soil Quality of Organic and Conventional Strawberry Agroecosystems." *PLoS ONE* 5, no. 9 (September 2010): e12346. doi:10.1371/journal.pone.0012346. www.plosone.org.

Roberts, William A., Jr. "Natural and Organic in the Marketplace." *Prepared Foods* 180, no. 6 (June 2011): 51.

# ORNISH, DEAN

Dr. Dean Ornish (born July 16, 1953, in Dallas) is a physician who has developed a system he maintains is scientifically proven to reverse heart disease without drugs or surgery, replacing those invasive techniques with a very-low-fat diet, exercise, and stress management. And unlike many diet book authors, Ornish has published research findings about his program in medical journals such as the *Journal of the American Medical Association* and the *American Journal of Cardiology*.

The doctor, whose best-selling books include *Dr. Dean Ornish's Program for Reversing Heart Disease: The Only System Scientifically Proven to Reverse Heart Disease without Drugs or Surgery* (1990); *Eat More, Weigh Less: Dr. Dean Ornish's Life Choice Program for Losing Weight Safely While Eating* (1993); *Stress, Diet and Your Heart* (1982), first gained attention from the medical community in 1989 when he released data showing a reduction in overall heart blockages in his patients. What was unusual was that the improvement came not from the standard treatment of drugs or surgery, but instead from a high-fiber, low-fat, vegetarian diet along with stress-management techniques.

His most recent book, *The Spectrum* (2007), is a lifestyle and diet program rather than a specific or strict diet plan. Ornish explains in the book there are no rules, forbidden foods, or guilt, just a blueprint to help individuals determine where they fit on a spectrum of healthy choices and how they can make healthy changes to reduce their risk of diseases often associated with obesity.

In 2008 Ornish published a randomized controlled trial in collaboration with Dr. Peter Carroll, Chair of Urology at the UCSF School of Medicine, and the late Dr. William Fair, Chair of Urologic Oncology at Memorial Sloan-Kettering Cancer Center, that indicated the progression of early-stage prostate cancer may be stopped or even reversed with diet and lifestyle changes. Additional studies listed on the Preventive Medicine Research Institute (PMRI) website and published in November 2008 in *The Lancet Oncology* showed that diet and lifestyle changes significantly increased telomerase and telomere length. Telomeres are located on the end of chromosomes and are thought to control longevity. According to the findings, this is the first time any type of lifestyle change had been shown to increase telomerase.

Founder and president of the Preventive Medicine Research Institute of the University of California at San Francisco, Ornish champions what other cardiologists at first labeled "radical" ideas. Many in the medical establishment still continue to insist Americans will never find a soy and plant diet acceptable.

Ornish wasn't always a maverick. Growing up in Dallas, he was a straight-A student in high school. While at Rice University, he came down with a case of mononucleosis and returned to his parents' home to recuperate. There he met the Swami Satchidananda, who was staying with the Ornish family during a lecture tour. Under the swami's influence, Ornish said in a *Discover* magazine interview (Grady, 1987) that he started to practice yoga, meditate, and eat a vegetarian diet. Following his recovery, Ornish transferred from Rice to the University of Texas at Austin and graduated first in his class in 1975.

His next move was to the Baylor College of Medicine in Houston, and it was there Ornish said he began questioning the standard treatment for heart patients. At the time, the Baylor-affiliated Texas Medical Center was a world leader in coronary-bypass operations. Yet years later Ornish told *Discover* that "having a bypass without changing your lifestyle is like trying to mop up the floor around an overflowing sink without turning off the faucet" (Grady, 1987, p. 55). In 1977 Ornish conducted his first medical experiment, a study titled "The Effects of Stress Management and a Low-Cholesterol Diet on Heart Disease." That study showed that after only 30 days on his plan, subjects said their chest pain was somewhat alleviated and more blood was flowing to their hearts. After graduating from Baylor, Ornish started his internship and residency at Massachusetts General Hospital, a Harvard University affiliate. By the time Ornish left Harvard in 1984, he had completed his internship and residency, conducted more original research, and published his first book, *Stress, Diet and Your Heart*.

In the summer of 1984 Ornish moved to San Francisco and established the Preventive Medicine Research Institute with Shirley E. Brown, whom he later married. The institute is based in Sausalito and is affiliated with the University of California at San Francisco, where Ornish joined the faculty as an assistant clinical professor of medicine. National recognition came in 1988 and 1989 following another Ornish study. He presented those results at a meeting of the American Heart Association and went on to win grants from the National Institutes of Health, among other major research organizations.

His work continued to achieve mainstream success when the Mutual of Omaha Insurance Company in 1993 agreed to provide full reimbursement to patients enrolled in Ornish's program for reversing heart disease. In the spring of 2000 the Health Care Financing Administration announced a demonstration project involving the Ornish program as an alternative to conventional medical treatments for selected Medicare patients. Meanwhile, dozens of health insurers now reimburse the cost of Dr. Ornish's program for selected patients. Today the idea of a low-fat diet is more acceptable to mainstream cardiologists who recommend that patients make food choices based on the U.S. Department of Agriculture Food Guide Pyramid or the so-called Mediterranean diet, which is rich in fruits, vegetables, and whole grains.

Ornish admits that there is nothing new about his approach that, in fact, is similar to the low-fat food plan developed in the 1970s by the late Nathan Pritikin, the California inventor, author, and founder of the Pritikin Longevity Center. In the late 1950s Pritikin was diagnosed with heart disease following an angina attack. Dissatisfied with the standard treatment for heart disease, Pritikin began to experiment with his diet. After seeing favorable results from his regime, he wrote several books, including his bestsellers, *The Pritikin Program for Diet and Exercise* (1979) and *The Pritikin Promise: 28 Days to a Longer, Healthier Life* (1983). Pritikin, like Ornish, promoted a diet filed with fresh fruits, vegetables, and whole grains, with only 10 percent of calories from fat. And like Ornish, Pritikin was also criticized by some doctors who called his diet unnecessarily severe.

Dr. John McDougall is another physician who developed a low-fat, vegetarian eating program, similar to the Ornish plan. McDougall established the St. Helena Health Center in 1987, located in California's Napa Valley. He is also the author of several best-selling diet books, including *The McDougall Plan* (1985), *The McDougall Program for Maximum Weight Loss* (1994), and *The McDougall Program for a Healthy Heart* (1996).

Ornish continues to break new ground in his research. In the 1998 book *Love and Survival: The Scientific Basis for the Healing Power of Intimacy,* he offers readers clinical and anecdotal evidence as well as research findings to support his newest theory that having deeply intimate, loving relationships can be invaluable in preventing and treating heart disease. The book classifies love broadly from the love of a mate to the love of family, friends, and God. But the overall message, along with his dedication to Molly, whom he married in 1998, remains that love and intimacy are among the most powerful factors in determining a person's health or illness.

*Marjolijn Bijlefeld and Sharon Zoumbaris*

*See also* Atkins, Robert C.; Pritikin, Nathan; Vegetarians.

## References

Brink, Susan. "The Low-Fat Life." *U.S. News & World Report,* July 12 1999, 56.

Condor, Bob. "Lifestyle Changes Can Go Right to the Heart." *Chicago Tribune,* February 13, 2000, 3.

Cowley, Geoffrey. "Healer of Hearts." *Newsweek,* March 16, 1998, 50–57.

"Dean Ornish." *Contemporary Authors Online.* Detroit: Gale, 2001.

Grady, Denise. "Can Heart Disease Be Reversed?" *Discover,* March 1987, 54–66.

Ornish, Dean. "Healing Broken Hearts." *Nutrition Action Healthletter* 26, no. 5 (June 1999): 1.

Ornish, Dean, J. Lin, J. Daubenmier, G. Weidner, E. Epel, C. Kemp, M.J. Magbanua, R. Marlin, L. Yglecias, P.R. Carroll, and E.H. Blackburn. "Increased Telomerase Activity and Comprehensive Lifestyle Changes: A Pilot Study." *Lancet Oncology* (November 9, 2008): 1048–57.

Perlmutter, Cathy. "Heal Your Heart with Love: America's Favorite Doctor Dean Ornish Gives Advice on Preventing Heart Attacks." *Prevention,* August 1998, 118–25.

## OSTEOPOROSIS

Osteoporosis, also known as "porous bones," causes bones to weaken and become susceptible to breaks and fractures. The root cause of the disorder is related to the process of how bones constantly remodel themselves. Osteoblasts create new bone in response to signals in the blood. Osteoclasts serve to break down bone, and they miraculously know when to stop. When this delicate dance becomes imbalanced, bone loss can exceed bone replacement, leading to osteoporosis.

In the United States alone, approximately 10 million people suffer from this bone disorder. Of those, approximately 8 million sufferers are women. In fact, women are four times as likely as men to develop osteoporosis. For another 44 million Americans, half of whom are over the age of 55, osteoporosis is a major public health threat. While being female and of advanced age are primary risk factors, the disease can strike at any age.

Certain groups of people are more likely than others to be affected by osteoporosis. These groups include women, older adults, people with a family history of the bone disorder, or those who have had broken bones; also, people with small, thin statures and people with low sex hormones are at a greater risk. Significant risk also has been found among people of all ethnic backgrounds. Factors that can be controlled, but also place individuals at risk for osteoporosis, include diets that lack adequate amounts of vitamin D and calcium and may contain too much protein and sodium; alcohol abuse and cigarette smoking; and health disorders such as anorexia, rheumatoid arthritis, and gastrointestinal diseases.

Occasionally, children and teens develop osteoporosis. When this happens, it's usually due to a medical condition or medication. These rare cases are called juvenile osteoporosis, and the condition can pose significant problems since it occurs during a young person's main years for bone development. Conditions that can cause juvenile osteoporosis include diabetes, cystic fibrosis, leukemia, and osteogenesis imperfecta or "brittle bone disease." Medications linked to juvenile osteoporosis include drugs used in chemotherapy for cancer, anticonvulsants for seizures, and steroids for arthritis.

Even rarer is idiopathic osteoporosis, which has no known cause. When this occurs, it happens more often in boys than in girls and it usually develops before the onset of puberty. While most of the bone density may return during puberty, children with juvenile osteoporosis usually have lower peak bone mass as adults than their peers who never experience the condition.

**Symptoms**  Symptoms of osteoporosis are not obvious. The condition has even been called "the silent disease." Many may not realize they have it until they experience a bone break. People with osteoporosis can break or fracture bones just by having a minor fall. In more extreme cases a sneeze can cause bones to break or fracture. In rarer cases, bones can break spontaneously. Sometimes spinal fractures can be felt in the form of severe back pain or seen in the form of stooped posture or height loss. Sometimes there is no pain.

Bone breaks and fractures are very debilitating occurrences that happen due to osteoporosis. They lower the quality of life and life expectancy. The rate of hip fractures is two to three times higher in women than in men; however, the one-year mortality following a hip fracture is nearly twice as high for men as for women. One in two women and one in four men over the age of 50 will experience an osteoporosis-related fracture in their lifetime. While fractures can happen in any bone, they are most likely to occur in the hip, spine, and wrist. By the year 2025, fractures due to the bone disorder are expected to rise to more than 3 million (National Osteoporosis Foundation).

There are other staggering statistics associated with this condition. Women who get hip fractures are four times more likely to experience a second one. While women experience more hip fractures than men, men are twice as likely as women to die within the year following a hip fracture. In women, the risk of hip fracture is equal to the combined risk of breast, uterine, and ovarian cancer. Caucasian women over the age of 65 are twice as likely to suffer from fractures as African American women.

Bone mineral density (BMD) refers to the amount of bone material present per square centimeter of bone. It also indicates the presence of osteoporosis or osteopenia, a precursor to osteoporosis. When physicians test for BMD the outcomes are described by two scores, the T-score and the Z-score. The T-score compares a patient's BMD to that of a healthy 30-year-old of the same gender and ethnicity. The Z-score measures the degree to which a patient's BMD deviates from the average BMD for his or her age, sex, and ethnicity.

A normal T-score is –1.0 or higher depending upon age. A T-score between –1.0 and –2.5 indicates the presence of osteopenia. Osteoporosis is defined by a T-score of –2.5 or lower. The T-score is used mostly for postmenopausal women and men over age 50 because it is a better predictor of future fracture risk. The Z-score is used primarily for premenopausal women, men under the age of 50, and children.

These results are gathered using specialized testing called dual energy x-ray absorptiometry (DXA). DXA can determine low bone density before a fracture can occur, if bones are losing density or staying the same, predict future fractures, and determine the need for treatment.

**Treatment**   While osteoporosis cannot be cured, it is treatable. Medications for the condition work to slow bone loss and improve bone density. These medications are classified as antiresorptive medications and bone-forming (anabolic) medications.

Antiresorptive medications go into bones and cling to the areas that are under attack. When osteoclasts try to break down parts of the bone, bisphosphonates interrupt the process so that more bone building can occur. Most medications fall under this category. Bone-forming (anabolic) medications are being looked to by researchers with increased interest. This type of therapy involves the parathyroid hormone (PTH). Currently, a form of PTH called teriparatide is used to help patients with osteoporosis. This approach works by stimulating osteoblasts. Some researchers believe this therapy is superior to others for the improvement of bone quality. However, a combination of the two types of therapies is recommended in order to maintain gains in bone density.

Estrogen loss is the main culprit behind the development of osteoporosis in women and can cause them to lose up to 20 percent of their bone mass in the five to seven years after the onset of menopause. Recommendations for prevention, detection, and treatment are especially important for this group. After menopause, the breakdown of bone becomes out of balance with the creation of new bone. Menopause occurring before the age of 45, extended periods of absent or infrequent menstrual flow, or low hormone levels can cause a reduction in bone mass.

A healthy, osteoporosis-reducing diet can go a long way in maintaining bone health. Adults up to age 50 require 1,000 milligrams of calcium per day. Women age 51 and older and men age 71 and over need 1,200 milligrams of calcium daily. Milk, whether skim, low fat, or whole, is one of the top sources of calcium. An 8-ounce glass contains 300 milligrams. For individuals concerned about lactose intolerance, cheese and yogurt are great substitutes. Greens and sardines also are good sources of calcium. Vitamin D, also a necessity, is contained in fatty fish such as salmon. Milk too can be fortified with vitamin D.

Lifestyle choices like exercise and sun exposure also affect osteoporosis risk. Getting about 15 minutes of sun per day allows the body to produce its own vitamin D. Weight-bearing exercises such as brisk walking, weight training, yoga, and even dancing put stress on bones that lead to the creation of more bone material and bone density improvement.

Men and women with osteoporosis need to prevent falling down. Some factors that lead to falls include poor vision and balance, diseases that can affect walking, and some medications. Men and women with the disease can prevent falls by using a cane or walker, wearing shoes with nonslip soles, avoiding slick sidewalks while outdoors, and using kitty litter or salt when icy conditions exist.

Falls can occur indoors as frequently as they can occur outdoors. Some ways to prevent indoor falls include removing clutter from rooms and floors, using plastic carpet runners for ease of walking, making sure that carpets have skid-proof backing, and wearing low-heeled shoes that provide support. Household accommodations such as stair rails, bathroom grab bars, and rubber bathmats also help prevent falls. When reaching for items in high places, individuals should use a sturdy step stool with wide steps. Buying a cordless phone can prevent having to rush to answer a call. Lighting is an important feature for avoiding falls in the home as well. Keeping a flashlight nearby can be handy for the unexpected loss of light.

*Abena Foreman-Trice*

*See also* Calcium; Exercise; Weight Training; Yoga.

## References

National Osteoporosis Foundation. "About Osteoporosis." www.nof.org/aboutosteoporosis.

PubMed.gov. "Parathyroid Hormone as an Anabolic Skeletal Therapy." www.ncbi.nlm.nih.gov/pubmed/16296873.

Richmond, B.J., M.K. Dalinka, R.H. Daffner, D.L. Bennett, J.A. Jacobson, C.S. Resnik, C.C. Roberts, D.A. Rubin, M.E. Schweitzer, L.L. Seeger, M. Taljanovik, B.N. Weissman, and R.H. Haralson. Expert Panel on Musculoskeletal Imaging. "Osteoporosis and Bone Mineral Density." [Online publication]. American College of Radiology (ACR). 2007. www.acr.org/SecondaryMainMenuCategories/Quality_safety/app_criteria/pdf/ExpertPanelonMusculoskeletalImaging/OsteoporosisandbonemineraldensityupdateinprogressDoc17.aspx.

WebMD. "Osteoporosis Guide." www.webmd.com/osteoporosis/guide/osteoporosis_symptoms_types.

WebMD. "Osteoporosis Medications: How They Work." www.webmd.com/osteoporosis/features/medications.